Y0-EGF-746

RESPIRATORY DISORDERS

RESPIRATORY DISORDERS
A PATHOPHYSIOLOGIC APPROACH

Benjamin Burrows, M.D.
Professor of Internal Medicine
Director, Division of Respiratory Sciences
and NHLBI Specialized Center of Research
University of Arizona College of Medicine
Tucson, Arizona

Ronald J. Knudson, M.D.
Professor of Internal Medicine
Director of Respiratory Services
Associate Director, Division of Respiratory Sciences
and NHLBI Specialized Center of Research
University of Arizona College of Medicine
Tucson, Arizona

Stuart F. Quan, M.D.
Assistant Professor of Internal Medicine
Director of Respiratory Therapy and of the
Medical Intensive Care Unit
Arizona Health Sciences Center
University of Arizona College of Medicine
Tucson, Arizona

Louis J. Kettel, M.D.
Dean, and Professor of Internal Medicine
University of Arizona College of Medicine
Tucson, Arizona

SECOND EDITION

YEAR BOOK MEDICAL PUBLISHERS, INC.
CHICAGO • LONDON

We wish to dedicate this book to our wives,
Nancy, Dwyn, Diana, and Lois
for their patience and support.

0 9 8 7 6 5 4 3 2

The first edition of this book was published under the title of:
Respiratory Insufficiency.

Copyright © 1983 by Year Book Medical Publishers, Inc. All rights reserved. No part of this publication may be reproduced, stored in a retrieval system, or transmitted, in any form or by any means, electronic, mechanical, photocopying, recording, or otherwise, without prior written permission from the publisher. Printed in the United States of America.

Library of Congress Cataloging in Publication Data
Main entry under title:

Respiratory disorders, a pathophysiologic approach.

   Rev. ed. of: Respiratory insufficiency / by Benjamin
Burrows, Ronald J. Knudson, and Louis J. Kettel.
1975.
   Includes index.
   1.   Respiratory insufficiency.   I.   Burrows, Benjamin.
[DNLM: 1.   Respiratory tract disease.   WF 140 R434103]
RC776.R4R46   1983   616.2   82-23745
ISBN 0-8151-1351-X

Contents

PART 1   NORMAL PHYSIOLOGY

PART II   PATHOPHYSIOLOGY

PART III   BRONCHOPULMONARY DISEASES

Preface

IT HAS BEEN MORE than seven years since the first edition of this book appeared under the title *Respiratory Insufficiency*. Since that time, there have been dramatic changes in the practice of chest medicine. To incorporate these changes, extensive revisions of the original text were required, particularly in regard to acute respiratory failure, ventilator care, and diseases affecting airways function. Since we now realize that the previous title of the book did not accurately reflect its scope and since the present text differs so greatly from the first, the previous title has been replaced by one which is similar to others in this Year Book Internal Medicine Series.

Morbidity and mortality from chronic respiratory diseases have increased notably during the past 25 years. A vast and often confusing literature on the pathophysiology, diagnosis, and treatment of these disorders has accumulated over the same period. The present volume attempts to review these subjects in simple, nonmathematical terms. It emphasizes the relationships of functional abnormalities to diagnosis, natural history, and therapy for respiratory diseases.

Following a glossary of commonly used symbols and terms, the volume is divided into three parts. The first presents a brief review of normal pulmonary physiology, emphasizing concepts that have direct clinical applications. In the second part, the pathophysiology, differential diagnosis, and management of various manifestations of bronchopulmonary dysfunction are discussed. The last part deals with categories of diseases which affect bronchopulmonary function. Since the type of dysfunction produced by a respiratory disease is generally more closely related to its anatomical location than to its specific etiology, this part is organized along anatomical lines. No attempt is made to provide a comprehensive survey of chest diseases. Specific pulmonary infections and neoplasms receive scant attention, and nonphysiologic diagnostic methods are largely ignored, despite their obvious importance in the diagnosis of pulmonary diseases. Disorders that manifest themselves primarily by the dysfunction they produce are given major emphasis. Their pathogenesis, diagnosis, physiologic consequences, and treatment are discussed.

Throughout we have directed the discussion to medical students and physicians who have had no special training in pulmonary diseases, and we have attempted to provide the basic knowledge of pathophysiology of the lung needed for diagnosis and management of most respiratory dysfunction.

BENJAMIN BURROWS
RONALD J. KNUDSON
STUART F. QUAN
LOUIS J. KETTEL

vii

Terminology, Abbreviations, and Symbols

IN THE FIELD of respiration there is a standard terminology, and certain conventions are recognized concerning symbols and abbreviations. In the interests of readability, definitions are given as terms appear in the text. For reference, however, the following glossary is provided. The terminology is based on recommendations published in the *American Thoracic Society News*, 3:6, 1977, and 4:12–15, 1978.

General Symbols

V	volume of a gas
F	fractional concentration of a gas
P	pressure
Q	volume of blood
C	content or concentration in blood
S	saturation of blood
%X	Percent sign preceding a symbol indicates percentage of the predicted normal value
X/Y%	Percent sign *after* a symbol indicates a ratio function with the ratio expressed as a percentage. Both components of the ratio must be designated; e.g., $FEV_1/FEV\% = 100 \times FEV_1/FVC$
f	Frequency of any event in time, e.g., respiratory frequency: the number of breathing cycles per unit of time
t	Time
anat	Anatomical
max	Maximum

A dot above a symbol indicates the time derivative of the value. (Thus V indicates volume, whereas $\dot{V}$ indicates volume per unit time, or flow.) A dash above the symbol indicates the mean value. In composite abbreviations, other letters appear as suffixes, either as small capital letters or subscripted symbols. These suffixes are as follows:

I	Inspired
E	Expired
A	Alveolar
T	Tidal
D	Dead space
B	Barometric
STPD	Standard temperature and pressure, dry. These are the conditions of a volume of gas at 0° C, at 760 torr, without water vapor
BTPS	Body temperature (37° C), barometric pressure at sea level (760 torr), and saturated with water vapor
ATPD	Ambient temperature and pressure, dry

ATPS	Ambient temperature and pressure, saturated with water vapor
L	Lung
b	Blood in general
a	Arterial. Exact location to be specified in text when term is used
v	Venous. Exact location to be specified in text when term is used
$\bar{v}$	Mixed venous
c	Capillary. Exact location to be specified in text when term is used
c′	Pulmonary end-capillary

Ventilation and Respiratory Mechanics

Volumes are expressed in liters (BTPS), flow in L/sec, and pressure in cm H_2O.

TLC	Total lung capacity: volume of gas in the lungs at maximum inspiration
RV	Residual volume: volume of gas remaining in the lungs at maximum expiration
VC	Vital capacity: maximum volume excursion of which the lungs are capable by voluntary effort (TLC − RV = VC)
IVC	Inspiratory vital capacity: vital capacity measured by maximal inspiration from residual volume
FVC	Forced vital capacity: vital capacity measured by rapid forced expiration from TLC to RV
FEV_1	Forced expiratory volume in one second: volume expired in the first second of the FVC maneuver
FRC	Functional residual capacity: volume of gas in the lung at the end of a normal tidal breath when respiratory muscles are relaxed
V_T	Tidal volume: volume of gas inspired or expired with each breath
V_D	Physiologic dead space: calculated volume (BPTS), which accounts for the difference between the pressures of CO_2 in expired gas and arterial blood. Physiologic dead space reflects the combination of anatomical dead space and alveolar dead space, the volume of the latter increasing with the importance of the nonuniformity of the ventilation/perfusion ratio in the lung
$V_{D_{anat}}$	Volume of the anatomical dead space (BTPS)
V_{D_A}	The alveolar dead-space (BTPS): $V_{D_A} = V_D = V_{D_{anat}}$
PEF	Peak expiratory flow (L/min or L/sec)
*$\dot{V}max_{XX\%}$	Maximum expiratory flow (instantaneous) qualified by the volume at which measured, expressed as percent of the FVC that has been exhaled. (Example: $\dot{V}max_{75\%}$ is the maximum expiratory flow after 75% of the FVC has been exhaled and 25% remains to be exhaled)
$\dot{V}max_{XX\%TLC}$	Maximum expiratory flow (instantaneous) qualified by the volume at which measured, expressed as percent of the TLC that remains in the lung. (Example: $\dot{V}max_{40\%TLC}$ is the maximum expiratory flow when 40% of the TLC remains in the lung)

---

*There has been confusion in the literature concerning this abbreviation. At times $\dot{V}max_{25\%}$ has been used instead of $\dot{V}max_{75\%}$ to indicate flow after exhalation of the first 75% of the FVC.

FEF$_{x-y}$ — Forced expiratory flow between two designated volume points in the FVC. These points may be designated as absolute volumes starting from the full inspiratory point or by designating the percent of FVC exhaled

FEF$_{.2-1.2L}$ — Forced expiratory flow between 200 ml and 1,200 ml of the FVC; formerly called maximum expiratory flow

FEF$_{25\%-75\%}$ — Forced expiratory flow during the middle half of the FVC; formerly called maximum midexpiratory flow

MVV — Maximum voluntary ventilation: maximum volume of air that can be breathed per min by a subject breathing quickly and as deeply as possible. The time of measurement of this tiring lung function test is usually between 12 and 30 sec, but the test result is given in L(BTPS)/min.

$\dot{V}_E$ — Expired volume per min (BTPS)

$\dot{V}_I$ — Inspired volume per min (BTPS)

$\dot{V}_{CO_2}$ — Carbon dioxide production per min (STPD)

$\dot{V}_{O_2}$ — Oxygen consumption per min (STPD)

R — Respiratory exchange ratio in general. Quotient of the volume of CO_2 produced divided by the volume of O_2 consumed

$\dot{V}_A$ — Alveolar ventilation: physiologic process by which alveolar gas is removed and replaced with fresh gas. The volume of alveolar gas actually expelled completely is equal to the tidal volume minus the volume of the dead space.

$\dot{V}_D$ — Ventilation per min of the physiologic dead space (BTPS)

$\dot{V}_{D_{anat}}$ — Ventilation per min of the anatomical dead space, that portion of the conducting airway in which no significant gas exchange occurs (BTPS)

$\dot{V}_{D_A}$ — Ventilation of the alveolar dead space (BTPS), defined by the equation:

$$\dot{V}_{D_A} = \dot{V}_D - \dot{V}_{D_{anat}}$$

Paw — Pressure at any point along the airways

Pao — Pressure at the airway opening; i.e., mouth, nose, tracheal cannula

Ppl — Pleural pressure: the pressure between the visceral and parietal pleura relative to atmospheric pressure, in cm H_2O

Palv — Alveolar pressure

PL — Transpulmonary pressure: transpulmonary pressure, PL = Palv − Ppl, measurement conditions to be defined

Pst(L) — Static recoil pressure of the lung; transpulmonary pressure measured under static conditions

Pbs — Pressure at the body surface

Pes — Esophageal pressure used to estimate Ppl

Pw — Transthoracic pressure: pressure difference between parietal pleural surface and body surface. Transthoracic in the sense used means "across the wall." Pw = Ppl − Pbs

Ptm — Transmural pressure pertaining to an airway or blood vessel

Prs — Transrespiratory pressure: pressure across the respiratory system. Prs = Palv − Pbs = PL + Pw

R — Flow resistance: the ratio of the flow-resistive components of pressure to simultaneous

	flow in cm H_2O/L/sec
Raw	Airway resistance calculated from pressure difference between airway opening (Pao) and alveoli (Palv) divided by the airflow, cm H_2O/L/sec
R_L	Total pulmonary resistance includes the frictional resistance of the lungs and air passages. It equals the sum of airway resistance and lung tissue resistance. It is measured by relating flow-dependent transpulmonary pressure to airflow at the mouth
Rrs	Total respiratory resistance includes the sum of airway resistance, lung tissue resistance, and chest wall resistance. It is measured by relating flow-dependent transrespiratory pressure to airflow at the mouth.
Rus	Resistance of the airways on the upstream (alveolar) side of the point in the airways where intraluminal pressure equals Ppl (equal pressure point), measured during maximum expiratory flow
Rds	Resistance of the airways on the downstream (mouth) side of the point in the airways where intraluminal pressure equals Ppl, measured during maximum expiratory flow
Gaw	Airway conductance, reciprocal of Raw
Gaw/V_L	Specific conductance expressed per liter of lung volume at which Gaw is measured
C	Compliance: the slope of a static volume-pressure curve at a point, or the linear approximation of a nearly straight portion of such a curve expressed in L/cm H_2O or ml/cm H_2O

Cdyn	Dynamic compliance: the ratio of the tidal volume to the change in intrapleural pressure between the points of zero flow at the extremes of tidal volume in L/cm H_2O or ml/cm H_2O
Cst	Static compliance, value for compliance determined on the basis of measurements made during periods of cessation of airflow
C/V_L	Specific compliance: compliance divided by the lung volume at which it is determined, usually FRC
E	Elastance: the reciprocal of compliance; expressed in cm H_2O/L or cm H_2O/ml

Gas Exchange, Transport, and Diffusion

Volumes are expressed in liters, flows in L/min, and gas pressures or tensions in torr.

$\dot{V}$	Total ventilation: The total volume of gas moved (inspired or expired) in the act of breathing during a given time interval, expressed in L/min
$\dot{Q}$	Blood flow or perfusion
DL_{CO}	Diffusing capacity of the lung for carbon monoxide
DL_{O_2}	Diffusing capacity of the lung for oxygen
PA_{O_2}	Alveolar oxygen tension (torr)
Pa_{O_2}	Arterial oxygen tension (torr)
PA_{CO_2}	Alveolar carbon dioxide tension (torr)
Pa_{CO_2}	Arterial carbon dioxide tension (torr)
Sa_{O_2}	Arterial oxygen saturation (%)

When chemical reactions are described, standard chemical symbols are used.

Respiratory Therapy Terms

GASES AND AEROSOLS

Aerosol: A suspension of fine particles of a liquid or solid in an atmosphere of gas.

Atomizer: An aerosol generator designed to produce a spray whose particle size is not maintained by baffling.

Nebulizer: An aerosol generator designed to produce particles within the therapeutic range for deposition along the airway.

Humidifier: A device used to increase water vapor content of air.

Low-Flow Oxygen System: A system in which the reservoir and total gas flow of the apparatus are insufficient to supply the entire inspired atmosphere, thus necessitating room air to comprise a portion of each tidal volume.

High-Flow Oxygen System: System in which the reservoir and total gas flow of the apparatus are sufficient to supply the entire inspired atmosphere; the ventilatory pattern should have no effect on the inspired oxygen concentration.

Nasal Cannula: A plastic appliance consisting of two tips about 1 cm in length arising from an oxygen supply tube and inserted into the anterior nares, used to deliver moderate concentrations of O_2.

Nasal Catheter (oropharyngeal catheter): A soft rubber or plastic catheter with several holes in its terminal 2 cm. The device is inserted into the oropharynx and is used to deliver moderate concentrations of oxygen.

T-piece (T tube): T-shaped tube designed to administer an aerosol and supplemental oxygen to patients with endotracheal or tracheostomy tubes.

Simple Mask: A face mask in which there is free mixing of both inspired and expired air.

Partial Rebreathing Mask: A face mask and a reservoir bag permitting a portion of the exhaled gas to enter the bag for mixing with source gas.

Nonrebreathing Mask: A face mask designed to separate flow of inspired and expired gases.

Venturi Mask: A face mask designed to entrain atmospheric air to provide a constant fractional dilution of a pressurized gas, most commonly oxygen. Within limits, the concentration of the gas delivered is independent of the gas flow.

CHEST PHYSICAL THERAPY

Postural Drainage (bronchial drainage): Positioning of a patient, usually during deep breathing and coughing, so that the drainage of secretions from various areas of the lungs is augmented by gravity.

Chest Wall Percussion: Clapping with cupped hands or with a mechanical device on the chest wall over draining areas of the lungs, usually performed with postural drainage.

Chest Wall Vibration: Manual or mechanical vibration and gentle application of pressure on the chest wall over draining areas of the lungs, usually performed with postural drainage.

MECHANICAL VENTILATION

Intermittent Positive-Pressure Breathing (IPPB): Pressure greater than atmospheric at the airway opening during inspiration, used to assist or support ventilation. During expiration, pressure returns to atmospheric.

Positive End-Expiratory Pressure (PEEP): A residual pressure greater than atmospheric maintained at the airway opening at the end of expiration.

Negative-Pressure Ventilation: A negative pressure applied to the thorax to assist or support ventilation.

Continuous Positive Airway Pressure (CPAP): A pressure greater than atmospheric, maintained at the airway opening throughout a spontaneous respiratory cycle.

Expiratory Positive Airway Pressure (EPAP): A pressure greater than atmospheric, maintained at the airway opening only during the expiratory phase of a spontaneous respiratory cycle.

Continuous Positive Pressure Ventilation (CPPV): Pressure greater than atmospheric at the airway opening during inspiration, used to support ventilation in conjunction with a pressure greater than atmospheric maintained at the airway opening at the end of expiration; i.e., IPPB plus PEEP.

Controlled Ventilation: Manual or mechanical ventilation in which the frequency of breathing is determined by a ventilator according to a preset cycling pattern without initiation by the patient.

Assisted Ventilation: Manual or mechanical ventilation in which the patient initiates inspiration and establishes the frequency of breathing.

Assist-Control Ventilation: Manual or mechanical ventilation in which the minimum frequency of breathing is predetermined by the ventilator controls, but the patient has the option of initiating inspiration to give a faster rate.

Intermittent Mandatory Ventilation (IMV): Periodic controlled ventilation with inspiratory positive pressure, with the patient breathing spontaneously between controlled breaths.

Synchronized Intermittent Mandatory Ventilation (SIMV): Periodic assisted ventilation with inspired positive pressure, with the patient breathing spontaneously between assisted breaths.

Volume-constant Ventilator: A device for delivering a preset inspired volume irrespective, within specified limits, of the pressure required to deliver that volume.

Pressure-limited Ventilator: A device designed to deliver inspired gas until a preset level of airway pressure is reached.

PART I

Normal Physiology

1

Overview of
the Respiratory System

THE HUMAN BODY may be regarded as a machine that requires energy to function. The energy is derived from the burning of fuel, a form of combustion that requires oxygen. Oxygen is obtained from the surrounding atmosphere and transported to the metabolizing cells within the body. The cells' combustion products are delivered, in turn, to the atmosphere. It is the primary function of the respiratory system to supply oxygen and to rid the body of carbon dioxide, the product of combustion. This process is complicated by the fact that man, as a whole organism, exists in a gaseous environment, breathing air, whereas the metabolizing cells function in a fluid milieu. Thus, the oxygen and carbon dioxide must be transferred between gas and liquid phases.

In order to accomplish its function, the respiratory system uses a reciprocating pump to move air into and out of the body. This pump has several interacting components. The air passes through a system of flexible, compliant branching tubes that offer resistance to air flow. The lung as a mechanical pump is a volume-elastic structure with certain physical characteristics. It is housed in a semi-rigid container, the thorax. This structure is acted upon by the respiratory muscles acting synchronously. The muscles driving the respiratory pump are under the control of the central nervous system, which, in turn, is responsive to the metabolic demands of the body. Within the lung, a large and vulnerable surface is exposed to the poten-

tially hostile external environment. Therefore, the lung possesses mechanisms to defend itself from injury.

To transfer oxygen and carbon dioxide between gas and liquid, the two phases must be brought into intimate contact while their separation is maintained by a thin membrane. The transfer of gas across the membrane is facilitated by an extensive pulmonary capillary bed, which provides a large surface for gas exchange; an alveolar anatomy, which provides a short path length for gas diffusion; and biochemical mechanisms, which allow the rapid movement of oxygen and carbon dioxide across the membrane. For maximum efficiency of gas exchange, blood flow and ventilation should be similarly distributed throughout the lung.

In the liquid or blood phase a transport mechanism for respiratory gases must be available that has a greater capacity than that provided by physical solution alone. Hemoglobin supplies this transport mechanism. An efficient circulatory pump, the heart, provides the mechanical apparatus to transport the respiratory gases between lungs and tissues.

In the following pages of this part, various facets of the normal respiratory system will be described. This is not intended to be a complete and detailed description of respiratory physiology. Rather, it is intended to provide a background that may form the basis for understanding and dealing with derangements in function caused by disease.

3

2

Lung Defense Mechanisms

THE RESPIRATORY SYSTEM, moving air into and out of the lung and presenting a large surface for gas exchange, is constantly and extensively exposed to a potentially hostile environment. Yet man can live in a variety of situations varying in temperature, humidity, and degree of atmospheric contaminants. Mechanisms exist that temper the air we breathe and defend the lung against insult or injury.

The Upper Airway

Whether we reside in a frigid or tropical clime, the inspired air reaching the lower respiratory tract is adjusted to a temperature close to 37 C. The nasal passages constitute an effective air conditioning unit. The rich vascular supply of the nasal turbinates coupled with the fact that the air-stream passing them is not much wider than 1 mm makes the turbinates an effective heat exchanger. Humidification of inspired air is also accomplished primarily in the nasal passages through an outpouring of nasal secretions. It is estimated that the volume of nasal secretion amounts to a liter or more per 24-hour period. The air reaching the lower air passages, therefore, is almost fully saturated as well as close to body temperature. In susceptible individuals bypassing or overwhelming the air conditioning function of the nasal passages by exercise or breathing cold air results in clinical bronchospasm (see chap. 27).

Each liter of urban air contains vast amounts of particulate matter. Various mechanisms are available to deal with such foreign material. The nasal passages constitute the first line of defense. The hairs of the nares filter out the larger particles. Most of the remaining particles greater than 10 μ in diameter settle or impact upon the mucus coating the nasal passages. As water is added to the inspired air, hygroscopic particles increase in size, rendering them more likely to deposit in the upper respiratory tract. Almost no particles larger than 10 μ and only 15% of those greater than 4.5 μ reach the level of the larynx.

The Mucociliary Escalator

The airways are lined with ciliated columnar epithelium. This epithelium is pseudostratified in large airways but becomes single-layered and finally cuboidal with subsequent generations of branching. The surface contains approximately five ciliated cells for each mucus-secreting goblet cell. The proportion of goblet cells diminishes in peripheral airways and they are altogether absent in terminal bronchioles. Ciliated cells may be found distally as far as in the respiratory bronchioles. Mixed serous and mucus-producing cells are seen in the bronchial glands. These glands are most numerous in medium bronchi, plentiful in the trachea and large bronchi, less numerous in small bronchi, and absent in bronchioles. These cellular elements and the secretions overlying them make up the mucociliary escalator.

Inhaled particles entering the trachea are for the most part smaller than 10 μ. Most of the particles greater than 2 μ deposit on the sticky mucus layer lining the tracheobronchial tree. Because of their inertia, particles tend not to follow flow stream lines at points of branching. As a result, particle deposition is greater at airway bifurcations. Only particles smaller than 2 μ are likely to reach the level of the alveoli.

It has been estimated that from 10 to 100 ml of tracheobronchial mucus is produced daily in the normal adult. This mucus blanket protects the underlying mucosa from dehydration as well as functions as an important cleansing mechanism. The mucus blanket is about 5 μ thick and appears to consist of a thin, watery solution covered by a more tenacious viscoelastic gel layer. The adhesive character of the gel layer enables it to trap and hold the particles that impinge upon it. The thinner solution layer has a high rate of shear, and it is within this layer that the cilia beat to move the mucus carpet upward toward the glottis.

Each ciliated cell bears about 200 cilia 5–7 μ long. The cilia beat in a synchronized fashion at a rate of between 1,000 and 1,500 times a minute. When the forward effective stroke achieves its maximum velocity, the tips of the cilia come in contact with the gel layer, moving it along. The recovery stroke is slower, taking three times as long as the forward stroke, and occurs in the solution layer. By this mechanism the mucus carpet is propelled upward at between 1 and 3 cm/min. Ultimately, the mucus bearing the captured particulates reaches the level of the pharynx, where it is swallowed. If the quantity is sufficient to stimulate the upper tracheobronchial tree, cough and expectoration may assist the removal of mucus.

This important and normally effective clearance mechanism may be altered by bacteriologic or chemical insults. Tobacco smoke and certain air pollutants have deleterious effects. Increase in mucus secretion or alteration of the character of mucus in response to such insults can diminish the effectiveness of this mechanism. Decrease in ciliary activity and damage to or even loss of ciliated cells further interferes with transport. Goblet cell hyperplasia or increase in number of bronchial glands contributes further secretions to the transport burden. Although increased stimulus to cough may assist in removal of these excessive secretions, mucus plugging may occur at a more peripheral level when the transport mechanism is overwhelmed.

Cough

Cough may result from mechanical irritation or chemical stimulation of the tracheobronchial tree. Cough due to chemical irritants occurs when the irritant is drawn deep into the lungs but exhibits ready tachyphylaxis on continued exposure. Mechanical irritation, however, continues to stimulate cough even on repetition. The larynx, tracheal bifurcation, and points of lobar branching are most sensitive to mechanical irritation. The sensory end-organs located here and in the posterior wall of the trachea transmit afferent impulses via the vagus to the medulla.

The cough sequence is a familiar one. Rapid inspiration is followed by generation of an expiratory effort against the closed glottis. At the peak of this effort, rapid opening of the glottis is followed by vigorous, almost explosive expiration. Frequently, a series of coughs may follow the initial inspiration, each one occurring at a progressively lower lung volume.

The intrathoracic or pleural pressure generated by the expiratory muscles during cough may be high, often in excess of 200 cm H_2O. When expiratory flow is permitted upon opening the glottis, the flow-limiting mechanisms described in chapter 6 come into play with establishment of equal pressure points, dynamic compression of large intrathoracic airways, and achievement of V̇max. That discussion of the dynamic properties of the respiratory system is concerned with airflow. Since the purpose of cough is to rid the tracheobronchial tree of excess secretions, we must now consider (1) the dynamics of liquid flow in relation to airflow as the two phases move in the same direction, and (2) the manner in which these liquid secretions are mobilized in this two-phase system.

If we consider the respiratory airways as analogous to a vertical pipe conducting upward flow in both liquid and gas phases, the patterns we observe are related to the linear velocity of the airflow. At low air velocities the gas rises as bubbles through the liquid. At slightly higher velocities the gas rises as large plugs. At even higher velocities annular flow is observed in which the liquid flows upward as a film along the wall of the tube. Finally, as sufficiently high gas velocities are achieved, droplets of liquid are sheared off and carried upward as mist. The latter three flow patterns are features of the cough process. Expectoration of mucus plugs is evidence that plug flow occurs. It is likely that annular flow occurs in some portions of the tracheobronchial tree. The spray of droplets observed during a cough make it apparent that mist flow must be achieved as well.

The viscosity of the liquid, as well as the air velocity, is an important factor in determining the upflow pattern. It has proved difficult, however, to determine the viscosity of tracheobronchial mucus. Furthermore, the viscosity may be considerably altered in disease states. The thick, viscid sputum of bronchitis will require higher air velocities for mobilization than will normal mucus. Nevertheless, the mechanics of the cough produce the substantial linear velocities required to mobilize secretions.

The linear velocity of air flowing through an airway depends on the cross-sectional area of the airway and the volume flow. The volume flow during cough is $\dot{V}$max, which is higher at large lung volumes. Therefore, the initial inspiration to a high lung volume permits a higher expiratory flow during the subsequent cough. If a relatively modest expiratory flow of 6 L/sec is achieved, for example, the air velocity in a trachea of 1.5 cm^2 relaxed cross-sectional area will be 4,000 cm/sec.

The dynamic compression during the forced expiratory phase of cough further increases linear velocity. As a result of the high intrathoracic pressures generated during cough, the trachea and main-stem bronchi may be compressed to one quarter to one sixth of their relaxed lumen area. The dynamic compression of upper intrathoracic airways and consequent reduction in cross-sectional area augments the linear velocities achieved for the same $\dot{V}$max. It has been

estimated that, as a result of these factors, the linear velocity generated in the trachea may even approach the speed of sound!

The total lumen area of the main-stem, lobar, and segmental bronchi differs little from that of the trachea. With the addition of expiratory dynamic compression, linear velocities sufficient to produce mist flow are achieved at least this far peripherally, and probably through a few of the subsequent generations of airway branching.

As serial coughing follows the initial deep inspiration, expulsive expiration occurs at lower and lower lung volumes, the equal pressure points move alveolar-ward and more of the tracheobronchial tree is subject to dynamic compression. Although $\dot{V}$max diminishes with volume, the end result is to extend the portion of the tracheobronchial tree in which high linear velocities are achieved. Through succeeding peripheral generations of branching, however, the total lumen area increases markedly, the velocity of flow diminishes accordingly. Although mist flow, therefore, is not achieved at the level of the smaller bronchioles, secretions can still be mobilized by the mechanism of plug flow in peripheral airways. Serial coughing following a single inspiration has an additional effect in loosening secretions in that the airways are alternately compressed during expiratory flow and reexpanded during the period of glottic closure. This in-and-out movement of the airway walls may serve to shake loose tenacious mucus secretions.

Other vibratory movements of airway walls have been observed during cough or forced expiration. These are of very high frequency, often above 300 cycles/sec. It seems likely that this vibratory phenomenon would assist in contributing droplets to the expulsive spray seen during a cough.

In patients with obstructive airways disease and diminished $\dot{V}$max, the dynamic compression of intrathoracic airways assumes a very important role. The reduction in airway cross-sectional area with dynamic compression permits development of the linear gas velocities essential to an effective cough even in the face of reduced $\dot{V}$max. Thus, to a considerable degree, cough may be regarded simply as a reflex device to achieve V̇max swiftly. It should be pointed out that glottic closure and reopening is helpful but not essential for production of an effective cough and mobilization of secretions. However, although patients with laryngectomies and tracheostomies are able to bring up secretions with rapid forced expirations through the same mechanisms described above in response to a cough stimulus, coughing may be more efficient when glottic closure is not impaired.

Phagocytes

The defense mechanisms of the lung are ultimately designed to protect the alveolar surface, a thin, highly vascular, epithelial surface of about 70 m^2. Inhaled particles and microorganisms smaller than 2 μ in diameter may be expected to reach the alveolar level. Here, the alveolar macrophage constitutes the final line of defense and the most important mechanism for preventing bacterial invasion of the lung.

The alveolar macrophage is a phagocytic cell of hematopoietic origin with unique migratory properties. Its defensive role of engulfing and digesting harmful particles is facilitated by the ability to move freely over the alveolar surface. Increased mobilization of macrophages follows inhalation of large amounts of particulates. The engulfed particulate matter may be carried by the migrating phagocytes to the respiratory bronchioles from which clearance is effected by the mucociliary escalator. Other macrophages migrate to lymphatics. Pigment particles not phagocytosed by macrophages may remain along alveolar septae and peribronchial or periarterial regions, or find their way via lymphatics to lymph nodes.

Particle clearance by macrophages is an understandably slow process. The clearance time is sufficiently long to allow multiplication of inhaled infectious microorganisms. Yet, sterility of the lung parenchyma is maintained. This is attributable to the antimicrobial function of alveolar macrophages. Upon engulfing a microbial particle, lysosomal enzymes are mobilized

within the phagocyte. These lytic enzymes kill and digest the microorganism. Thus, the microbial particles are already subject to degradation before clearance occurs. Phagocytosis is an active process reflected by an increase in oxygen consumption and other changes indicative of increased cellular metabolic activity. For complete effectiveness against a specific microorganism, the macrophage system depends on a variety of associated immunologic mechanisms.

These scavenger cells wandering over the alveolar surface epithelium normally provide an effective alveolar defense against inhaled inert or microbial particulates. Certain circumstances may interfere with this defense mechanism, however. Bacterial clearance by alveolar macrophages has been shown to be diminished following ethanol ingestion. Corticosteroids stabilize lysosomal membranes, and their administration may diminish the release of lysosomal enzymes, reducing the antimicrobial activity of these cells. Cigarette smoke, oxidant gases, and radiation also adversely affect macrophage activity. These recent observations may help explain the high frequency of respiratory infections noted in alcoholics and after exposure to certain types of polluted air.

When particles of crystalline silica are ingested by alveolar macrophages, the cellular defense mechanism fails. Silica produces damage to the lysosomal membrane. The resultant mobilization of lysosmal enzymes results in autodigestion of the macrophage itself with cell death and release of the silica particle, which is then free to repeat the cycle in subsequent generations of macrophages. Ultimately, the fibrosis characteristic of silicosis occurs. The inhibition of lysosomal activity by cortisone can diminish the fibrogenic process induced by silica.

It is possible that other pulmonary diseases may also be related to inappropriate responses of the alveolar macrophage.

The circulating blood polymorphonuclear leukocyte (PMN) is also an important phagocyte during an inflammatory response within the lung. Although the PMN is not normally present in large numbers in the lung parenchyma, in response to acute inflammation it migrates to the affected area. With evolution of the inflammatory response, it is gradually replaced by mononuclear cells.

Immunologic Defense Mechanisms

Recent evidence indicates that immunologic responses are important contributors to the lung's defense mechanisms. Secretory IgA is produced by plasma cells located in the submucosa lining the airways. The presence of secretory IgA in respiratory secretions provides an immunologic defense against invasion of the lung by many respiratory viruses. In addition, small amounts of IgG, IgE, and complement are also found in lavage specimens from the lower respiratory tract. Their contribution, if any, to local humoral immunity is unclear.

The lung may also possess local cell-mediated immunity. Focal lymphoid aggregates are present in the airway submucosa, and bronchoalveolar washings normally contain small numbers of B- and T-lymphocytes. Production of macrophage inhibition factor in response to introduction of microorganisms into the lower respiratory tract suggests the existence of cell-mediated immunity. Furthermore, activation of alveolar macrophages may require production of lymphokines such as macrophage inhibition factor by sensitized T-lymphocytes. Abnormal numbers of lymphocytes have also been detected in lung washings in patients with various interstitial lung diseases (see chap. 25). Lymphocytes may therefore contribute to their pathogenesis, but their exact role in these diseases remains an important area of further investigation.

READING LIST

Brain J.D., Proctor D.F., Reid L.M. (eds.): *Respiratory Defense Mechanisms (Parts I and II)*. New York and Basel, Marcel Dekker, Inc., 1977.

A recent thorough review of the subject.

Green G.M., Jakob G.J., Low R.B., et al.: Defense mechanisms of the respiratory membrane. *Am. Rev. Respir. Dis.* 115:479–480, 1977.

An extensive review of the cellular and humoral aspects of lung defense mechanisms.

Hocking W.G., Golde D.W.: The pulmonary alveolar macrophage. *N. Engl. J. Med.* 301:580–587;639–645, 1979.

The function of the alveolar macrophage is discussed.

Leith D.E.: Cough. *J. Am. Phys. Ther. Assoc.* 48:439–447, 1968.

A review of the function and physiology of coughing.

Macklem P.T.: Physiology of cough. *Ann. Otol.* 83:761–768, 1974.

The role of dynamic compression of the airways in generating an effective cough is emphasized.

3

Control of Ventilation

THE ACT OF BREATHING is spontaneous in that it is accomplished without conscious effort or awareness but, unlike automatic functions such as myocardial contraction or peristalsis, it involves skeletal muscles and is susceptible to voluntary interference. At rest, normal breathing has a nearly sinusoidal rhythmicity, but the frequency is readily altered, not only by physiologic demands but also by cortical influences such as anxiety or anticipation. Furthermore, this normal rhythmic pattern may be interrupted by conscious effort or subconsciously altered during common acts such as laughing or talking.

The following brief description of respiratory control mechanisms is only a cursory summary of a complex subject in which investigation is continuing. Four aspects are to be considered: (1) respiratory centers, which impart rhythmicity to the act of breathing; (2) sensorimotor mechanisms, which provide fine regulation of respiratory muscle tension and give rise to sensations related to breathing; (3) chemical or humoral regulation of ventilation, which maintains arterial blood gas tensions within narrow normal limits; and (4) changes which occur in ventilation during sleep. The interaction of these various control mechanisms are represented diagrammatically in Figure 3–1.

Respiratory Centers

Groups of nerve cells dispersed throughout the reticular formation of the brain stem have been identified as respiratory "centers" responsible for rhythmic respiration. Information concerning central control of respiration and the location and function of these control centers has been derived primarily from animal experiments.

In the medulla oblongata two groups of respiratory neurons, the dorsal respiratory group (DRG) and the ventral respiratory group (VRG), have been identified as appearing to be primarily responsible for respiratory rhythmicity. Although the specific mechanism of rhythmicity is still not clear, the prior concept of reciprocal inhibition between separate inspiratory and expiratory centers is probably not accurate. Instead, both groups of respiratory neurons appear to be important in determining respiratory rhythmicity simultaneously. The DRG processes afferent respiratory inputs carried in the ninth and tenth cranial nerves. It also projects to the motor neurons of the phrenic nerve and to the VRG. The VRG is controlled by the DRG and has a primary function to project to motor neurons of the intercostal muscles, upper airway musculature, and the accessory muscles of respiration (see chap. 4).

Although the medullary respiratory centers are the principal determinants of respiratory rhythmicity, the pontine centers may also be important in producing a normal respiratory rhythm. Within the pons two centers have been identified which are associated with control of respiration. Stimulation of the apneustic center, located in the middle and caudal pons, results in

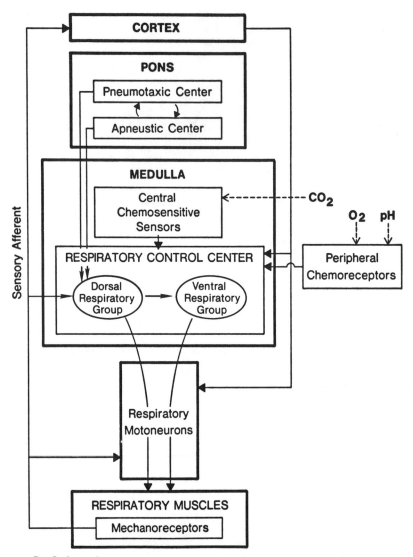

Fig 3–1.—Schematic representation of ventilatory control mechanism.

respiratory arrest in the maximal inspiratory position, or apneusis. It appears that the apneustic center may be the location of a normal inspiration termination switch. Located in the rostral pons is the pneumotaxic center. Stimulation of this center leads to an increase in respiratory frequency with an inspiratory shift, whereas ablation of the center leads to a slowing of respiration. Although the pneumotaxic center has no intrinsic rhythmicity, it probably acts on the apneustic and medullary centers to modulate precisely respiratory timing. In animal models total

removal of the pons does not eliminate respiratory rhythmicity, although breathing under these experimental circumstances is not well coordinated.

Sensorimotor Mechanisms

Respiratory muscles, like other skeletal muscles, possess muscle spindles, which by sensing length form a part of a reflex loop that insures that the muscle contraction is appropriate to the anticipated respiratory load and required effort.

Afferent impulses from respiratory mechanoreceptors are transmitted to the brain stem respiratory centers via the vagus nerve. This servomechanism facilitates fine regulation of respiratory movements and may, for example, stabilize the tidal volume (VT) in spite of changes in mechanical loading of the respiratory system. Breathing is automatic when the respiratory load is constant or when changes in load are subconsciously anticipated. Thus, because it is anticipated, we are not consciously aware of the increase in expiratory resistance during phonation. Under such circumstances, the increase in effort is not sensed because it is appropriate to the expected load. When there occur unexpected changes in mechanical loading of the respiratory system, e.g., sudden addition or subtraction of resistance to breathing, we become aware that the result of the effort does not correspond to the demand, and breathing is no longer a subconscious act. It has been suggested that signals from respiratory muscle and joint mechanoreceptors are integrated to produce a sensation that may reach consciousness when there is this "length-tension inappropriateness." Mechanisms of the sensation of shortness of breath—dyspnea—are discussed further in chapter 19.

Humoral Regulation

Of great clinical significance is the interaction between ventilation and blood oxygen tension, carbon dioxide tension, and pH. Humoral regulation of the medullary centers is mediated by chemosensitive areas in the medulla itself and through peripheral chemoreceptors.

Peripheral chemoreceptors are primarily responsible for the hypoxic drive to respiration. These receptors are highly vascular structures located at the carotid bifurcation and arch of the aorta.

In man, the actions of the aortic chemoreceptors are principally to mediate circulatory rather than ventilatory changes. The mechanism by which chemical stimuli are transformed into neural impulses within the carotid body is still not known, although it has been suggested that changes in metabolism within a special oxygen-sensitive cytochrome system is an important factor. The carotid bodies are highly vascular structures with an extremely high rate of blood flow. Although they have one of the highest metabolic rates in the body, their arterial-venous oxygen content difference is very small (approximately 0.15 ml O_2/100 ml blood). They are thus very sensitive to changes in arterial oxygen tension (Pa_{O_2}), but not to a reduction in oxygen content alone. Therefore, an increase in ventilation may not be seen with anemia, since in this condition there is a decrease in oxygen content but not in oxygen tension. Progressive increases in carotid sinus nerve activity are noted as the Pa_{O_2} decreases from 500 torr, with a marked increase occurring when the Pa_{O_2} falls below 60 torr. This results in an exponential rise in ventilation with a decreasing Pa_{O_2}. However as a result, the relationship between increasing ventilation and hemoglobin desaturation is linear.

A decrease in arterial pH and an increase in arterial carbon dioxide tension (Pa_{CO_2}) also stimulate the peripheral chemoreceptors and result in an increase in ventilation, although the principal effect of changes in Pa_{CO_2} and pH is determined by the central chemoreceptors. The stimulation produced by an increase in Pa_{CO_2} is mediated primarily by a secondary decrease in pH. The independent effect of pH and Pa_{CO_2} to increase ventilation also amplifies the carotid body response due to hypoxia. Denervation of the carotid body abolishes the hypoxic drive to ventilation, but has little effect on the influence due to Pa_{CO_2} or pH. A decrease in perfusion to the carotid body also stimulates ventilation and may be responsible for the ventilatory changes seen in shock states.

Changes in Pa_{CO_2} have a profound effect on central chemoreceptors located in the medulla. These are primarily responsible for mediating the hypercapneic respiratory drive. The chemosensitive areas appear to be directly responsive to hydrogen ions rather than to carbon dioxide per se. Carbon dioxide, which diffuses readily into the cerebrospinal fluid, combines with water to release hydrogen ions. Thus, while central chemoreceptors are sensitive to changes in pH, through this mechanism they appear to be specifically responsive to Pa_{CO_2}. Hydrogen ions themselves do not readily traverse the blood-brain barrier.

The ventilatory response to changes in a single humoral stimulus may be examined experimentally by studies in which all other potential stimuli are held constant. Except in such experimental situations, however, ventilatory responses occur as a result of combinations and interrelationships of stimuli. For example, a decrease in arterial pH increases ventilation, but this additional ventilation results in a fall in carbon dioxide tension and an increase in oxygen tension, which attenuate the ventilatory response. Similarly, the net increase in ventilation induced by breathing a hypoxic gas mixture is limited because any increase in ventilation also produces hypocapnia and respiratory alkalosis, which inhibit ventilation.

Under normal circumstances, carbon dioxide plays the primary role in chemical control of ventilation while Pa_{O_2} and extracellular pH have lesser roles. Normal subjects increase their ventilation more than twofold while breathing a 5%

carbon dioxide gas mixture. More precise measurements of ventilatory response to carbon dioxide are obtained by plotting minute ventilation against Pa_{CO_2} while breathing varying carbon dioxide gas concentrations (Fig 3–2). The relationship of increase in ventilation to increase in Pa_{CO_2} is nearly linear.

Although the ventilatory response to carbon dioxide or hypoxia is primarily a measurement of central control of respiration, airways obstruction or deranged ventilatory mechanics also may affect minute ventilation. Direct measurement of ventilatory drive, such as with diaphragmatic electromyography, is often impractical and technically complex. Alternatively, mouth occlusion pressure, the pressure at the mouth measured 0.1 second after initiation of a normal tidal inspiration against an occluded airway ($P_{0.1}$), has been proposed as a simple index of central drive. This pressure is measured before the subject senses and can respond to an unanticipated inspiratory occlusion. It therefore directly reflects phrenic discharge during what is essentially an isometric contraction of the dia-

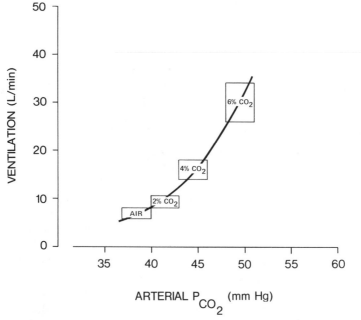

Fig 3–2.—Normal ventilatory response to increasing Pa_{CO_2}. The variability in data obtained while breathing air and 2%, 4%, and 6% carbon dioxide is indicated. (Modern terminology would express carbon dioxide tension in terms of torr rather than mm Hg.)

phragm at functional residual capacity (FRC). Inasmuch as there is no airflow and only a negligible change in lung volume, increased airway resistance or altered compliance of the respiratory system should not affect the measurement. Simple to obtain, occlusion pressure may prove to be a useful index of respiratory center output (see chap. 20).

Chronic elevation of Pa_{CO_2} (hypercapnia) is found in patients having certain respiratory diseases. For reasons that are not entirely clear, the ventilatory response to carbon dioxide appears to have become markedly diminished in these patients, and they depend to an unusual degree on their diminished Pa_{O_2} (hypoxemia) for respiratory drive. Overly exuberant oxygen administration in an effort to correct hypoxemia may have dire consequences by removing the dominant respiratory stimulus. This and other matters of clinical relevance are discussed in chapter 17.

Control of Ventilation During Sleep

Sleep is not a homogeneous state, but constantly fluctuates every 90–120 minutes between two distinct conditions: non-rapid eye movement (non-REM) sleep and rapid eye movement (REM) sleep. Non-REM sleep is divided into four stages representing increasingly deeper levels of sleep. The stages are characterized by a progressive decrease in frequency and increase in amplitude of electroencephalographic (EEG) waves. Stages 3 and 4 of non-REM sleep are also termed "slow-wave sleep" (SWS). In REM sleep, the EEG pattern is distinguished by a rapid, low-voltage wave similar to that occurring during wakefulness, and it is punctuated with short periods of REM. REM sleep is asso-ciated with dreaming, and is a state of general activation of the autonomic nervous system as manifested by large fluctuations in blood pressure, heart rate, and breathing pattern. There are also two forms of REM sleep: tonic—characterized by suppression of skeletal muscle tone; and phasic—marked by periods of REM, irregular respiratory activity, and muscle movement.

During light non-REM sleep (stages 1 and 2), periodic breathing and episodes of apnea lasting as long as 15 seconds may occur. With the transition from wakefulness to sleep, the stimulus of the awake state on breathing diminishes. This leads to a decrease in the sensitivity of the feedback mechanism which insures that ventilation is adequate to maintain a normal Pa_{CO_2}. The resulting manifestations are a periodicity in breathing pattern and wider variability in the Pa_{CO_2}. With the onset of SWS, a higher threshold for CO_2 is established, and breathing becomes regular. During SWS, the ventilatory responses to both hypercapnia and hypoxia remain intact, although the effect of hypercapnia is diminished.

Phasic REM sleep is marked by irregular breathing, with short periods of apnea occurring in conjunction with bursts of REM and skeletal muscle activity. In contrast, breathing is more regular during tonic REM sleep. However, because of loss of skeletal muscle tone including the intercostal groups, there may be paradoxical motion of the rib cage and a decrease in FRC (see chap. 6). As a result of marked fluctuations in the level of ventilation during REM sleep, the ventilatory responses to hypoxia and hypercapnia are difficult to determine. However, it appears that the hypercapnic response is less in REM sleep than in SWS, whereas the hypoxic response may be normal.

READING LIST

Berger A.J., Mitchell R.A., Severinghaus J.W.: Regulation of respiration. *N. Engl. J. Med.* 297:92–97;138–143;194–201, 1977.

This article is a comprehensive review of the neural and chemical stimuli which normally control ventilation.

D'Angelo E.: Control of breathing: central mechanisms and peripheral inputs. *Bull. Eur. Physiopathol. Respir.* 16:111–122, 1980.

This article presents some recent hypotheses regarding mechanisms which control ventilation in the pons and medulla.

Hornbein T.F. (ed.): *Regulation of Breathing, Part I & II*. New York and Basel, Marcel Dekker, Inc., 1981.

A two-volume thorough review of the subject.

Irsigler G.B., Severinghaus J.W.: Clinical problems of ventilatory control. *Annu. Rev. Med.* 31:109–126, 1980.

This review combines a brief synopsis of the physiology underlying the control of ventilation and the pathophysiology of some common clinical disorders.

Milic-Emili J., Whitelaw W.A., Derenne J.Ph.: Occlusion pressure—a simple measure of the respiratory center's output. *N. Engl. J. Med.* 293:1029–1030, 1975.

A short review and description of occlusion pressure measurements with references to other papers.

Milic-Emili J.: Clinical methods for assessing the ventilatory response to carbon dioxide and hypoxia. *N. Engl. J. Med.* 293:864–865, 1975.

A brief review of methods used to assess ventilatory drive.

Phillipson E.A.: Control of breathing during sleep. *Am. Rev. Respir. Dis.* 118:909–939, 1978.

In this comprehensive review is a description of normal sleep architecture and the changes in ventilatory control which occur during sleep.

4

The Thoracic Cage

THE MUSCLES OF RESPIRATION generate the force to produce a deformation of the chest wall and, at the same time, are an integral part of the chest wall. To understand their function, we must first consider the design and kinematics of the bony thorax upon which the respiratory muscles act.

Thoracic Skeleton

The thoracic skeleton consists of 12 thoracic vertebrae, 12 pairs of ribs, the sternum, and fibrocartilaginous or ligamentous connections between the bony structures. Even excluding the musculature and soft tissue, this structure possesses a considerable degree of elastic tension, being semi-rigid but capable of deformation. In configuration it resembles a truncated cone, somewhat dorsoventrally flattened in man. There are 10 costal rings, the last three having a common sternal connection through their costal cartilages. Straightening of the thoracic spinal column from its normal, slightly dorsal convexity results in spreading of the ribs and some increased thoracic volume, but movement of the ribs around their costovertebral joints, effected by the respiratory muscles, produces the volume changes necessary to ventilation.

Two points of articulation exist between the ribs and the vertebrae, one between the head of the rib and the body of the vertebra, the other between the costal tubercle and the vertebral transverse process. A line drawn from the head of the rib to the tubercle defines the axis of the neck of the rib, which is also the axis of motion

of the rib. This is illustrated in Figure 4–1. The transverse process of the first thoracic vertebra is placed nearly frontally but, with succeeding vertebrae, deviates progressively from the frontal plane. As a result, the axes of rotation of the ribs also deviate progressively. With inspiration, the ribs move upward. The first rib, rotating on an axis only slightly deviated from the frontal plane, moves forward as well as upward. This forward and upward displacement has been called the "pump handle" movement. As the axis of rotation approaches a more dorsoventral direction in succeeding lower ribs, the displacement becomes upward and outward—the "bucket handle" movement. During inspiration (see Fig 4–1), this shift in axis of rotation from the first to the twelfth rib causes an increase in antero-posterior diameter of the upper thorax and an increase in transverse diameter of the lower thorax.

The abdomen also moves with respiration and therefore functions as a part of the chest wall. Displacements of the abdominal wall are related not only to movement of the diaphragm but also to thoracoabdominal mechanics. The relationship of transdiaphragmatic pressure to diaphragmatic muscle activity constitutes a realm of complex relationships that are still under investigation.

Diaphragm

The diaphragm is the principal muscle of inspiration. Its muscular components may be ana-

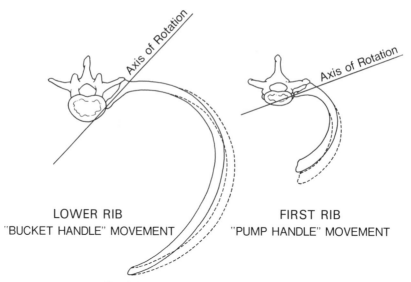

Fig 4–1.—Rib motion with respiration.

tomically subdivided according to their attachments to the bony thorax; *vertebral fibers* attach to the second and third lumbar vertebrae and the medial and lateral arcuate ligaments; *sternal fibers* to the lower xiphoid process and *costal fibers* to the lower six ribs, interdigitating with fibers from the transversus abdominis. The efferent innervation of the diaphragm is the phrenic nerve. The innervation ratio, or number of muscle fibers per motor unit, of the diaphragm is surprisingly small for such a large skeletal muscle. Small innervation ratios are characteristic of muscles performing fine movements, whereas large skeletal muscles usually have high innervation ratios. The diaphragm, having few muscle spindles and tendon organs, exhibits a paucity of proprioceptors. As expected, therefore, stretch reflex is minimal. The afferent innervation is also supplied by the phrenic nerve, with some small contribution from T_6 through T_{12}.

The mechanical effects of diaphragmatic contraction are complex. Contraction causes the dome of the diaphragm to descend, with resulting decrease in intrathoracic pressure and increase in lung volume. However, the diaphragm has a complex geometry and does not act as a simple piston. Since the costal muscle fibers are directed somewhat vertically, their contraction

lifts the lower ribs and rotates them outward around their axes. The mechanical advantage enjoyed by the diaphragm at low lung volumes is lost at high lung volumes when the costal fibers assume a more horizontal direction. Hyperinflation with a low, flattened diaphragm is often observed in patients with chronic airways obstruction. Contraction of the diaphragm in this position may actually oppose further enlargement of the lower thorax. Transdiaphragmatic pressure, taken as an index of the effectiveness of diaphragmatic contraction, decreases with increasing lung volume at the same level of electromyographic activity, illustrating this loss of mechanical advantage with increasing volume.

The electrical activity of the diaphragm increases progressively during quiet inspiration and decreases or vanishes during expiration. During sustained phonation or singing, the diaphragm is electrically inactive. During expulsive efforts the diaphragm is electrically active, assisting the abdominal muscles in raising intra-abdominal pressure.

Intercostal Muscles

Although the role of the intercostal muscles in respiration has been a subject of controversy, it is generally accepted that the external intercostals are muscles of inspiration, and the internal intercostals those of expiration. Their additional role as muscles of posture often supersedes their respiratory function. Nevertheless, contraction of intercostal muscles stabilizes the intercostal spaces, preventing their movement with changes in intrathoracic pressure. They are well supplied with muscle spindles and tendon organs and are innervated through intercostal nerves.

The external intercostals occupy the intercostal spaces from the costal tubercles posteriorly to the costochondral junction anteriorly. Their fibers slope obliquely from each rib downward and forward to insert on the rib below. As a result of this arrangement, contraction of an external intercostal muscle produces a force tending to raise the lower rib.

The internal intercostal muscles lie beneath the external intercostals from the sternum to the angles of the ribs. Their fibers slope obliquely from each rib upward and forward to their insertion on the rib above. Contraction of these muscles has a net effect of lowering the ribs on expiration.

Accessory Muscles

Many muscles of the shoulder girdle and back have been thought to act as accessory muscles of inspiration. Only the scaleni and sternoclei-domastoids serve effectively as inspiratory muscles, however.

The scaleni take their origin from the transverse processes of the lower five cervical vertebrae and insert on the upper surface of the first two ribs. They function to elevate or fix the first two ribs. Although their total contribution to inspiration is small, they may be used at high lung volumes when the contribution of the upper thorax to expansion is greatest.

The sternocleidomastoids originate from the manubrium and medial part of the clavicle and insert on the mastoid process and occipital bone. Contraction elevates the sternum, increasing the anteroposterior diameter of the thorax but contributing nothing to rotation of the ribs and lateral expansion. The contraction of the sternocleidomastoids, commonly seen in patients with severe obstructive diseases, suggests that these may be the most important accessory muscles of inspiration.

The muscles of the abdominal wall—rectus abdominis, transversus abdominis, and internal and external obliques—are powerful expiratory muscles. They may be brought into play when ventilation is voluntarily increased. Normally, however, they play little role in respiration except to generate the expulsive pressure preceding a cough or during maximum expiratory effort.

5

The Pleural Space

THE PLEURA is the continuous, thin mesothelial membrane covering the surface of the lung, superior aspect of the diaphragm, lateral aspects of the mediastinum, and interior aspect of the thoracic wall. Separation into right and left pleural cavities is complete in man, the mediastinal structures filling the central portion of the thoracic cavity. Normally, the remainder of the thoracic cavity is filled by the expanded lung. As a result, there exists only a potential space lined by visceral and parietal pleura, the two pleural surfaces in continuous apposition, gliding over each other during respiratory movements. Beneath the visceral pleura is a network of capillaries derived from the pulmonary circulation. The parietal pleura has a somewhat less extensive capillary network, which is part of the systemic circulation.

As will be described, the lung, being a volume-elastic structure, exerts an elastic force, as does the chest wall. At the resting end-tidal lung volume position, the elastic force of the chest wall directed outward is balanced by the inward elastic forces of the lung. Ignoring gravitational effects, the result is a negative pressure in the potential pleural space of about -5 cm H_2O, reflecting the opposing forces tending to separate the lung from the chest wall. Neither adhesion, cohesion, nor surface forces of attraction explain the failure of the visceral and parietal surfaces to separate. Two plates of glass separated by a thin film of liquid may be held together by such physical forces. Unlike glass, however, the pleura is permeable to fluid and

gas, and other mechanisms must exist to keep the pleural surfaces in contact, the potential space free of air, and the amount of pleural fluid at a minimum. The apposition of parietal and visceral pleuras is attributable to the subatmospheric gas pressure in systemic venous blood.

The total gas tension in arterial blood is close to atmospheric. As blood traverses the tissue capillary bed, each 100 ml gives up approximately 5 ml of oxygen and takes up about 4 ml of carbon dioxide. The loss of oxygen is associated with a 60 torr fall in oxygen tension, but because of the greater solubility of carbon dioxide, the carbon dioxide tension increases only 6 or 7 torr with the increase in carbon dioxide content. The result of gas exchange between blood and tissues, therefore, is a net decrease in total gas pressure in mixed venous blood compared with arterial blood or atmosphere. Thus, the venous blood perfusing the parietal pleura is able to remove gas from the pleural cavity and, under normal circumstances, prevents spontaneous gas accumulation. The clinical significance of this mechanism in the case of spontaneous resolution of pneumothorax is discussed in chapter 23.

The balance of hydraulic and colloid osmotic pressures across the pleural membranes (summarized in Table 5–1) determines the passage of protein-free liquid through them. The presence of a pleural space hydraulic pressure of -5 cm H_2O due to opposing elastic forces has already been noted. This force tends to pull fluid toward the pleural space. The pulmonary capillary

TABLE 5–1.—PRESSURES REGULATING PLEURAL
FLUID*

Pressures Regulating Fluid Flow Across Parietal Pleura
Pleural hydraulic pressure	−5 cm H_2O
Pleural fluid osmotic pressure	−8 cm H_2O
Systemic capillary hydraulic pressure	−30 cm H_2O
Systemic capillary osmotic pressure	+34 cm H_2O
TOTAL PRESSURE	−9 cm H_2O

Pressures Regulating Fluid Flow Across Visceral Pleura
Pleural hydraulic pressure	−5 cm H_2O
Pleural fluid osmotic pressure	−8 cm H_2O
Pulmonary capillary hydraulic pressure	−11 cm H_2O
Pulmonary capillary osmotic pressure	+34 cm H_2O
TOTAL PRESSURE	+10 cm H_2O

*All pressures tending to cause fluid to flow *into* the pleural cavity are designated as minus, and pressures tending to cause fluid to flow *out* of the pleural space as positive.

blood pressure *adds* about 11 cm H_2O to the hydraulic pressure, increasing the tendency for fluid to move across the visceral pleura into the pleural space. The pleural liquid contains protein and exerts a colloid osmotic pressure of 8 cm H_2O. Thus, the total pressure tending to drive fluid into the pleura from the pulmonary circulation is approximately 24 cm H_2O. This is *opposed* by the pulmonary capillary colloid osmotic pressure of about 34 cm H_2O. The result of the combination of osmotic and hydraulic forces is a net pressure of almost 10 cm H_2O, tending to move protein-free liquid *out* of the pleural space across the visceral pleura.

On the chest wall side of the pleural space, the mean blood pressure of systemic capillaries of the parietal pleura is about 30 cm H_2O. This is a hydraulic pressure tending to drive fluid into the pleural space. Added to this is the 5 cm H_2O hydraulic pressure due to elastic forces and the 8 cm H_2O colloid osmotic pressure of pleural fluid, resulting in a total pressure of 43 cm H_2O driving fluid across the parietal pleura into the pleural space. This is opposed by the plasma colloid osmotic pressure of 34 cm H_2O in the parietal pleura capillaries. The result is a net

pressure of 9 cm H_2O, driving fluid *into* the pleural space from capillaries in the parietal pleura. Thus, the tendency of pleural fluid to be absorbed by the pulmonary circulation is nearly balanced by a tendency for fluid to escape from systemic capillaries, allowing the pleural surfaces to stay moist and well lubricated. The greater vascularity and absorptive power of the visceral pleura maintain the pleural liquid at a minimum.

The pleural space is maintained free of gas because the total gas pressure of mixed venous blood is less than atmospheric, and it is free of fluid accumulation because the combination of hydraulic and osmotic forces results in a net pressure tending to fluid absorption. Thus, the lung is held against the chest wall, changes in thoracic volume are transmitted to the lung, and a discontinuous film of pleural liquid remains to function as a lubricant, allowing pleural surfaces to glide over one another.

Careful measurements of true intrapleural pressure in animals have revealed that the pressure is not constant over the entire surface of the lung. In the upright posture pleural pressure exhibits a vertical gradient that is gravity-dependent. Intrapleural pressure is most negative at the apex of the lung and becomes progressively less negative down the lung, revealing a gradient of about 0.3 cm H_2O/cm vertical distance. This suggests that the weight of the lung is supported within the thorax primarily at the pleural surface and to an insignificant degree by the hili. Other studies have revealed that alveoli at the apex of the lung are inflated to a greater degree than those at the base and that inspired air is distributed sequentially from apex to base rather than uniformly. These gravity-dependent phenomena related to the gradient of transpulmonary pressure have important implications in the regional distribution of ventilation discussed in chapter 10.

READING LIST

Black L.F.: Subject Review. The pleural and space and pleural fluid. *Mayo Clin. Proc.* 47:493–506, 1972.

Setnikar I., Agostoni E.: Factors keeping the lung expanded in the chest. *Proc. Int. Union Physiol. Sci.* 1:281–286, 1962.

These two articles deal with pleural fluid and factors influencing pleural pressure.

Hoppin F.G., Jr., Green I.D., Mead J.: Distribution of pleural surface pressure in dogs. *J. Appl. Physiol.* 27:863–873, 1969.

McMahon S.M., Proctor D.F., Permutt S.: Pleural surface pressure in dogs. *J. Appl. Physiol.* 27:881–885, 1969.

Proctor D.F., Caldini P., Permutt S.: The pressure surrounding the lungs. *Respir. Physiol.* 5:130–144, 1968.

The preceding articles describe experimental evidence for a gravity-dependent gradient of pleural pressure.

Mechanics of
the Respiratory System

THE RESPIRATORY SYSTEM behaves mechanically as a pump consisting of a volume-elastic component and a flow-resistive component connected in series. The volume-elastic component is capable of deformation and volume change. A change in volume is accompanied by a flow of gas through the airways, a system of branching collapsible tubes that exhibit resistance to flow. In analyzing this or any mechanical system, we may use a form of Newton's Third Law of Motion relating the forces applied to the system to the opposing forces within the system.

The respiratory muscles generate pressures that produce mechanical alterations in the respiratory system. To produce these alterations, opposing forces must be overcome. The pressure (P), the action resulting from the application of this pressure, the opposing forces, and their relationship to one another are summarized in Table 6–1.

Thus, the pressure applied must overcome elastic forces to produce a volume change, resistive forces to produce volume flow ($\dot{V}$), and inertial forces to produce volume acceleration ($\ddot{V}$). These relationships may be combined to form an *equation of motion* for the respiratory system:

$$P = \left(\frac{1}{C} \times V\right) + (R \times \dot{V}) + (I \times \ddot{V})$$

At normal breathing frequencies, inertance is small and may be neglected. Each of the static elastic and dynamic resistive properties of the system will be discussed, along with a consideration of the work required to overcome these forces.

Static Elastic Properties and Lung Volumes

The physical properties of a linear elastic structure, such as a spring, may be described by the relationship of change in applied force to change in length. The elastic characteristic of the three-dimensional respiratory system is described by the relationship of pressure to volume. Measurements of elastic characteristics must be made under static conditions in which pressures required to overcome flow resistance or inertance need not enter into consideration.

The respiratory pump has two elastic components, the lung itself and the chest wall surrounding the lung. The latter consists not only of the skeleton and tissues of the thoracic cage, but also of the diaphragm, abdominal contents, and abdominal wall. Both the lung and chest wall have elastic characteristics of their own, the characteristic of the total respiratory system being the sum of the two.

The air-filled lung, upon opening the thorax, tends to collapse to a certain minimal volume, but does not become totally airless. Therefore, it is apparent that the lung exerts a force which, when unopposed, tends to reduce its volume, and that force, measured as the pressure differ-

TABLE 6–1.—RESPONSE OF THE RESPIRATORY
SYSTEM TO MECHANICAL FORCES

ACTION	OPPOSING FORCE	EQUATION
Deformation = volume change (V)	Elastic $\left(\dfrac{1}{C}\right)$	$P = \dfrac{V}{C}$
Rate of deformation = volume flow ($\dot{V}$)	Resistive (R)	$P = R\dot{V}$
Rate of change of flow = volume acceleration ($\ddot{V}$)	Inertial (I)	$P = I\ddot{V}$

ence between the interior and exterior of the lung, can be related to the lung volume. When measured in a stepwise fashion under static conditions, the transpulmonary pressures and corresponding lung volumes can be used to describe the elastic characteristic of the lung. In the pulmonary laboratory, an esophageal balloon can be used to measure a close approximation of pleural pressure, and, when related to mouth pressure measured with glottis open to derive alveolar pressure, one can obtain transpulmonary pressure together with corresponding lung volume on a living human subject. The static pressure-volume characteristic is constructed from a series of simultaneous pressure and volume measurements made at different volumes under static conditions. The resulting pressure-volume (P-V) curve during deflation from total lung capacity (TLC) to residual volume (RV) is shown in Figure 6–1.

The static deflation P-V curve has been used to describe the effects of aging on the lung and to assess changes in lung mechanics associated with disease processes. Utilization of such measurements is complicated by the nonlinearity of the relationship of pressure to volume as well as by the variability in lung volumes between individuals. The problem has been essentially one of describing and comparing the shapes of curves. In recent years, such comparisons have been facilitated by mathematical techniques. At least at volumes above functional residual capacity (FRC), P-V data can be fitted to an exponential equation in which a constant appears as the exponent. This constant is, in effect, a descriptor of the shape of the curve and can be used to distinguish normal from abnormal P-V

curves. This derived number better describes the entire curve than does a value for compliance (see below) which describes only a segment of the curve.

Because the P-V characteristic is nonlinear, it is apparent that a single number will not describe the elastic properties of the lungs. Yet, because it is convenient to use, the term " pulmonary compliance" has gained acceptance. Compliance is defined as the change in volume for a given change in pressure:

$$C = \frac{\Delta V}{\Delta P}$$

It is expressed in liters per cm H_2O but, since the characteristic is clearly curvilinear, C is the *slope* of this curve at a point and is therefore volume-dependent. As can be seen from Figure 6–1, the lung is least compliant at high lung volumes. According to convention, compliance has come to mean the slope of the static deflation P-V curve over the tidal volume (V_T) range, a short segment of a curve being treated as a straight line (see Fig 6–1). However, if so de-

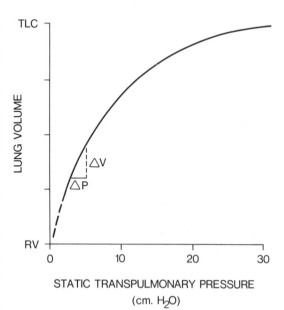

Fig 6–1.—The static deflation pressure-volume (P-V) curve for the lung. The conventional definition of compliance is the ratio of change in volume to change in pressure over the tidal volume range, as illustrated here.

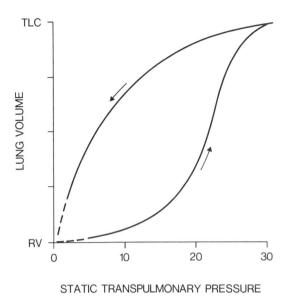

STATIC TRANSPULMONARY PRESSURE (cm. H₂O)

Fig 6–2.—Static deflation and inflation pressure-volume curves for the lung. The deflation and inflation curves differ. The complete P-V loop, therefore, exhibits hysteresis.

fined, compliance may remain unchanged even if there are marked changes in lung elastic properties, resulting in a shift of the P-V curve to the left or right, particularly if the volume at which tidal breathing occurs is also changed. Thus, changes in lung recoil, i.e., the recoil pressure at some state of lung inflation, should be distinguished from changes in compliance.

Not only is the elastic characteristic of the lung nonlinear, it also exhibits hysteresis. A structure is said to exhibit hysteresis if, when a force is withdrawn, the path of deformation differs from that described as a force is applied. If measurements of pressure and volume are made during lung inflation, the curve takes on a different configuration from that observed during deflation, higher pressures being required to achieve a given lung volume in inflation compared with deflation. The complete P-V loop, demonstrating hysteresis, is shown in Figure 6–2. From this it is apparent that compliance and lung recoil pressure are not only dependent on the volume at which they are determined, but on volume history as well.

Three factors contribute to the elastic characteristic of the lung and its hysteresis. First, the tissue elements of which the lung is constructed have their own elastic properties which demonstrate hysteresis. Perhaps more important, however, is the architectural arrangement of the elements within a structure. Because of the arrangement of threads in a nylon stocking, for example, the stocking has a different elastic characteristic from the nylon strands themselves. The lung is a complex three-dimensional mesh-like structure, with approximately 300 million alveoli, many thousands of alveolar ducts, respiratory bronchioles, and multiple branching airways, blood vessels, and collagen and elastic fibers. The "nylon stocking elasticity" resulting from lung architecture contributes to the elastic retraction force of the lung. Disruption of lung architecture resulting, for example, from the destructive process seen in emphysema can markedly alter the elastic characteristic of the lung.

A second factor contributing to the elastic characteristic, pulmonary hysteresis, and alveolar stability appears to be the presence of a film of surface-active material (surfactant) lining the alveoli. Pulmonary surfactant, a phospholipid

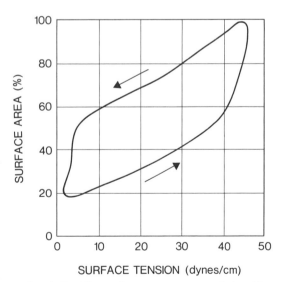

SURFACE TENSION (dynes/cm)

Fig 6–3.—The surface tension-area relationship for a film of pulmonary surfactant. The surface tension varies with the area over which the surfactant film is distributed, and the relationship exhibits hysteresis.

rich in lecithin, is produced by the alveolar type
II cell. The surface tension of a surfactant film
is not fixed, but varies with the area of the surface over which the liquid is distributed. In addition, the area-tension characteristic of a surfactant film itself exhibits hysteresis, as shown
in Figure 6–3. The possible physiologic significance of this alveolar lining layer becomes apparent when the LaPlace relationship is applied
to the alveolus, which in this discussion is assumed to be spherical. The LaPlace relationship
states that the pressure (P) within an elastic
sphere is directly proportional to the tension (T)
of the wall and inversely proportional to the radius of curvature (r):

$$P = \frac{2T}{r}$$

The liquid that lines the alveolus must exert a
surface tension. If surfactant were not present in
this liquid, the surface tension would be fixed,
and greater pressure would be required to keep
an alveolus open as its radius of curvature diminished with decrease in volume. Small alveoli
would empty into larger ones, atelectasis would
regularly occur at low lung volumes, and large
expanding pressures would be required to reopen collapsed lung units. This is prevented by
the presence of surfactant in alveolar lining film.
As the radius of curvature of alveoli diminishes,
so does the area over which the surfactant film
is stretched. This causes a reduction in the surface tension exerted by the surfactant film, allowing the air spaces to remain open at low
transpulmonary pressure. In this way, surfactant
plays an important role in imparting stability to
alveoli in the normal lung.

The area-tension hysteresis of surfactant also
contributes to the lung P-V hysteresis. When the
effect of surface forces is eliminated experimentally by filling the lung with saline instead of
air, the resulting P-V loop exhibits little hysteresis. Furthermore, as shown in Figure 6–4, the
saline curves are shifted to the left, since less
pressure is required to expand and fill the lung.
From this it is apparent that surface forces make
a major contribution to the lung's elastic retractive force. It is also evident that the elastic prop-

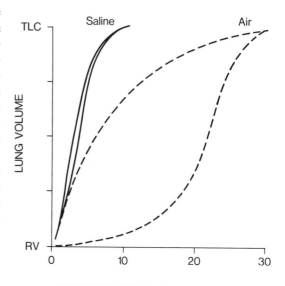

STATIC TRANSPULMONARY PRESSURE
(cm. H_2O)

Fig 6–4.—Pressure-volume curves for the lung:
air-filled and liquid-filled. The difference between
the curves is the contribution of surface tension to
the lung elastic characteristic.

erties of the lung are dependent upon production
of this unique surface-active substance. Respiratory system disorders that involve destruction,
inactivation, or insufficient production of surfactant are characterized by marked changes in the
P-V characteristic of the lung, even without
structural changes in the lung parenchyma. Examples of such disorders are described in chapter 28.

Alveoli are not spherical but are closely
packed, irregularly faceted polyhedral structures
which change shape and configuration as lung
volume changes. The elastic interdependence of
adjacent structures imparts an additional degree
of alveolar stability. The alveoli, alveolar ducts,
and respiratory bronchioles of a single acinus
are served by one terminal bronchiole of 0.5 to
0.6 mm in diameter. There is evidence to suggest that at low lung volumes, these terminal
airways may undergo functional closure. The
lung units peripheral to these closed airways will
then cease to participate in the change in lung
volume and will not inflate until these airways
open again. The pressure required to reopen

these closed airways may be considerably greater than the pressure at which they closed. Only when this critical opening pressure is achieved can these airways reopen and the lung units served by them be recruited to participate in volume change. This recruitment on inflation and derecruitment on deflation is the third factor contributing to the elastic characteristic and hysteresis of the P-V loop. These terminal bronchioles are also lined with pulmonary surfactant. The variable surface tension of surfactant lining terminal airways is of great importance in stabilizing their behavior and maintaining their patency. In the absence of this stabilizing surfactant lining layer, these airways would close more readily and require higher pressures to reopen, and the work of breathing would be increased. Indeed, pulmonary surfactant may play its most important role at the level of terminal airways.

The many disorders associated with altered compliance and lung elastic recoil and with abnormalities in lung volumes are described in Part III. Several mechanisms may be responsible for these abnormalities. Disruption of lung architecture, with destruction of alveolar walls and formation of large intraparenchymal air spaces (pulmonary emphysema), is accompanied by loss of lung recoil and increased compliance. The lung may be stiff, with a decrease in compliance, when there is surfactant deficiency, interstitial fibrosis, diffuse parenchymal disease, or a decrease in the number of functioning lung units. The influence of the number of functioning units on compliance becomes apparent if we consider the acute effect of lung resection. If each lung expands 100 ml/cm H_2O of applied transpulmonary pressure, the compliance of each lung is 0.1 L/cm H_2O, and the compliance of the total system 0.2 L/cm H_2O. Removal of one lung would reduce the compliance of the total system by 50%. For the same reason, an intact small lung would appear to be stiffer than a large one simply because it is smaller. An infant must generate almost the same intrapleural pressure to take in a tidal breath as an adult does to produce a much larger V_T. To take these size differences into account, the term "specific

compliance," or "compliance per liter of lung volume," is sometimes used. Here, exponential analysis offers certain advantages. In these examples, if volume is expressed as a percent of TLC, the overall *shape* of the P-V curve may be the same, and consequently the shape constant derived from exponential analysis would also be the same.

The elastic properties of the chest wall are more difficult to characterize, since muscular tone is often an undefined variable in this component of the respiratory pump. However, the elastic characteristic of the chest wall may be approximated by obtaining pressure and volume measurements during voluntary relaxation. Because its structural components are semi-rigid, the thoracic cage alone, when unstressed, assumes the volume it usually achieves when the lung is approximately two thirds of its maximum capacity. The P-V characteristic of the thorax is shown in Figure 6–5.

In vivo the lung and chest wall must act in concert. The elastic characteristic of the total respiratory system, therefore, is the algebraic sum of the characteristics of its two components. This combined P-V characteristic is referred to as the *relaxation pressure curve* in Figure 6–5. In this figure, pressures tending to reduce lung volume are positive in sign; pressures tending to increase lung volume are negative in sign.

Changes of lung volume are produced by the forces generated by the respiratory muscles. At resting end-tidal volume, or FRC, however, the respiratory muscles are relaxed, and volume is determined by a balance of elastic forces. The elastic retractive properties of the lung exert a force tending to reduce lung volume. The chest wall, on the other hand, is below its resting volume and exerts a force tending to increase lung volume. At FRC these forces in opposite directions are exactly in balance, establishing this as the resting volume of the respiratory system (see Fig 6–5). Tidal inspiration requires muscular activity; tidal expiration is normally passive. It can be seen from the relaxation pressure curve for the respiratory system that, over the tidal volume range, less change in pressure is required

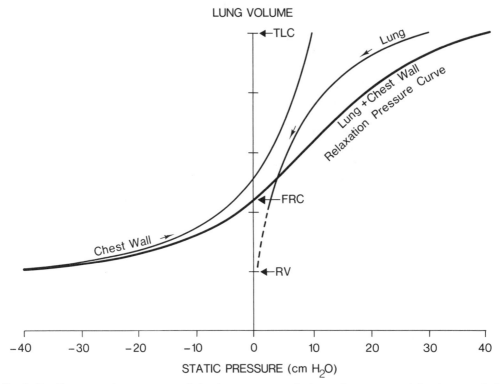

LUNG VOLUME

TLC

Lung

Lung + Chest Wall
Relaxation Pressure Curve

FRC

Chest Wall

RV

STATIC PRESSURE (cm H$_2$O)

Fig 6–5.—Pressure-volume curves of the lung, chest wall and combined respiratory system. The latter is the algebraic sum of the first two and is often called the relaxation pressure curve. Functional residual capacity is determined by the bal-ance of elastic forces exerted by lung and chest wall when no muscular forces are applied. Positive pressures on this diagram represent pressures tend-ing to decrease lung volume; negative pressures increase lung volume.

for a comparable change in volume than else-where on the curve. In terms of energy expen-diture, optimum efficiency is obtained by breathing in this volume range.

The static determinants of the TLC and RV, and hence of the vital capacity (VC), are also the result of a balance of forces. In this instance, the sum of elastic forces is balanced by maxi-mum muscle forces. The extremes of pressure generated by respiratory muscles may be mea-sured, relative to lung volume, by making max-imum inspiratory and expiratory efforts against an obstructed airway (Fig 6–6). Such maximum pressures, measured under static conditions, cannot be achieved when flow is permitted. However, at the extremes of lung volume (RV and TLC), static conditions are achieved. The elastic forces of the respiratory system at TLC are balanced by the maximum inspiratory mus-cle forces. Similarly, at RV, the elastic forces, contributed primarily by chest wall tending to expand, are balanced by the maximum expira-tory muscle forces. Thus, the limits of volume excursion are determined by a balance of static elastic and muscle forces. The volume excursion defined by these limits is, of course, the VC. The important point to remember is that these lung volume measurements—RV, TLC, VC, and FRC—do not refer to fixed, anatomically determined spaces. Rather, they are determined by elastic charcteristics of the respiratory sys-tem and by the muscle forces applied to that system.

Because TLC, RV, and VC are determined by a balance between elastic and muscle forces, lung volume changes will occur as a result of changes in the compliance of lungs or chest wall or weakness of respiratory muscles. A wide va-

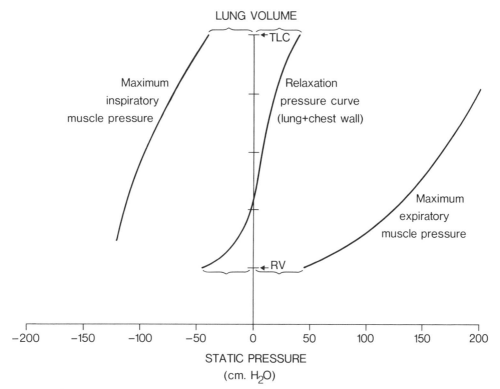

Fig 6–6.—The relaxation pressure characteristic of the respiratory system (lung + chest wall) compared to static maximum pressures generated by inspiratory and expiratory muscles. Total lung capacity **(TLC)** and residual volume **(RV)** are determined by the balance of elastic and muscular forces. Positive pressures decrease lung volume; negative pressures increase lung volume.

riety of conditions, such as chest wall deformity, pulmonary fibrosis, and poliomyelitis, may reduce VC and TLC.

Dynamic Resistive Properties and Maximum Expiratory Flow

The second term in the equation of motion for the respiratory system deals with resistive forces, dynamic phenomena encountered when pressure is applied to generate flow. A mechanical equivalent of Ohm's law defines resistance (R) as the relationship between pressure (P) and flow ($\dot{V}$):

$$R = \frac{P}{\dot{V}}$$

Resistance is expressed in units of cm H_2O per liter per second. This relationship is sometimes

expressed as conductance, the reciprocal of resistance.

There are marked differences in the contributions of various portions of the tracheobronchial tree to total pulmonary resistance. When breathing is through the nose, nasal resistance contributes at least 50% of the total resistance and may be quite variable, as anyone suffering from nasal congestion can testify. If resistance is measured during mouth breathing, the mouth, pharynx, glottis, larynx, and upper extrathoracic trachea account for at least one third of the total resistance.

The intrathoracic airways go through many generations of branching from the trachea through the alveolar ducts. With succeeding generations of branching, the total cross-sectional area of the tracheobronchial tree increases, and each individual airway conducts

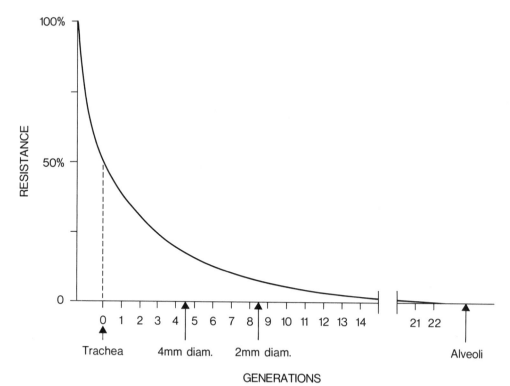

Fig 6–7.—The distribution of airway resistance. Succeeding generations of branching of the tra- cheobronchial tree contribute a diminishing proportion of the total resistance to flow through airways.

less and less of the total flow. As a result of this design, the large upper airways from the trachea through segmental bronchi contribute a substantial portion of the remainder of the total resistance, whereas the smaller peripheral airways contribute very little to total resistance. At a given lung volume, the approximate relationship between resistive contribution and generation of branching may be depicted as shown in Figure 6–7.

Resistance varies with lung volume, diminishing with increasing volume. In order to take lung volume into consideration, the term "specific conductance," defined as conductance per unit of lung volume, has been used. The influence of lung volume on resistance stems from the elastic interaction of lung parenchyma and intrapulmonary airways. The intrapulmonary airways depend upon lung recoil for their external support. As lung elastic recoil increases with increasing lung volume, the radial traction ex- erted on the walls of intrapulmonary airways increases. With increasing airway caliber, the resistance to flow decreases. This increase in airway diameter, as well as length, with increase in volume is readily seen fluoroscopically during bronchography.

The airways themselves have intrinsic properties that influence their caliber. Thus, the tone of bronchial smooth muscle, thickness of bronchial mucosa, or the amount of bronchial secretions also contributes to airway resistance. These factors are of particular significance in disease states.

Although resistance can be measured directly, the most common method of assessing airway function involves analysis of the forced vital capacity (FVC) maneuver. In most laboratories this is accomplished by obtaining during forced expiration a spirometric recording of volume in time, as depicted in Figure 6–8. In addition to providing a measurement of the res-

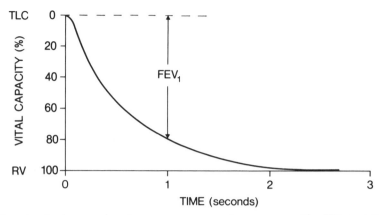

Fig 6–8.—The standard normal spirogram, a plot of expired volume in time during a forced vital capacity maneuver. The **FEV₁** is defined as the volume expired during the first second.

piratory system's maximum volume excursion, this curve also provides measurements of maximum expiratory flow ($\dot{V}$max). Many methods have been used to quantitate the maximum flow, including peak flow rate, maximum expiratory flow rate (MEFR, forced expiratory flow or $FEF_{200-1200}$), maximum midexpiratory flow (MMF or $FEF_{25-75\%}$), and forced expiratory volumes over different time intervals. The most widely used of these is the forced expiratory volume in the first second (FEV_1), which is an expression of the average flow during the first second of exhalation. At any point on the volume-time spirogram, the slope of the curve is an expression of the instantaneous flow at that volume. That maximum expiratory flow, $\dot{V}$max, can be plotted against volume as the maximum expiratory flow-volume (MEFV) curve illus-

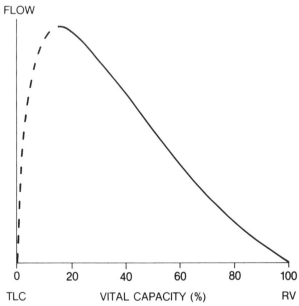

Fig 6–9.—The maximum expiratory flow-volume curve. The solid descending portion of the curve is independent of effort in excess of the minimum effort required to achieve maximal flow. The abscissa represents the percent of the forced vital capacity exhaled at the time flow is measured.

trated in Figure 6–9. From such a curve, the flow after 50% ($\dot{V}max_{50\%}$) or 75% ($\dot{V}max_{75\%}$) of the VC has been expired is often reported.

From the MEFV curve shown in Figure 6–9, it is apparent that there is a unique relationship between $\dot{V}max$ and lung volume. Once $\dot{V}max$ has been achieved at a given lung volume, it cannot be exceeded regardless of further increases in expiratory effort on driving pressure. Thus $\dot{V}max$ is said to be "effort-independent."

The effort independence of $\dot{V}max$ can be demonstrated by having a subject repeat an expiratory maneuver with graded efforts, increasing the effort and expiratory flow with subsequent maneuvers. In so doing, a series of flow-volume curves is generated, as shown in Figure 6–10. Let us now examine the relationship of effort, or driving pressure, and flow at a single lung volume. In Figure 6–10 a line ZZ is drawn at an arbitrary lung volume; in Figure 6–11, the pressure-flow relationships at that lung volume

are described. From this isovolume pressure-flow curve, it may be seen that flow increases with driving pressure only up to the point at which $\dot{V}max$ is attained, after which flow does not increase, remaining independent of further increases in driving pressure. This "effort-independent" plateau of flow occurs at all lung volumes except those near TLC. Thus, the first 25% of an MEFV curve is said to be "effort-dependent."

The role of the several factors which determine $\dot{V}max$ at a given lung volume can be understood by considering the schematic model of the respiratory system depicted in Figure 6–12. In this model of a normal lung, where ventilation is assumed to be evenly distributed, we may consider flow-resistive and volume-elastic components as elements connected in series within the thorax. If we take the pressure at the outlet of the airway as the zero reference point, the total driving pressure down the airway is equal to alveolar pressure (P_{alv}). At a given lung vol-

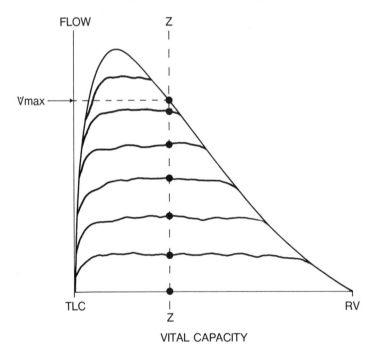

Fig 6–10.—A series of expiratory vital capacity maneuvers with sequentially increasing effort would result in this series of flow-volume curves culminating with the maximum expiratory flow-volume curve, which cannot be exceeded. By examining pressure and flow during these graded efforts at any specific volume, indicated by line ZZ, we can construct the curve shown in Figure 6–11.

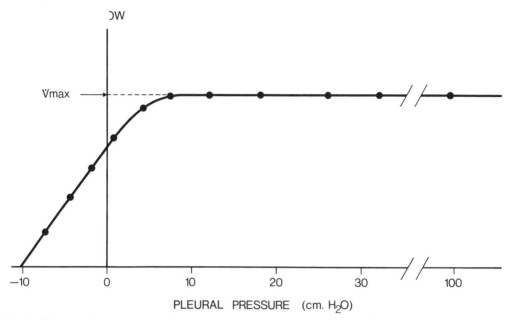

Fig 6–11.—Isovolume pressure-flow curve. Pressure and flow are plotted against each other for the graded expiratory efforts at a specific volume, as shown in Figure 6–10.

ume during forced exhalation, P_{alv} is the sum of two components, lung recoil pressure, $P_{st}(L)$, and pleural pressure, P_{pl}:

$$P_{alv} = P_{pl} + P_{st}(L)$$

Because there is a gradient of diminishing pressure down the airway from the alveolus to the outlet, there are points within the airways at which the pressure drop from P_{alv} will be equal to $P_{st}(L)$. These points, at which the lateral airway pressure is exactly equal to P_{pl}, are referred to as the equal pressure points (EPP). For airways upstream of the EPP, the driving pressure is equal to $P_{st}(L)$, the pressure drop from alveolus to EPP. $\dot{V}max$, then, is determined by the relationship:

$$\dot{V}max = \frac{P_{st}(L)}{Rus}$$

where Rus is the resistance of the airways upstream from the EPP. At any given lung volume, $P_{st}(L)$ is fixed, being uniquely related to lung volume by the P-V characteristic of the lung. However, during forced expiration, P_{pl},

which is the driving pressure for the segment of airways downstream from the EPP, is not fixed. It varies with the expiratory effort being generated. Whereas the pressure within airways upstream from the EPP is greater than P_{pl}, the pressure within airways downstream is everywhere less than P_{pl}. Since the airways are nonrigid tubes, they are subject to dynamic compression. The greater the P_{pl} generated, the greater the degree of dynamic compression. For this reason, the resistance of the airways downstream from the EPP (Rds) increases in direct proportion to P_{pl}:

$$Rds = \frac{P_{pl}}{\dot{V}max}$$

These airways function as a Starling resistor, limiting expiratory flow. As a result of these mechanisms, further effort beyond the minimum necessary to achieve $\dot{V}max$ will result in no further increase in flow, and $\dot{V}max$ may be considered to be effort-independent.

The topographic locations of the EPP within the tracheobronchial tree have been determined

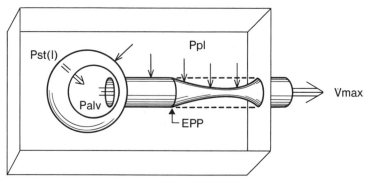

Fig 6–12.—A schematic model of the respiratory system. Pleural pressure (**P$_{pl}$**) is applied equally to the system. The driving pressure down the system is alveolar pressure (**P$_{alv}$**), the sum of **P$_{pl}$** and the elastic recoil pressure of the lung (**P$_{st}$(L)**) at that lung volume. At the equal pressure point (**EPP**), lateral pressure in the airway is equal to **P$_{pl}$**. The EPP divides the airway into two segments, one upstream and one downstream from that point. When maximal flow (V̇max) is achieved, the resistance for each segment may be separately defined. The downstream segment is subject to dynamic compression during forced expiration.

by empirical observations. At high lung volumes, the EPP are located in large upper airways. The cross-sectional area of large airways assumes significance here, when we also must consider the pressures required to accelerate gas molecules from the alveoli, where linear velocities are small, to the large airways, where linear velocities are significantly large. At lower lung volumes, V̇max diminishes and the EPP move toward the alveoli. Under these circumstances, accelerative losses become less significant, whereas frictional resistance of smaller, more peripheral airways assumes a more important influence on V̇max.

According to this analysis, V̇max is determined by the driving pressure, P$_{st}$(L), down the airways from the alveoli to the EPP, and the resistance, Rus, of those airways. The resistance of airways is a function of their geometry. Changes in airway caliber may be intrinsic. However, many of the airways upstream from EPP are intrapulmonary, depending upon lung recoil for part of their support. Thus, P$_{st}$(L) may affect Rus by its extrinsic influence on airway caliber. The cross-sectional area of large airways also affects V̇max.

Ultimately, flow is limited regardless of further increase in driving pressure when a critical velocity is achieved at some point within the airways. If we consider the analogy of a rigid tube

in which was incorporated a plug with a pinhole orifice, flow through the tube would be limited to that achieved when gas molecules moved through the orifice at the speed of sound. Because the speed of sound is the critical velocity which cannot be exceeded, once that velocity is achieved, further increase in driving pressure would not result in further increase in flow. In flexible tubes, however, the critical velocity is the wave speed, the maximum speed at which a pressure pulse would be propagated through the tube, and the first point down the airways at which that velocity is achieved is the choke point. Wave speed is determined by the balance between the inertia of the fluid, or gas density (ρ), and the elastic characteristic of the airway at the choke point. The latter is expressed as the change in airway transmural pressure, dPtm, producing a given change in area, dA, and in turn determines the area, A, at the choke point under flow-limiting conditions. Thus,

$$\text{wave speed} = \left(\frac{1}{\rho} \times \frac{dPtm}{dA} \times A\right)^{0.5}$$

Inasmuch as flow is the product of the area and the velocity, the flow at wave speed, or V̇max, can be expressed by the equation:

$$\dot{V}max = \left(\frac{1}{\rho}\right)^{0.5} \left(\frac{dPtm}{dA}\right)^{0.5} A^{1.5}$$

From this it follows that flow will be greater if the gas is less dense, if the tube is stiffer, or if the cross-sectional area is greater.

Thus, $\dot{V}$max is determined by a number of complexly interrelated factors. Timed spirograms, which yield measurements of average flows over increments of expired volumes, have been widely used in clinical practice to assess ventilatory function and instantaneous measurements of $\dot{V}$max breathing air or breathing gas mixtures of different densities are coming to be regarded as useful. It is clear that $\dot{V}$max would be expected to be reduced in any disorders associated with decreased lung elastic recoil or with airway narrowing from whatever cause.

Work of Breathing and Patterns of Respiration

The act of breathing requires that the muscles of respiration perform work. This work is a product of the pressure generated by muscular forces and the motion or volume change that results. To achieve a given level of ventilation, the work performed must be sufficient to overcome opposing forces and thus will vary with the rate and depth of respiration and the lung volume at which the breathing cycles occur.

Work must be expended to overcome elastic forces of the respiratory system. The amount of elastic work, therefore, is related to the V_T and the lung volume at which we breathe. It is modified by alterations in the elastic properties of the lung or chest wall. Work is also required to overcome the resistance to airflow presented by the respiratory airways. The amount of such resistive work is related to flow and is modified by anything that affects airway caliber or patency. An additional small amount of work is required to rearrange the molecular orientation of thoracic tissues as the system assumes an altered configuration. This is the nonelastic work necessary to overcome tissue viscous resistance. Finally, work is required to overcome inertia. At normal breathing frequencies inertial work is minimal, but at very high frequencies it may be significant.

It is interesting to consider the effect of breathing pattern on work of breathing. With each breath about 150 ml of ventilation is "wasted" on the anatomical dead space; i.e., the conducting airways where no gas exchange occurs (see chap. 8). Thus, a greater *total* ventilation is required to maintain a given level of *alveolar* or *effective* ventilation as the respiratory rate increases. An increase in total ventilation per minute implies a higher average flow rate. Since resistive work is a function of flow rate, resistive work also must increase. Thus, to maintain a given level of alveolar ventilation, resistive work is minimized by a slow, deep breathing pattern and increases with respiratory frequency.

An opposite effect is noted on elastic work. Elastic work is roughly proportional to the square of the V_T. Thus, slow deep breathing greatly increases work needed to overcome elastic forces. The relationship of elastic and resistive work to breathing frequency in resting normal subjects is shown in Figure 6–13. It should be noted that the total work of breathing (the sum of resistive and elastic work) is minimal with respiratory frequencies near 14 per minute. It is near this frequency that the least average force is required of the respiratory muscles to achieve a particular level of alveolar ventilation.

Abnormalities of respiratory mechanics will result in altered breathing patterns. If flow resistance is increased, a slow, deep breathing pattern will be adopted, whereas a rapid, shallow pattern may be optimal when compliance is decreased. The pattern adopted will be that requiring the least respiratory work, but the total work will still be greater than it would have been had the mechanical abnormality not developed. For this reason, increased work of breathing is a common feature of most respiratory disorders, the amount of increase depending on the severity of the disorder.

The performance of work requires the expenditure of energy, which, in turn, is reflected by the consumption of oxygen. The oxygen consumed by respiratory muscles in a normal healthy person is extremely small at rest (approximately 5% of the total metabolic rate) and increases moderately with increase in ventila-

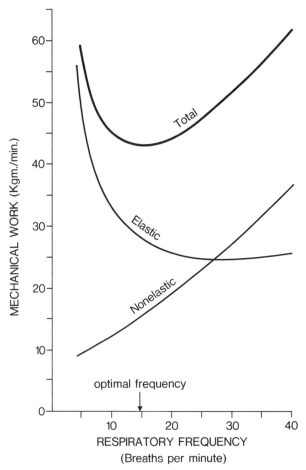

Fig 6–13.—The relationship between mechanical work and respiratory frequency. Elastic work is expended to overcome elastic forces. Nonelastic work is required to overcome flow resistance and tissue viscous resistance. The sum of these two components is the total work of breathing and varies with breathing frequency. Breathing frequency is optimal when the work required is least.

tion. However, if the work of breathing is increased because of a disorder affecting the respiratory system, the oxygen cost of breathing will be markedly elevated. The oxygen cost of breathing at rest in a patient with emphysema, for example, may be as great as ten times the normal value and becomes a significant factor limiting increases in ventilation.

READING LIST

Fry D.L.: Theoretical considerations of the bronchial pressure-flow-volume relationships with particular reference to the maximum expiratory flow volume curve. *Phys. Med. Biol.* 3:174–194, 1958.

Fry D.L., Ebert R.V., Stead W.W., et al.: Review: The mechanics of pulmonary ventilation in normal subjects and in patients with emphysema. *Am. J. Med.* 16:80–97, 1954.

Fry D.L., Hyatt R.E.: Reviews: Pulmonary Mechanics—a unified analysis of the relationship between pressure, volume and gasflow in the lungs of normal and diseased human subjects. *Am. J. Med.* 29:672–689, 1960.

Hyatt R.E.: The interrelationships of pressure, flow, and volume during various respiratory maneuvers in normal and emphysematous subjects. *Am. Rev. Respir. Dis.* 83:676–683, 1961.

Hyatt R.E., Schilder D.P., Fry D.L.: Relationship

between maximum expiratory flow and degree of lung inflation. *J. Appl. Physiol.* 13:331–336, 1958.

These early articles dealing with pressure-flow-volume relationships form the basis for subsequent work in this area and may be considered classics.

Dayman H.: The expiratory spirogram. *Am. Rev. Respir. Dis.* 83:842–843, 1961.

This is a classic early paper on analysis of the FVC maneuver.

Mead J., Turner M.M., Macklem P.T., et al.: Significance of the relationship between lung recoil and maximum expiratory flow. *J. Appl. Physiol.* 22:95–108, 1967.

Pride N.B., Permutt S., Riley R.L., et al.: Determinants of maximal expiratory flow from the lungs. *J. Appl. Physiol.* 23:646–662, 1967.

These two papers discuss the determinants of maximum expiratory flow from different viewpoints. The first describes the equal pressure point concept.

Green M., Mead J., Hoppin E., et al.: Analysis of the forced expiratory maneuver. *Chest* 36:335–355, 1973.

Hyatt R.E., Black L.F.: The flow-volume curve: a current perspective. *Am. Rev. Respir. Dis.* 107:191–199, 1973.

The flow-volume curve is discussed in general terms in these two papers.

Dawson S.V., Elliott E.A.: Use of the choke point in the prediction of flow limitation in elastic tubes. *Fed. Proc.* 39:2765–2770, 1980.

Dawson S.V., Elliott E.A.: Wave-speed limitation on expiratory flow—a unifying concept. *J. Appl. Physiol.* 43:498–515, 1977.

Elliott E.A., Dawson S.V.: Test of wave-speed theory of flow limitation in elastic tubes. *J. Appl. Physiol.* 43:516–522, 1977.

Mead J.: Expiratory flow limitation: a physiologist's point of view. *Fed. Proc.* 39:2771–2775, 1980.

These papers describe in considerable detail the wave speed theory of flow-limitation. They are highly technical.

Colebatch H.J.H., Greaves I.A., Ng C.K.Y.: Exponential analysis of elastic recoil and aging in healthy males and females. *J. Appl. Physiol.* 47:683–691, 1979.

Gibson G.J., Pride N.B., Davis J., et al.: Exponential description of the static pressure-volume curve of normal and diseased lungs. *Am. Rev. Respir. Dis.* 120:799–811, 1979.

Knudson R.J., Kaltenborn W.T.: Evaluation of lung elastic recoil by exponential curve analysis. *Respir. Physiol.* 46:29–42, 1981.

The pressure-volume curve can be described by a mathematical expression. That technique is described in the preceding articles.

7

The Pulmonary Circulation

NORMAL RESPIRATORY FUNCTION, as reflected by the level of arterial oxygenation, depends upon the interaction of both the ventilatory and circulatory mechanisms of the respiratory system. Pa_{O_2} is not only related to ventilation but is also affected by the supply of blood to the lung, pressure-flow relationships of the pulmonary circulation, distribution of perfusion in relation to ventilation in the lung, and presence or degree of arterial-venous admixture.

Blood Supply to the Lung

The lung has a dual blood supply, receiving nonoxygenated blood via the pulmonary arteries and oxygenated blood through the bronchial circulation. Early in gestation, the embryonic lungs, trachea, and esophagus are supplied by branches of the paired dorsal aortas. The pulmonary arteries develop from the sixth aortic arches, and the remaining systemic blood supply to the lung normally atrophies. Failure to atrophy may result in an aberrant systemic blood supply to a portion of lung. With further embryonic lung growth, the bronchial arteries develop as new systemic vessels, which then grow as the cartilaginous airways develop. Although they exhibit considerable anatomical variation, the bronchial arteries most often are three in number, arising from the cephalad portion of the thoracic aorta or upper intercostal arteries. Supplying oxygenated arterial blood from the systemic circulation, they are the nutrient vessels

for the lower trachea and for the bronchi as far as the respiratory bronchioles. They also supply the vasa vasorum of the large pulmonary vessels. The venous drainage of the circulation supplying the major bronchi uses the azygous vein, returning to the right atrium. Anastomoses with pulmonary veins provide the route of venous return for the bronchial vessels supplying the smaller peripheral airways.

Although the bronchial circulation is capable of expanding its role under pathologic circumstances, it normally receives only a small portion of the output of the left ventricle. Through the pulmonary circulation, however, the lung receives all of the right ventricular output. Unlike the systemic circulation, the pulmonary circulation is a low-pressure system capable of much greater distensibility than the systemic vascular bed. Approximately 10% to 20% of the total circulating blood volume is found in the lungs, subject to variation with posture and other conditions. Of the volume of blood in the pulmonary circulation at any instant in time, about 10% is present in the pulmonary capillaries in a resting subject. Another 60% of pulmonary blood volume may be found in pulmonary veins. Systemic venous return is under the influence of intrathoracic pressure. As a result, right ventricular output varies with the rate or depth of respiration. The substantial pulmonary venous reservoir supplying the left ventricle permits maintenance of left ventricular output in the face of these variations in right ventricular output.

Vascular Pressure-Flow Relationships

The same mechanical equivalent of Ohm's law according to which respiratory resistance was described may be applied to a vascular system to relate driving pressure to blood flow:

$$\text{Vascular resistance} = \frac{\text{driving pressure } (\Delta P)}{\text{blood flow } (\dot{Q})}$$

Driving pressure across the pulmonary vasculature equals the difference in pressure between the pulmonary artery and the left atrium. Although this pressure may be properly expressed as force per unit area (dyne/cm^2), it is more convenient to express it in the units in which blood pressure is usually measured, mm Hg. When pulmonary blood flow is expressed in liters per minute, the normal pulmonary vascular resistance is approximately 1.6 mm Hg/L/min, about one tenth of the resistance to flow presented by the systemic circulation. Since the same flow of blood is conducted by both pulmonary and systemic circulations, this marked difference in resistance reflects the lower pressure required to drive the blood through the pulmonary vasculature. The difference between the normal mean pulmonary artery pressure of 14 mm Hg and mean left atrial pressure of 5 mm Hg is 9 mm Hg, the driving pressure across the pulmonary vascular bed. Pulmonary arterioles contribute most of the pulmonary vascular resistance. The contribution of pulmonary capillaries is relatively small, and the venous system between pulmonary capillaries and the left atrium adds only about 1 mm Hg to the total flow-resistive pressure drop.

The amount of oxygen taken up by the blood in its passage through the lung is reflected by the difference in oxygen content between arterial and mixed venous blood. This provides a convenient method of measuring pulmonary blood flow by the direct Fick method. Measurements of oxygen uptake and of oxygen concentrations of arterial and mixed venous blood are related by the equation:

$$\text{Pulmonary blood flow (L/min)} = \frac{O_2 \text{ uptake (ml/min)}}{a - v \; O_2 \text{ difference (ml/L)}}$$

Flow data derived from this or other available techniques, when combined with direct pressure measurements made during cardiac catheterization, provide the information needed to calculate pulmonary vascular resistance.

The pulmonary arteries are much more compliant than comparable systemic vessels. Furthermore, the pulmonary capillary bed is capable of considerable volume distensibility by opening of closed channels and by passive dilatation. The pulmonary vasculature, because of this distensibility, is able to accommodate variations in circulatory load with little change in pressure. Thus, dilatation of vessels serves to decrease resistance to flow as blood flow increases. Ultimately, however, when flow has increased by approximately 250%, maximum pulmonary vascular distensibility is achieved, and further increases in flow are accompanied by increases in pressure, as shown in Figure 7–1. An increase in resistance should be differentiated from an increase in tone of the pulmonary ves-

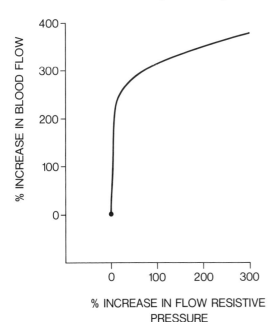

Fig 7–1.—Pressure-flow relationships in the pulmonary vascular bed.

sels. Certain stimuli decrease the distensibility of the vascular bed, causing pulmonary artery pressure (PAP) to increase in response to an increasing blood flow. Since the increase in PAP may not exceed an increase in flow, no change in resistance need occur. The increased vascular tone is then manifested only by a failure to achieve a normal decrease in resistance with increasing cardiac output.

Alterations in pulmonary vascular tone have been observed in response to hypoxia and acidemia. The increase in vascular tone induced by hypoxia apparently involves both precapillary and postcapillary vessels. Hypoxia also leads to an increase in cardiac output. The combination of increased pulmonary blood flow and increased vascular tone results in an elevation of PAP. Oxygen breathing readily reverses acute hypoxic pulmonary hypertension. Hypercapnia is associated with pulmonary vasoconstriction only in the presence of acidemia, suggesting that hypercapnia alone has little effect on pulmonary vascular tone. Acidemia, however, can result in increased vascular tone and accentuates the effect of hypoxia on the pulmonary vascular bed. Chronic stimulus to increase vascular tone can lead to anatomical changes in the pulmonary vessels, aggravating pulmonary hypertension (see chap. 29).

Whereas the driving pressure, or pressure difference across the pulmonary vascular bed, is significant in determining resistance to flow, the absolute intravascular and transmural pressures are significant for other reasons. A balance of hydraulic and colloid osmotic pressures similar to the mechanism that keeps the pleural space fluid free also serves to keep the alveoli free of fluid. The low pulmonary capillary hydraulic pressure (approximately 11 cm H_2O) is more than balanced by plasma osmotic pressure (approximately 34 cm H_2O). Not only does this mechanism prevent transudation of fluid into alveoli, it also effects rapid absorption of fluid from alveoli. At the limits of pulmonary vascular distensibility, however, added load may result in an increase in transmural vascular pressure. When the transmural capillary pressure exceeds the plasma colloid osmotic pressure, pulmonary edema can result. This may occur when both pulmonary artery and left atrial pressures increase with no change in the driving pressure, as in mitral stenosis. On the other hand, the driving pressure may be increased with no increase in capillary transmural pressure if the pulmonary arterioles present increased resistance to flow. The latter situation may result in right ventricular failure with no evidence of pulmonary edema, as in primary pulmonary hypertension.

The above explanation refers to average conditions in the lung. As we shall see, capillary hydraulic pressures at the base of the lung are normally higher than at the apex. At least at the lung bases, some fluid loss from capillaries occurs even in normal lungs. Furthermore, the full effect of capillary colloid osmotic pressure is lost if there is damage to the capillary wall with extravasation of proteinaceous fluid, and many factors may impair the integrity of the capillary wall. Normally, the lung is kept free of edema as a result of an effective lymphatic system, and fluid accumulation can occur only when the rate of fluid loss from capillaries exceeds the capacity of lymphatic channels to remove it. Thus, maintenance of an edema-free lung depends on: (1) relatively low pulmonary capillary pressures, (2) relatively high colloid osmotic pressure in the blood, (3) integrity of the pulmonary capillary wall, and (4) an effective pulmonary lymphatic drainage system.

Distribution of Pulmonary Blood Flow

Pulmonary blood flow is not uniformly distributed throughout the lung, but exhibits a gravity-dependent gradient related to regional differences in pulmonary vascular pressure and resistance. In the pulmonary vascular bed, absolute intravascular pressure, relative to atmospheric, exhibits a vertical hydraulic gradient. In a man of average height, the distance from the apex of the lung to the base is about 30 cm. In upright man the pulmonary vasculature represents a column of fluid 30 cm high, with the main pulmonary artery entering at approximately its midpoint. To perfuse the apex of the lung, PAP must be great enough to overcome a hydraulic pressure of 15 cm of fluid, or about 11 mm Hg. There is adequate pressure to perfuse the apex during systole when pulmonary artery pressure is 22 mm Hg, but not during diastole when the pressure is 9 mm Hg. Below the entrance of the pulmonary artery, the hydraulic pressure is added to the pulmonary artery pressure. As a result, due to the effect of gravity, absolute intravascular pressure increases progressively down the lung from the hilus. Since the added hydraulic pressure in the artery is balanced by the same added pressure in the veins, the driving pressure is unchanged, although the vascular transmural pressure increases down the lung. For this reason, when pulmonary capillary pressures are abnormally increased, fluid transudation will be greater in the dependent zones of the lung.

The vertical gradient of flow resistance is also

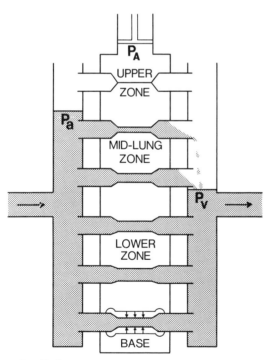

Fig 7–2.—Vertical gradient of flow resistance depicted as a function of capillary transmural pressure.

a function of capillary transmural pressure. The pulmonary capillaries are, in effect, collapsible tubes exposed to surrounding P_{alv}. Flow is determined by the relative magnitude of arterial pressure (P_a), P_{alv}, and venous pressure (P_v) in a manner analogous to that observed in a parallel series of Starling resistors, as depicted in Figure 7–2. Whereas P_{alv} is assumed to be uniform throughout the lung, P_a and P_v exhibit a gravity-dependent gradient down the lung. In the upper zones, where P_{alv} exceeds P_a, the vessels will collapse, and no flow will occur. In the mid-lung zone, P_{alv} is less than P_a but greater than P_v. Some capillary compression results and, throughout this zone, the magnitude of flow will be related to the difference between P_a and P_{alv}. In the lower zone, where both P_a and P_v exceed P_{alv}, no capillary compression occurs, and flow will be a function of the difference between P_a and P_v. The result of this mechanism is a gravity-dependent gradient of perfusion, the blood flow per unit lung volume increasing down the lung from apex to base. Very near the base of the lung, however, flow again diminishes somewhat, probably as a result of higher perivascular pressures and reduced regional lung expansion.

Shunts

True venous admixture resulting from an anatomical right-to-left shunt occurs when venous blood with low oxygen tension bypasses the lung and mixes with oxygenated arterialized blood, reducing its oxygen tension. Some true venous admixture occurs normally. A portion of the venous return of the bronchial circulation is added to oxygenated blood in the pulmonary veins. Thebesian veins drain the myocardium directly into the left side of the heart. As a result, the oxygen tension measured in arterial blood is slightly less than the pulmonary end-capillary oxygen tension. However, the magnitude of this shunt is normally small, constituting no more than 2.5% of the cardiac output and reducing Pa_{O_2} by only a few torr. Larger shunts resulting in arterial hypoxemia occur in a number of disease states, a subject discussed in chapter 29.

READING LIST

Von Hayek H.: *The Human Lung.* New York, Hafner Publishing Co., 1960.

On the subject of lung morphology, including the pulmonary circulation, this is an excellent reference work.

Harris P., Heath D.: *The Human Pulmonary Circulation.* Edinburgh and London, E & S Livingstone, 1962.

This book remains a useful reference.

West J.B.: *Ventilation/Blood Flow and Gas Exchange,* ed. 3. Oxford, London, Edinburgh, Melbourne, Blackwell Scientific Publications, 1977.

Though more has been written on the subject since the first edition of this slim volume appeared, it remains a useful introduction to the subject.

8

Respiratory Gas Exchange

RESPIRATORY GAS EXCHANGE involves the movement of gas between the atmosphere and the alveoli and, at the alveolar surface, between alveolar air and pulmonary capillary blood. In considering gas exchange and, in the next chapter, gas transport, we must deal with gas tensions and physicochemical reactions of gases in the blood. Therefore, a brief discussion of certain basic physical principles may be appropriate.

Physical Principles

The earth's atmosphere is composed of 79.03% nitrogen, 20.93% oxygen, and small quantities of carbon dioxide and rare gases. These gas molecules are in a state of continuous random motion. Placed in an enclosed container, the gases will occupy all available space, distributing themselves uniformly with no detectable inhomogeneity. Being in constant motion, the gas molecules collide with each other and with the walls of the container, thereby exerting a pressure. The pressure exerted by a given number of molecules of a gas, or mixture of gases, is related to the volume of the container and to the temperature of the gas. Boyle's law states that, at a constant temperature, the pressure varies inversely with the volume occupied by a given number of gas molecules. As the volume is reduced, collisions with the wall of the container increase and the pressure becomes greater. If temperature is increased, the molecules will move faster, and the number of

collisions with the wall will increase. The result will be an increase in pressure if the volume is held constant, or an increase of volume if pressure is held constant. This relationship is expressed by the laws of Charles and Gay-Lussac.

The pressure exerted by a mixture of gases is the sum of the pressures exerted by the individual components of the mixture. According to Dalton's law, the pressure of each component is independent of other gases in the mixture. The pressure exerted by one component defines the partial pressure or tension of that particular gas. The total pressure of air in the atmosphere is the atmospheric pressure, 760 torr at sea level. The partial pressure of a component depends upon the fraction of the total mixture occupied by the component. Thus, oxygen, which makes up 20.93% of the air we breathe, exerts a partial pressure of 20.93% of 760 torr or 159 torr at sea level. Although the fractional composition does not change with altitude, the absolute number of molecules in a given volume, and hence the barometric pressure, decreases with altitude. Therefore, at an altitude of 5,000 feet, where the atmospheric pressure is 632 torr, the partial pressure of ambient oxygen is 20.93% of 632, or 132.5 torr.

Water vapor obeys the same gas laws, but the number of molecules entering the gas phase is a function of the temperature. The air in the lower respiratory passages is fully saturated with water vapor. Regardless of altitude or atmospheric pressure, the vapor pressure of water varies directly with temperature and exerts a pressure of

41

47 torr at 37 C. Thus, the remaining components of the water vapor-saturated inspired gas mixture reaching the bronchi exert a pressure at sea level of 760 − 47, or 713 torr and the partial pressure of oxygen has been reduced to 20.93% of 713, or about 149 torr.

At the end of expiration, gas from which some oxygen has been removed and to which carbon dioxide has been added remains in the lungs and airways. The inspired air, in addition to becoming saturated with water vapor, is mixed with and diluted by this gas so that the oxygen tension of air in the alveolar spaces is about 105 torr at sea level. This is the gas that is in contact with pulmonary capillary blood at the site of alveolar-capillary gas exchange.

Ventilation and Dead Space

The respiratory pump has as its sole function ventilation, the repetitive inspiration and expiration that exchanges volumes of gas between alveoli and atmosphere. Because this cyclic volume exchange has as its purpose the replenishment of alveolar oxygen and the elimination of carbon dioxide, only ventilation of adequately functioning alveoli may be considered physiologically useful. Because it is not useful but "wasted," ventilation of spaces that do not contribute to this gas exchange has been called "dead space" ventilation.

The conducting airways down to the level of respiratory bronchioles are essential elements in the structure of the tracheobronchial tree but do not participate in gas exchange. Since these airways constitute an anatomically defined space that still must be ventilated, this space has been called the "anatomic dead space." Because gas must be moved in and out of the anatomic dead space with each breath, the resulting volume of wasted ventilation is the product of the volume of the dead space and the respiratory frequency. The volume of the anatomical dead space is virtually fixed and is approximately 150 to 200 ml, depending on body size. Since the magnitude of wasted ventilation is directly related to the respiratory rate, it is clear that a breathing pattern of slow, deep breaths is less wasteful of ventilation than one of rapid, shallow breaths.

If there are alveoli that continue to be ventilated although deprived of blood flow, they too contribute nothing to gas exchange and constitute "alveolar dead space." In addition, and more commonly, rather than being totally deprived of blood flow, some alveoli are overventilated in relation to their blood flow. Because the ventilation to these lung units is in excess of its contribution to gas exchange, some of this ventilation is wasted and is also considered alveolar dead space ventilation.

The respiratory or physiologic dead space is the total ventilation that is wasted on each breath. It is the sum of the anatomic and alveolar dead space ventilations. The terminology used to describe wasted ventilation is unfortunate and often confusing. Except for conducting airways, dead space is a concept rather than an anatomically defined portion of lung. It is perhaps most accurate to think of the physiologic dead space as that volume of gas that is inhaled in excess of the volume sufficient to account for the observed carbon dioxide gas exchange. Likewise, the "effective alveolar ventilation" is the ventilation that would have been needed to account for the observed carbon dioxide exchange if all of the inspired air had reached normally functioning alveoli. The total minute ventilation is the sum of the effective alveolar and physiologic dead space ventilations.

Oxygen Transfer and Diffusing Capacity

The size of an alveolus changes with lung volume. There is also a gravity-dependent gradient of alveolar size (see chap. 5 and 10). The average diameter of an alveolus in an adult human lung is of the order of 250 μ. Because there are about 300 million alveoli in the lung, the total alveolar surface area is approximately 70 m^2, many times the body surface area. This is the surface available for gas exchange. However, only a portion of this surface is occupied by pulmonary capillaries and, at any instant in time, the capillaries are not totally occupied by red blood cells. Thus, the *effective* surface area available for gas exchange is probably of the order of 35 to 40 m^2. During exercise, when more of the alveolar capillary bed is used and there are more red blood cells in the capillaries, the effective alveolar surface area may increase to 60 m^2. Compared with the amount of blood in the pulmonary circulation at any given instant in time, the volume of blood in the capillaries actually in contact with alveolar air is small, perhaps less than 100 ml. This may be increased with exercise. A red blood cell passing through the pulmonary circulation is in proximity to alveolar air for only 0.75 seconds at rest and for an even shorter time during exercise. During this brief interval, gas exchange must take place.

Oxygen uptake must be sufficient to meet tissue metabolic demands. Oxygen is removed from the alveolus to be carried in the blood to its site of utilization. For this to occur, the oxygen molecule must first cross the alveolar-capillary membrane, traverse the plasma, enter the erythrocyte, and chemically combine with unsaturated hemoglobin. These constitute the barriers or resistances to oxygen transfer or diffusion. The difference in partial pressure of oxygen between the alveolus and the capillary ($A - c\ O_2$ gradient) must be sufficient to drive the oxygen across the barriers resisting oxygen transfer. The diffusion resistance depends upon five factors: (1) membrane area, (2) distance that must be traversed or membrane thickness, (3) diffusing characteristics of the intervening tissue, (4) quantity of hemoglobin available in the capillaries at the time, and (5) rate of reaction between hemoglobin and oxygen. Though more than diffusion is involved in the process, the relationship of oxygen transferred to the $A - c\ O_2$ gradient is designated as the diffusing capacity of the lung for oxygen (DL_{O_2}):

$$DL_{O_2} = \dot{V}_{O_2}/\text{mean } A - c\ O_2 \text{ gradient}$$

Since this is, in effect, a flow-pressure relationship, it expresses conductance, the reciprocal of resistance. Thus, the resistance to diffusion is $1/DL_{O_2}$, and the five factors named above determine this resistance.

Blood entering a pulmonary capillary has a low oxygen tension, which then increases during its transit past an alveolus. To determine the diffusion of oxygen during this transit, it is necessary to know the alveolar and mean capillary oxygen tensions. Available techniques allow accurate estimates of PA_{O_2}, but no convenient direct or indirect methods are available for estimating $P\bar{c}_{O_2}$. For this reason, the DL_{O_2} is usually not measured.

Carbon monoxide has diffusing characteristics similar to oxygen, and its mean capillary tension may be determined with reasonable ease and accuracy. Therefore, routine clinical determinations of diffusing capacity are usually performed using carbon monoxide rather than oxygen as the test gas. This technique, involving inhalation of very low concentrations of carbon monoxide in air, takes advantage of not only the normal absence of carbon monoxide in pulmonary capillary blood but also its marked affinity for hemoglobin. Thus, diffusing capacity is usually expressed as DL_{CO} rather than DL_{O_2}.

The concept that $1/DL$ is an expression of resistance to diffusion permits us to consider separately the resistance to oxygen transfer offered by the alveolar capillary membrane and the component contributed by the blood.

The resistance to diffusion contributed by the membrane, $1/DM$, is a function of membrane area available for diffusion and refers to the blood-gas interface provided by functioning capillaries and adequately ventilated alveoli. Inadequate pulmonary perfusion; deficient alveolar ventilation; destruction of alveolar walls, as in emphysema; or loss or replacement of alveoli by disease will reduce the area available for gas exchange. Membrane resistance is also related to the thickness of the physical barrier through which the gas molecule must pass. This barrier consists of alveolar epithelium, basement membrane, interstitial fluid, and capillary endothelium. Normally less than 0.5 μ thick, the diffusion resistance contributed by the membrane may be increased when the alveolar wall is thickened, if interstitial fluid is excessive as in interstitial edema, or if intra-alveolar edema fluid is present. The gas molecule must also traverse capillary plasma to reach the red blood cell. This intracapillary path length may be increased with hemodilution and capillary dilatation. Finally, the diffusing characteristics of the tissue components themselves contribute to membrane resistance.

Intravascular factors affecting resistance to gas transfer are the quantity of blood available in the pulmonary capillary bed and the rate of the reaction of gas with that blood. The latter, θ, is expressed as the number of milliliters of gas taken up per milliliter of blood per minute per torr pressure gradient. This, combined with the pulmonary capillary blood volume, Vc, yields the value θVc, the "diffusing capacity" of the blood in the capillaries at any instant. The magnitude of the intravascular resistance to diffusion will depend on the number of red cells in the capillary bed and their hemoglobin content.

Since the membrane and intravascular resistances to diffusion act in series, their sum is the total resistance:

$$\frac{1}{D_L} = \frac{1}{D_M} + \frac{1}{\theta Vc}$$

The value of θ for carbon monoxide may be predictably altered by changes in oxygen tension. By measuring D_{LCO} under different conditions of P_{O_2} and applying the above equation, assessments of D_M and Vc have been made. Such data suggest that normally approximately one half of the resistance to diffusion is at the membrane and the remainder within the blood itself. Normal capillary blood volumes are in the range of 70–100 ml.

Each functioning lung unit, or acinus, is served by one terminal bronchiole. Within each acinus, the terminal bronchiole gives rise to respiratory bronchioles which bear alveoli and which in turn give rise to alveolar ducts. The latter, after several branchings, finally terminate in alveolar sacs. The distance a gas molecule must traverse from its entrance into the acinus at the end of the terminal bronchiole to a gas exchanging surface is, in effect, another barrier which can affect the measured diffusing capacity. Normally, the mean distance from the terminal bronchiole to the end of an alveolar sac is

about 7 mm, but, because there are alveoli throughout the acinus, the mean path length to be traversed by gas diffusion is only about 2 mm. To traverse this distance takes a very short but finite time. It has been shown that the diffusion distances may be increased to 7 mm in centrilobular emphysema and to more than 10 mm in panacinar emphysema, compared with the normal distance of 2 mm. This anatomical derangement of normal lung architecture coupled with loss of gas-exchanging surface contribute to the reduced value for diffusing capacity observed in emphysema.

Unfortunately, the methods used in clinical practice for determination of D_{LCO} involve certain assumptions that may detract from the validity of the measurement, especially in abnormal lungs. Because of these assumptions, different methods for D_{LCO} measurement may give different results in the presence of disease. Caution must be exercised in interpretation of a D_{LCO} measurement in an abnormal lung.

Erythrocyte Transit Time

As mentioned above, blood passing through the lung is in a pulmonary capillary for only about 0.75 seconds. Oxygen transfer is not instantaneous. During this brief interval, oxygen must pass through the alveolar capillary membrane, enter the blood, and combine with a hemoglobin molecule. The amount of oxygen taken up depends upon the A−c tension gradient. As the blood first comes in contact with the alveolar surface, the oxygen tension gradient is the difference between the $P_{A_{O_2}}$ of about 105 torr and the mixed venous oxygen tension of 40 torr. Because of this large A−c O_2 gradient, oxygen transfer is initially rapid. But as the blood takes up oxygen in its course through the capillary, the A−c tension gradient diminishes and the rate of oxygen uptake decreases progressively, as shown in Figure 8–1. Nevertheless, when room air is breathed at sea level, virtual equilibrium between alveolar air and blood is reached in about 0.3 seconds. Even when the transit time is reduced, as in exercise, adequate oxygenation can occur. When the diffusing ca-

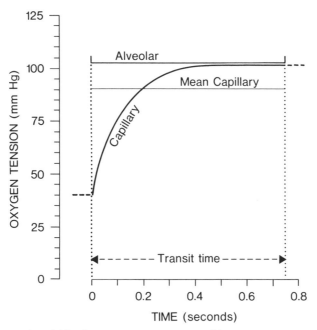

Fig 8–1.—Oxygen uptake of blood in its transit through a pulmonary capillary. (Modern terminol-ogy would express oxygen tension in terms of torr rather than mm Hg.)

pacity, the amount of gas taken up per torr A − c gradient, is reduced, the rate of oxygen equilibration is diminished. It is also diminished when a gas mixture low in oxygen is breathed and the A − c O_2 gradient is thereby reduced. If ambient oxygen tension is low enough, complete equilibration may not occur within the erythrocyte transit time, particularly if transit time is also reduced. Therefore, any combination of reduced transit time, low diffusing capacity, and a low ambient oxygen tension may result in an increase in the difference between alveolar and end-capillary oxygen tensions, which, if pronounced, results in arterial hypoxemia.

Transfer of Carbon Dioxide

The specific mechanisms governing the movement of carbon dioxide between pulmonary capillary blood and alveolar air cannot be completely separated from those involved in gas transport, the subject of the chapter to follow. Carbon dioxide and oxygen face the same physical barriers to diffusion at the alveolar-capillary interface. Whereas the pulmonary capillary-mean alveolar carbon dioxide gradient is smaller than the A-c O_2 gradient, the membrane diffusing capacity for carbon dioxide is much greater, a result of its 20-fold greater solubility. The diffusion transfer of carbon dioxide has therefore been considered to be many times more rapid than the equivalent transfer of oxygen. However, the membrane and transcapillary diffusion path of carbon dioxide must be considered, together with the transfer across several cell membranes of the various molecules and ions involved in the carbon dioxide transport reactions. The carbamino-hemoglobin mechanism of carbon dioxide transport is intimately associated with oxygenation of hemoglobin and accounts for a significant portion of the venoarterial difference in carbon dioxide content. As a result, total equilibration of carbon dioxide does not occur much more rapidly than oxygen equilibration at the alveolar-capillary interface. Nevertheless, although the transfer of carbon dioxide may not be as rapid as once thought, it is still unlikely that clinically significant resistance to carbon dioxide diffusion can occur.

READING LIST

Forster R.E.: Diffusion of gases. Interpretation of measurements of pulmonary diffusing capacity, in Fenn W.O., Rahn H. (eds.): *Respiration,* vol. 1 and 2, sec. 3. *Handbook of Physiology.* Washington, D.C., American Physiological Society, 1965, pp. 839–872; 1453–1468.

These two chapters in the Handbook of Physiology *provide a thorough review of the subject of gas exchange and diffusing capacity.*

Hills B.A.: *Gas Transfer in the Lung.* Cambridge, Cambridge University Press, 1974.

As the title indicates, the general topic of gas transfer is covered in this slim volume.

9

Transport of Respiratory Gases
in the Blood

WHEN AIR AND LIQUID are in contact, a gas will diffuse from one phase to the other until equal gas tensions are achieved. When this gas transfer occurs at the alveolar-capillary interface, a series of physicochemical reactions occurs in the blood that contributes to transport of respiratory gases. In the tissue capillaries, similar reactions are involved in the transfer of oxygen and carbon dioxide between blood and tissues.

Oxygen Transport

Inspired air is saturated with water vapor in the conducting airways, slightly lowering its oxygen tension. In the alveoli it mixes with oxygen-depleted, carbon dioxide-enriched gas remaining in the alveoli at the end of the previous expiration. As a result, the oxygen tension of alveolar air is considerably lower than that of the ambient atmosphere. Blood traversing the alveolar capillaries achieves an oxygen tension close to that of alveolar air, but, because of a normal small amount of venous admixture, the oxygen tension of arterial blood is slightly lower. In its passage through tissue capillaries, the blood gives up oxygen with the result that the oxygen tension of mixed venous blood returning to the lung is about 40 torr. These changes in oxygen tension are depicted graphically in Figure 9–1.

The amount of oxygen carried in physical solution by plasma is linearly related to oxygen tension and also depends on the solubility factor for oxygen in plasma. By this mechanism each 100 ml of blood could carry only 0.003 ml O_2/torr oxygen tension. Even breathing 100% oxygen, the amount of oxygen carried in physical solution would be inadequate for metabolic needs.

Most of the oxygen in the blood is carried in chemical combination with hemoglobin. One gram of hemoglobin is capable of carrying 1.34 ml of oxygen in chemical combination. Thus, with a normal blood hemoglobin content of 15 gm/100 ml, the blood, fully saturated with oxygen, carries approximately 20 ml O_2/100 ml blood, an efficient mechanism of oxygen transport.

Hemoglobin is composed of a globulin molecule, globin, bound to four heme molecules. Each heme molecule is made up of four pyrrole groups and one atom of iron, which may react with one molecule of oxygen. The ferrous iron of the heme molecule does not change its valence in combining with oxygen. The reaction is therefore *oxygenation* rather than *oxidation* and is readily reversible. In vitro studies have shown that the reversibility of this reaction is a phenomenon conferred upon the heme molecule through its association with the protein globin.

The actual amount of oxygen carried in chemical combination with hemoglobin is related in a nonlinear fashion to the partial pressure of oxygen in the blood (Pa_{O_2}). This nonlinear relation-

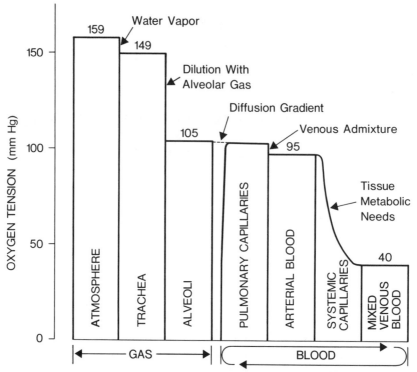

Fig 9–1.—Normal oxygen tension in gas and blood phases from atmosphere to mixed venous blood. (Modern terminology would express oxygen tension in terms of torr rather than mm Hg.)

ship between oxyhemoglobin and Pa_{O_2} is described by the *oxyhemoglobin dissociation curve*. This curve, shown in Figure 9–2, is derived empirically and does not express a mathematical relationship between saturation and Pa_{O_2}. If a sample of blood is equilibrated with 100% oxygen, its hemoglobin is considered to be fully saturated. The maximum amount of oxygen carried per unit volume of blood is the *oxygen capacity*. The *oxygen content* of samples equilibrated with gases of lower oxygen tension are compared with this to obtain the percentage of saturation. After subtracting the quantity of oxygen dissolved in the plasma (0.3 ml/100 torr O_2 tension) from both oxygen content and oxygen capacity:

$$\% \text{ saturation} = \frac{O_2 \text{ content}}{O_2 \text{ capacity}} \times 100$$

The saturation expresses the amount of oxygen chemically bound to hemoglobin in relation to the maximum amount of oxygen the hemoglobin is capable of carrying. When hemoglobin is fully saturated, the total amount of oxygen in the blood can be increased only by the addition of physically dissolved oxygen to the plasma.

The sigmoid configuration of the oxyhemoglobin dissociation curve describes the remarkable properties of hemoglobin as a carrier of oxygen and is of great physiologic significance. At the oxygen tensions normally found in alveolar air, hemoglobin becomes oxygenated at a very rapid rate, quickly becoming highly saturated. At the flat upper portion of the curve, large changes in oxygen tension are associated with small changes in oxygen content or saturation. Thus, relatively constant quantities of oxygen can be maintained in the blood at various levels of atmospheric oxygen tension, even at moderately high altitudes. Although the Pa_{O_2} is normally 105 torr at sea level, it can be as low as

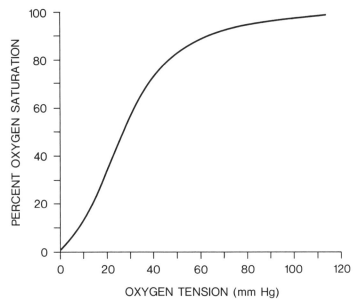

Fig 9–2.—Oxyhemoglobin dissociation curve. (Modern terminology would express oxygen tension in terms of torr rather than mm Hg.)

60 torr, and blood leaving pulmonary capillaries will still be 89% saturated.

The subsequent release of oxygen to the tissues is augmented by the relationship of saturation to Pa_{O_2} along the steep portion of the dissociation curve. The difference between the saturation, or oxygen content, of arterial blood and the saturation, or content, of venous blood leaving the tissues is the amount of oxygen given up by the blood to meet the metabolic needs of the tissues. Along the steep portion of the curve, large changes in oxygen content are associated with relatively small changes in Pa_{O_2}. The Pa_{O_2} of mixed venous blood is about 40 torr, corresponding to a saturation of 75%. Of course, tissues vary in their metabolic needs and oxygen demands. For example, venous blood leaving an exercising limb muscle may have an oxygen tension as low as 5 torr.

The sigmoid configuration of the oxyhemoglobin dissociation curve describes only one property of hemoglobin. In addition, the amount of oxygen combined with, or released by, hemoglobin may vary with other factors that accompany tissue metabolism. Thus, oxygen binding shifts under the influence of pH, carbon

dioxide tension, and temperature. With a decrease in pH, elevation of Pa_{CO_2}, or elevated temperature, the dissociation curve shifts to the right. When the blood reaches the tissues that it supplies, the tissue capillary blood sees a more acid environment and an increase in carbon dioxide tension, resulting in a shift of the dissociation curve which facilitates the unloading of oxygen. When the tissues increase their metabolic activity, their increased oxygen demands are met in part by further shift in the dissociation curve as carbon dioxide and hydrogen ions are produced. An increase in temperature, which may accompany exercise; increased metabolism; and hence increased oxygen needs will have a similar effect.

The influence of carbon dioxide tension on the dissociation curve (the Bohr effect) also operates as the blood passes through the lungs. Here, a fall in carbon dioxide tension shifts the curve to the left so that hemoglobin is now able to take up more oxygen at a given oxygen tension. The effect of changes of pH, carbon dioxide tension, and temperature on the oxyhemoglobin dissociation curve are shown in Figure 9–3.

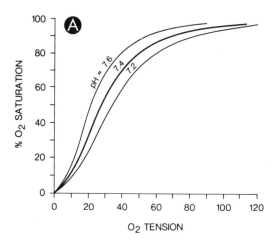

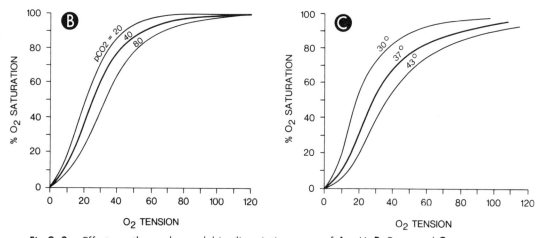

Fig 9–3.—Effects on the oxyhemoglobin dissociation curve of **A**, pH; **B**, P_{CO_2}; and **C**, temperature.

The amount of 2,3-diphosphoglycerate (DPG) in the erythrocyte also affects the oxygen-carrying capacity of hemoglobin. This organic phosphate decreases the affinity of hemoglobin for oxygen, thereby increasing the amount of oxygen released to the tissues. Red cell 2,3-DPG levels have been observed to be increased in anemia or as a response to hypoxia. The consequence of this is to reduce the degree of tissue hypoxia by shifting the oxyhemoglobin dissociation curve to the right. In addition, this serves to compensate in part for the shift of the curve in the opposite direction occasioned by the respiratory alkalosis seen on moving to an altitude.

With an increase in pH, 2,3-DPG levels decrease markedly. This decrease in erythrocyte 2,3-DPG may be viewed as a compensatory mechanism opposing the shift of the dissociation curve to the right with fall in pH. Thus, in the face of acid-base changes tending to shift the oxyhemoglobin dissociation curve or in the presence of diminished blood oxygen content, maintenance of optimum tissue oxygenation is facilitated by appropriate changes in red blood cell 2,3-DPG.

Carbon Dioxide Transport

While ambient air is virtually free of carbon dioxide, the carbon dioxide tension of alveolar

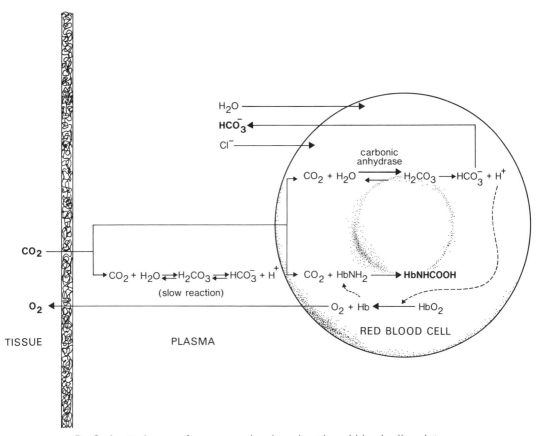

Fig 9–4.—Exchange of oxygen and carbon dioxide red blood cell and tissue.

air (PA_{CO_2}) is normally about 40 torr. Since blood leaving the pulmonary capillaries has come into equilibrium with alveolar air, the Pa_{CO_2} is also 40 torr. Mixed venous blood has a carbon dioxide tension of about 46 torr. The difference between mixed venous and arterial carbon dioxide tensions is a reflection of the elimination through the lung of the approximately 210 ml CO_2/min produced in the tissues.

Carbon dioxide may be carried in dissolved form or in chemical combination with the amino groups of nonoxygenated hemoglobin. Arterial blood entering tissue capillaries normally has a Pa_{CO_2} of 40 torr. Since the carbon dioxide concentration in tissue cells is higher than that in arterial blood, carbon dioxide diffuses into the blood, bringing the carbon dioxide tension of blood leaving the tissue capillary bed up to about 46 torr.

The physicochemical reactions involved in carbon dioxide transfer and transport are summarized in Figure 9–4. Carbon dioxide from the tissues enters the plasma and subsequently the red blood cells. In plasma, some of this gas goes into solution and a small amount of carbon dioxide combines with water to form carbonic acid.

$$CO_2 + H_2O \leftrightarrows H_2CO_3$$

In plasma, this is a relatively slow reaction. Carbonic acid then dissociates to form bicarbonate and hydrogen ions; the H^+ is buffered primarily by plasma proteins:

$$H_2CO_3 \leftrightarrows HCO_3^- + H^+$$

Carbon dioxide entering the red cell is rapidly hydrated to form carbonic acid through the action of an enzymatic catalyst, carbonic anhydrase. The carbonic acid formed in the red cell then dissociates. The resulting H^+ is buffered by basic groups provided by hemoglobin. The increase in pH and the reaction of H^+ with hemoglobin promotes the release of oxygen to the tissues. The oxygen release enhances the buffering capacity of hemoglobin inasmuch as reduced hemoglobin is a better H^+ acceptor. Because of the absence of carbonic anhydrase in plasma, little HCO_3^- is produced there. Thus, the concentration gradient of HCO_3^- between red cells and plasma results in diffusion of HCO_3^- out of the cells into the plasma. Electric neutrality is maintained by an equivalent movement of Cl^- ions from plasma into the cells, the "chloride shift." Osmotic equilibrium is preserved by movement of water into the red cells, increasing their volume. Although little HCO_3^- is produced in the plasma, most of it is carried there after being produced in the red cell. Through this mechanism and the presence in the red blood cell of carbonic anhydrase, most of the carbon dioxide is transported in this ionic form.

The association of oxygen with hemoglobin is a loose one, and oxygen is readily given up to the tissues in the presence of a blood-tissue oxygen gradient favoring its release. The loss of oxygen from hemoglobin facilitates another reaction in carbon dioxide transport. Carbon dioxide reacts with the amine groups of nonoxygenated hemoglobin to form carbamino-hemoglobin:

$$HbNH_2 + CO_2 \rightleftarrows HbNHCOOH$$
$$\leftrightharpoons HbNHCOO^- + H^+$$

Although a relatively small fraction of the total blood carbon dioxide is carried in this carbamino form, it is an important transport mechanism through its intimate association with the oxygenation and deoxygenation of hemoglobin. It accounts for almost one quarter of the veno-arterial difference in carbon dioxide content.

While oxygen is being released to the tissues, oxyhemoglobin converted to reduced hemoglobin, and carbon dioxide entering the blood from the tissues, hydrogen ions are being released in various reactions. Although several effective buffering systems are in operation, the net result

is a slight excess in hydrogen ion concentration. Therefore, the pH of venous blood leaving the tissues is slightly lower than that of arterial blood.

In the pulmonary capillary bed the processes described are reversed. A reverse chloride shift facilitates the movement of bicarbonate into the red cell where carbonic anhydrase promotes rapid dehydration of carbonic acid to carbon dioxide and water. The carbamino-hemoglobin association is reversed as hemoglobin takes up oxygen. Carbon dioxide is liberated and rapidly diffuses from capillary to alveolus as capillary blood becomes slightly more alkaline. The rapidity of the reactions assumes importance in the pulmonary capillary, since a red cell remains there for less than one second. Only the dissociation of H_2CO_3 into carbon dioxide and water in the plasma, where carbonic anhydrase is absent, is slow, and this constitutes a relatively insignificant facet of the carbon dioxide transport mechanism.

As with oxygen, the amount of carbon dioxide carried by the blood is related to its partial pressure. This is expressed by the carbon dioxide dissociation curve shown in Figure 9–5. Although the relationship is clearly curvilinear, the physiologic range of carbon dioxide tensions is so narrow that, within that range, it may be regarded as linear. The relationship between carbon dioxide content and tension is influenced by oxygen tension (Haldane effect). This confers a physiologic advantage similar to the effect of carbon dioxide tension on the oxyhemoglobin dissociation curve (Bohr effect). Thus, the unloading of oxygen at the tissue level facilitates the loading of carbon dioxide, the opposite phenomenon occurring in the lung.

Changes in Pa_{CO_2} have profound effects on blood pH. A reduction in Pa_{CO_2} leads to an increase in pH, whereas an increase in Pa_{CO_2} increases the acidity of the blood. This effect is advantageous in compensating for acid-base abnormalities of metabolic origin. With metabolic acidosis, an increase in ventilation and increased elimination of carbon dioxide corrects toward normal the excessively low pH. On the other hand, changes in alveolar ventilation in respira-

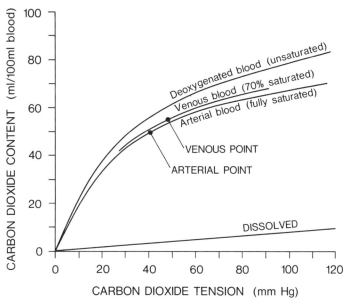

Fig 9–5.—Carbon dioxide dissociation curve. (Modern terminology would express carbon dioxide tension in terms of torr rather than mm Hg.)

tory diseases lead to inappropriate changes in arterial carbon dioxide and consequent acid-base abnormalities. These are discussed more fully in chapter 14.

Tissue Demands

The partial pressure of oxygen or carbon dioxide within tissue cells has been difficult or impossible to measure with accuracy and varies with the tissue in question. However, by measuring gas tensions in the blood entering and leaving an organ and the blood flow through the organ, the rate of utilization of oxygen or production of carbon dioxide can be determined. Obviously, oxygen use will depend on the aerobic metabolic activity of the tissue at the time. The arteriovenous difference in gas tensions of a skeletal muscle, for example, will be quite different when the muscle is at rest or active. An active muscle may remove almost all of the oxygen from the blood circulating through it. The decrease in tissue oxygen tension and increase in carbon dioxide tension that accompany increased metabolic activity have a local effect on smooth muscle of tissue blood vessels. The re-

sulting vasodilatation promotes local increase in blood flow. During exercise the cardiovascular responses increasing cardiac output augment the increase in blood flow to the active tissues.

To meet the metabolic needs of the tissues, both adequate Pa_{O_2} and adequate blood flow are necessary. Tissue hypoxia may result from deficiencies in either the amount of oxygen carried in the blood or reduced flow of blood to the tissue. The latter condition, referred to as stagnant or circulatory hypoxia, may occur locally due to vascular disease or, generally, due to cardiac failure or vasomotor collapse. The Pa_{O_2} is normal under such conditions but, since more oxygen is extracted as the blood flows more slowly through the tissues, the oxygen saturation of venous blood draining the area will be lower than normal. The increased deoxygenation of hemoglobin may reveal itself as localized so-called venous cyanosis.

On the other hand, available oxygen supply may be deficient, even in the absence of cyanosis, when the oxygen-carrying capacity of the blood is reduced. In anemia, for example, the amount of arterial oxygen may be inadequate without the presence of enough unsaturated hemoglobin to produce cyanosis. In carbon monoxide poisoning severe reduction in arterial oxygen content occurs without cyanosis. Carbon monoxide has an affinity for hemoglobin many times greater than that of oxygen, supplanting oxygen and forming cherry red carboxyhemoglobin.

From the above discussion, it may be seen that tissue hypoxia can be the result of (1) inadequate oxygen in inspired air, (2) failure of the respiratory system adequately to oxygenate arterial blood, (3) venous admixture producing severe arterial hypoxemia, (4) deficient flow of blood to the tissues, or (5) reduced oxygen-carrying capacity of the blood. Though it is not related to any of the above, there is one additional classification of tissue hypoxia that should be mentioned: (6) histotoxic hypoxia. Certain toxic substances, notably cyanide, can interfere with the ability of the tissues to use the oxygen available to them. Since the tissues cannot utilize the oxygen, their venous oxygen saturation will be higher than normal. In histotoxic hypoxia, therefore, the site of the abnormality is in the tissues, rather than in the respiratory or circulatory systems.

READING LIST

Roughton F.J.W.: Transport of oxygen and carbon dioxide, in Fenn W.O., Rahn H. (eds.): *Respiration,* vol. 1, sec. 3. *Handbook of Physiology.* Washington, D.C., American Physiological Society, 1974, pp. 767–825.

A thorough review by a pioneer in the field.

Hlastala M.D.: Interactions between O_2 and CO_2: the blood. *Semin. Respir. Med.* 3:70–74, 1981.

A brief and useful review.

10

Distribution of Lung Function

EFFECTIVE GAS EXCHANGE depends upon relatively uniform distribution of function throughout the lung. In an ideal lung all parts would be uniformly and adequately ventilated and just as uniformly perfused, behaving as if they were a single unit. In actuality, the lung is a complex structure. Ventilation must be distributed to 300 million alveoli through 23 generations of branching airways and the blood distributed through myriad capillaries. It is therefore not surprising that, even in the normal lung, distribution of function is not uniform.

Distribution of Ventilation

The regular application and withdrawal of inspiratory muscle forces generate semi-sinusoidal changes in intrapleural pressure that produce the cyclic volume excursions of tidal ventilation. Although inspiratory pressure is applied over the entire lung, the distribution of inspired volume and therefore of ventilation is not uniform.

Experimentally, an isolated excised lung is seen to expand uniformly, indicating that the structure and physical properties of the lung may be presumed to be uniform. However, in the living subject with lung and thorax intact, there is a gravity-dependent gradient of pleural pressure in the upright lung of about 0.3 cm H_2O/cm vertical distance. The pleural pressure over a normal adult lung 30 cm in height is about 9 cm H_2O more negative at the apex than at the base. Since under static conditions alveolar pressure is uniform throughout the lung, lung units near the apex are distended by a greater transpulmonary pressure and hence are more fully inflated than are those near the base. Units near the apex, therefore, are functioning along the upper, least compliant portion of their pressure-volume curve, while units near the base function along the most compliant part of the curve. When subjected to cyclic changes in pleural pressure, volume changes of the apical lung units will be less than those of basal units. The end result is a gradient of ventilation increasing down the lung from apex to base. Since the least ventilated units are also largest in volume, there is also a gravity-dependent gradient of the ratio of alveolar ventilation to volume ($\dot{V}_A/V_A$) down the lung.

The nonuniformity of $\dot{V}_A/V_A$ ratios is commonly demonstrated by the use of inert gas equilibration or washout studies. During the measurement of lung volumes by the helium equilibration technique, equilibration is normally quickly achieved. A mathematical expression for helium mixing efficiency has been employed in the past, but is no longer used in most laboratories. In general, if it takes longer than three minutes to achieve a constant helium concentration during this test, it is suggestive of abnormal distribution of ventilation.

Ventilation distribution may be examined more systematically by the multiple-breath nitrogen washout curve, which is obtained by monitoring expired nitrogen concentration as a subject breathes 100% oxygen. At the end of seven minutes of breathing 100% oxygen, the nitrogen

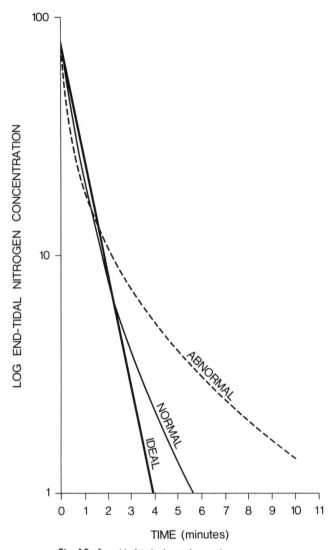

Fig 10–1.—Multiple-breath washout curve.

concentration of a gas sample obtained at the end of maximal expiration, representative of alveolar air, should not exceed 2.5%. From the nitrogen washout test, one may calculate a lung clearance index, the volume of oxygen breathed required to wash 90% of the FRC free of nitrogen divided by FRC. In effect, this is the volume of oxygen expressed in FRCs to reduce the alveolar N_2 concentration to 2%.

If $\dot{V}_A/V_A$ ratios were uniformly distributed, nitrogen elimination from the ideal lung would follow a course of simple exponential decay, as shown in Figure 10–1. However, the plot of log-expired nitrogen concentration in time departs from such a course, reflecting the normal degree of nonuniformity. The distribution of $\dot{V}_A/V_A$ ratios may become markedly abnormal in disease states and will be reflected by an increased curvilinearity of the nitrogen washout curve. Complex exponential analyses have been employed, but such analyses are seldom used in clinical testing. As an alternative, one can assess the curvilinearity of the nitrogen washout curve by examining the ratio of the ventilation re-

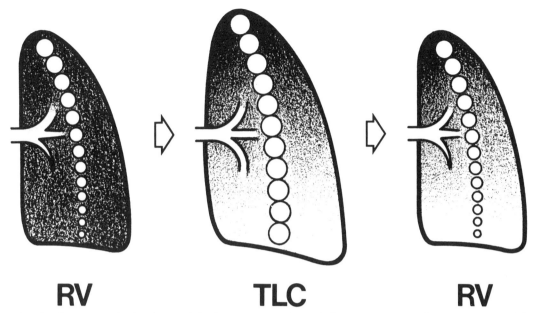

RV   TLC   RV

Fig 10–2.—At residual volume *(left)* there is a gravity-dependent gradient of alveolar size, and nitrogen is uniformly distributed. When one inspires 100% oxygen and all lung units have achieved their maximum volume at TLC *(middle panel)*, the nitrogen *(shaded)* is more dilute in lower regions. To complete the test, one then expires again to RV *(right)*.

quired to make the nitrogen concentration fall from 9% to 3% N_2 divided by that required to decrease it from the original 81% to 27% N_2. If the relationship of log N_2 to ventilation (see Fig 10–1) is ideal, this ratio will be 1, and normally it should not exceed 3.

The gravity-dependent gradient of pleural, and hence transpulmonary, pressure affects the distribution of inspired gas as a subject fully inspires from residual volume. This is illustrated diagrammatically in Figure 10–2, in which is represented the gravity-dependent gradient of alveolar size at residual volume and the changes which occur upon inspiration to total lung capacity (TLC). With complete expiration, only the most dependent regions are truly at their residual volume (RV); the most superior regions are at a higher regional volume. During the subsequent inspiration, the more superior regions receive the first gas inspired. The most dependent regions inflate along the inflation curve of the P-V loop shown in Figure 6–2 for which a substantial increase in transpulmonary pressure is required before volume increases appreciably.

Here a critical pressure must be attained to reopen closed terminal airways in dependent regions. Finally, when all regions have attained their TLC, the dependent regions have undergone a greater volume change than the superior regions.

These phenomena have been cited to explain the results of the single-breath nitrogen washout, or "closing volume," test. If 100% oxygen is inspired from RV, when TLC is achieved the resident nitrogen in dependent regions is more diluted by the inspired oxygen (see Fig 10–2). Then, during the subsequent expiration as expired nitrogen concentration is plotted against expired volume (Fig 10–3), the expired gas concentration changes sequentially as one again expires slowly to RV. The first gas expired, phase I, comes from the anatomical dead space which was filled with oxygen and is nitrogen-free. This is followed by a rapid increase in nitrogen concentration, phase II, as alveolar gas is mixed with dead space gas. During the next phase, phase III or the alveolar plateau, nitrogen concentration slowly increases with expired

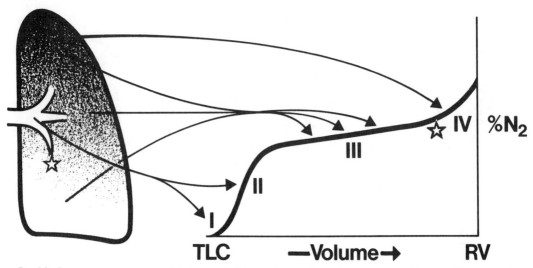

Fig 10–3.—As one expires to RV after a full inspiration of 100% oxygen (see Fig 10–2), expired N_2 concentration is plotted against expired volume. For explanation, see text. Stars indicate onset of phase IV or "closing volume" and presumed closure of airways in dependent lung regions.

volume. Finally, the nitrogen concentration abruptly begins to increase near the end of expiration, phase IV.

To explain this final phase IV increase in nitrogen concentration, it has been postulated that terminal airway closure occurs, beginning in the most dependent regions and progressing upward as the lung volume decreases. As a consequence, the last gas expired comes primarily from the superior zones of the lung, rich in nitrogen. Though the first oxygen to be inspired reached the superior regions, it was preceded by the nitrogen resident in the conducting airways. To achieve TLC these superior regions underwent a lesser volume change than more dependent regions. Therefore, the resident nitrogen is diluted to a lesser degree near the top of the lung. Because airway closure is thought to occur, the volume which remains to be exhaled when the change of slope from phase III to phase IV occurs (indicated by the star in Fig 10–3) has been called the closing volume. The volume remaining in the lungs at the onset of phase IV—i.e., closing volume plus RV—is the closing capacity.

Closing volume normally increases progres-

sively with age in adults (see chap. 11). Because closure occurs in very peripheral airways, probably at the level of terminal bronchioles, an abnormal increase in closing volume has been thought to indicate small airway dysfunction. The clinical utility of this measurement, however, remains to be demonstrated.

The slope of the alveolar plateau, phase III, expressed as the change in percent nitrogen per liter, is an index of uniformity of gas distribution or the lack thereof. An increase in the slope above values of about 2% N_2/L suggests an abnormality in inspired gas distribution, or interregional inhomogeneity. However, inasmuch as the test maneuver is done slowly, intraregional or stratified inhomogeneity may also affect the slope. Pathologic enlargement of intraacinar airspaces, as in emphysema, may result in increased slope. Active gas exchange, by changing the relationship between oxygen uptake and carbon dioxide production, will also affect the nitrogen concentration and, hence, the slope of phase III. An increase in the slope of phase III is a nonspecific finding, the diagnostic or prognostic significance of which is uncertain (see chap. 13).

Distribution of Ventilation-Perfusion Relationships

In the discussion of pulmonary blood flow (see chap. 7), a gravity-dependent gradient of pulmonary perfusion was described. Blood flow, like ventilation, is least at the apex and increases down the lung. However, alveolar ventilation and perfusion are not evenly matched, so that the gradient of perfusion is steeper than the gradient of ventilation. The relationship between the two is described in terms of the ventilation-perfusion ($\dot{V}A/\dot{Q}$) ratio. The average $\dot{V}A/\dot{Q}$ for the lung as a whole is approximately 0.8. The distribution of ventilation, blood flow, and $\dot{V}A/\dot{Q}$ are shown in Figure 10–4. It should be pointed out that, because of the nonuniform distribution of ventilation, perfusion, and $\dot{V}A/\dot{Q}$, the composition of alveolar gas and the pulmonary capillary oxygen and carbon dioxide tensions are also not uniform throughout the lung. Thus, the values defined for PA_{CO_2} or calculated for alveolar oxygen tension (PA_{O_2}) are mean values representative of the lung as a whole, not of any specific lung regions.

Ideal gas exchange depends on matching adequate ventilation with adequate perfusion. The physiologic consequences of regions of increased and decreased $\dot{V}A/\dot{Q}$ will be considered separately.

INCREASED $\dot{V}A/\dot{Q}$.—In regions of the lung where the $\dot{V}A/\dot{Q}$ ratio is increased above normal, wasted ventilation occurs. This has the effect of adding a space that is ventilated but does not participate adequately in gas exchange. An extreme example is the situation that can occur when perfusion is virtually eliminated, as by a blood clot or following ligation of a pulmonary artery. Alveoli served by the occluded vessels will no longer participate in gas exchange. The Pa_{CO_2}, which is normally assumed to represent PA_{CO_2}, now represents only adequately perfused alveoli. Under normal circumstances, end-expiratory carbon dioxide tension, monitored during tidal breathing, approximates PA_{CO_2} and is about the same as Pa_{CO_2}. But under the abnormal circumstances described above, the end-tidal carbon dioxide tension will be much lower than the Pa_{CO_2}, since carbon dioxide-free gas from unperfused alveoli reduces the carbon dioxide tension of the end-tidal air.

In the discussion of dead space ventilation (see chap. 8), it was noted that ventilation of regions of the lung with high $\dot{V}A/\dot{Q}$ ratios is

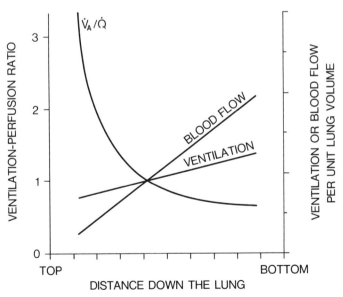

Fig 10–4.—Gravity-dependent distribution of blood flow and ventilation in the lung.

partly wasted and contributes to alveolar dead space ventilation. Although such a phenomenon exists in the normal lung (see Fig 10–4), its effect is relatively small. Under the abnormal conditions of many disease states, however, this effect may be quite pronounced.

To compensate for this wasted ventilation and yet maintain normal Pa_{O_2} and Pa_{CO_2}, total ventilation must be increased. If the wasted dead space ventilation is of such a magnitude that effective alveolar ventilation cannot be maintained by increasing total ventilation, carbon dioxide retention may ensue. The cost of compensatory hyperventilation is an increase in the work of breathing. As noted in chapter 6, the increased oxygen cost of breathing that attends many respiratory disorders may set limits to the increase in total ventilation that may be attained.

DECREASED $\dot{V}_A/\dot{Q}$.—When regional ventilation is impaired without concomitant decrease in blood flow or, in the extreme case, when perfusion continues to nonventilated regions of lung, as in atelectasis, there is a decrease in $\dot{V}_A/\dot{Q}$. Gas exchange is inadequate in such regions or totally absent in the extreme case. The blood perfusing such regions is poorly oxygenated and, when mixed with blood from adequately ventilated regions, leads to arterial hypoxemia. Hyperventilation of normally functioning regions of the lung can compensate for whatever

hypercapnia is contributed by areas of low $\dot{V}_A/\dot{Q}$, but not for the hypoxemia. If compensatory hyperventilation of adequately perfused portions of the lung does not occur, carbon dioxide retention will also result.

The addition of poorly oxygenated blood from areas of low $\dot{V}_A/\dot{Q}$ to normally oxygenated blood *acts* like a right-to-left shunt. Though the physiologic end result, arterial hypoxemia, is the same, this shunt-like effect ("physiologic" shunting) must be differentiated from true venous admixture produced through an "anatomical" shunt. This differentiation may be accomplished by having the patient breathe 100% oxygen. Ultimately, the oxygen tension of all air-containing alveoli, even the poorly ventilated ones, will be increased to the point at which adequate capillary oxygenation will occur, and the shuntlike effect, reflected by a wide alveolar-arterial oxygen tension gradient, will appear to vanish. However, true venous admixture will not be changed by breathing 100% oxygen and can be distinguished by failure to correct the wide alveolar-arterial oxygen gradient. From the data obtained in such a study, the magnitude of the blood flow that does not pass air-containing alveoli can be estimated. Though such flow defines the anatomical shunt, it also includes pulmonary blood flow through totally airless lung.

READING LIST

Fowler W.S.: Intrapulmonary distribution of inspired gas. *Physiol. Rev.* 32:1–20, 1952.

This is a classic early review of the subject of distribution.

Bates D.V., Christie R.V.: Intrapulmonary mixing of helium in health and in emphysema. *Clin. Sci.* 9:17–29, 1950.

The helium mixing index is described in this article.

Becklake M.R.: A new index of the intrapulmonary mixture of inspired air. *Thorax* 7:111–116, 1952.

The nitrogen lung clearance index was first described in this article.

Glazier J.B., Hughes J.M.B., Maloney J.E., et al.: Vertical gradient of alveolar size in lungs of dogs frozen intact. *J. Appl. Physiol.* 23:694–705, 1967.

Gravity-dependent gradient of alveolar size was proved morphometrically in this study.

Rahn H., Farhi L.E.: Ventilation, perfusion, and gas exchange—the $\dot{V}_A/\dot{Q}$ concept. *Respiration,* vol. I, sec. 3. *Handbook of Physiology.* Washington, D.C., American Physiological Society, 1964, pp. 735–766.

The $\dot{V}_A/\dot{Q}$ concept is reviewed in this chapter of the Handbook of Physiology.

West J.B.: *Regional Differences in the Lung.* New York, San Francisco, London, Academic Press, 1977.

The general topic of regional differences in lung function is covered in this book.

For references on the single-breath nitrogen or "closing volume" test, see chapter 13.

11

Effects of Age on Lung Function

LUNG FUNCTION IS AFFECTED by age even in healthy individuals. These changes in lung function reflect growth and development in children, further maturation in young adults, and finally the decline with senescence in aging adults. Exposure to disease, insult, and injury are a part of life, and their accumulated effects also adversely affect lung function. If further decline in lung function results from a disease process, it becomes important to distinguish such changes from those produced by the normal aging process. To assess whether a measurement of lung function in a given individual is abnormal, we compare the measurement with a predetermined normal value, usually derived from a prediction equation. Normal values are based on data from large numbers of people of different size and various ages who have been free of cardiorespiratory disease and who do not smoke cigarettes. Age, of course, enters into these prediction equations.

Blood Gas Measurements

The ultimate function of the respiratory system is to effect gas exchanges, the transfer of oxygen and carbon dioxide between the liquid blood phase and the gas phase at the alveolar surface. This function is assessed by measurement of arterial blood gas tensions and pH. Compensatory mechanisms normally maintain pH within a narrow range of variability around a mean of 7.40, and departure from that range is of physiologic significance regardless of age.

Arterial carbon dioxide tension (Pa_{CO_2}) should not vary with age and would be expected to vary little from the normal value of 40 torr at sea level. Residence at altitude, however, would be expected to reduce the normal value for Pa_{CO_2}.

Alteration in lung mechanics and increasing imbalance in ventilation-perfusion relationships in the lung are a normal consequence of advancing age in the adult. Consequently, the normal value for arterial oxygen tension (Pa_{O_2}) can be anticipated to decrease with age. There are data to suggest that the normal decrease of Pa_{O_2} can be expressed by the equation:

$$Pa_{O_2} = 100.1 - 0.323 \times \text{age in years}$$

It is reasonable to consider a value below 90% of this predicted value for Pa_{O_2} as suggestive of abnormality. True abnormality in Pa_{O_2} also exists when the value is low enough to be of physiologic significance, regardless of predicted limits. In the interpretation of Pa_{O_2} values, one may wish to distinguish grades of hypoxemia. In Figure 11–1, three grades of hypoxemia are defined. Values for Pa_{O_2} below 90% of predicted for age and altitude or below 65 torr but above 55 torr define mild hypoxemia; values between 55 and 40 torr, moderate hypoxemia; and values below 40 torr, severe hypoxemia. These limits, although somewhat arbitrary, have proved to be useful guides in blood gas analysis interpretation.

The above equation for predicting age-specific Pa_{O_2} applies only to adults at sea level. Because ambient oxygen tension decreases with altitude,

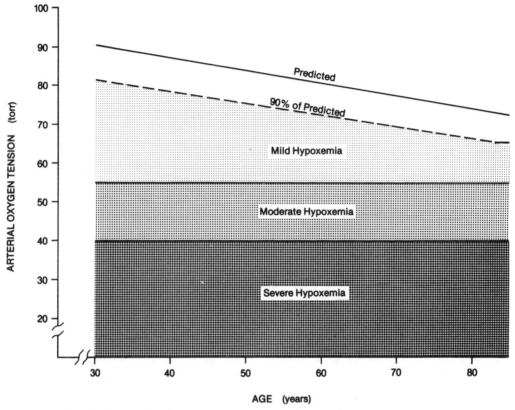

Fig 11–1.—Predicted arterial oxygen tension for healthy adults at sea level. Grades of hypoxemia are indicated.

the anticipated normal Pa_{O_2} in high-altitude residents would be lower than predicted by that equation. Faced with decreased ambient oxygen tension, human beings compensate by increasing ventilation. One cannot simply calculate what the Pa_{O_2} would be, therefore, but it is a useful approximation to assume that the normal Pa_{O_2} would decrease by almost 2.24 torr for each 1,000 ft of altitude above sea level. This factor should also be considered when interpreting blood gas values. When both age and altitude are considered, a very elderly, normal, healthy person at altitude may have Pa_{O_2} levels below 65 torr, in the range interpreted as mild hypoxemia.

It is important to note that the above prediction equation for Pa_{O_2} does not apply to infants or to children. In infants and very young children, the Pa_{O_2} tends to be low and increases with growth and development.

Lung Mechanics

The changes in lung mechanics in the aging adult are relatively subtle compared with the changes in the same direction which can be caused by disease processes, from which they must be distinguished. With advancing age, lung elastic recoil diminishes, maximum expiratory flow decreases, and the lung volume at which small airway closure occurs appears to increase.

The static deflation pressure-volume curve, which describes the elastic characteristic of the lung (discussed in chapter 6), is altered with advancing age. There is loss of lung elastic recoil which is greatest at high lung volumes but becomes insignificant at lung volumes below functional residual capacity (FRC). The result is a change in the shape of the P-V curve (Fig 11–2). The changes are small in magnitude and well

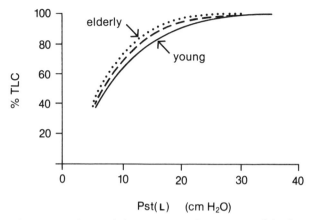

Fig 11–2.—Changes in shape of the pressure-volume curve of the lung with age.

tolerated. These changes, however, must be distinguished from the similar but more marked changes which are considered to be the physiologic hallmark of emphysema.

Maximum expiratory flow (Vmax) decreases with advancing age. When flow is expressed as TLC/sec to compensate for differences in lung size and volume expressed as percent expired VC, as shown in Figure 11–3, it is apparent that the decrease in Vmax is greatest at lower lung volumes, and the shape of maximum expiratory flow becomes increasingly concave in the direction of the volume axis with aging.

If, as described in chapter 6, Vmax is largely

determined by lung elastic recoil, the preservation of size-compensated flows in the face of loss of lung recoil at high lung volumes seems paradoxical. Flow is also a function of the resistance of intrapulmonary airways, which depend on lung recoil for their support. It is likely that these airways themselves lose recoil at a rate commensurate with the loss of parenchymal recoil and that resistance to flow does not therefore increase with aging. The decrease in Vmax at lower lung volumes, where lung recoil is relatively well preserved, may be the consequence of a more central location of equal pressure points (see chap. 6) in the elderly or, more

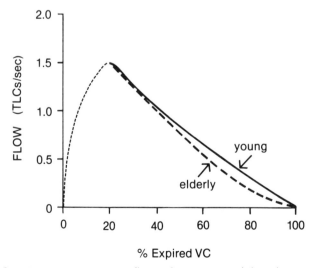

Fig 11–3.—Maximum expiratory flow-volume curve exhibits decrease in flow at lower lung volumes with advancing age.

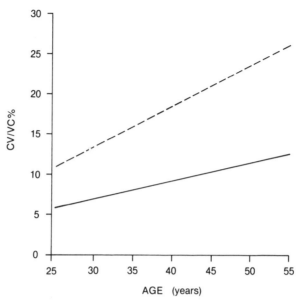

Fig 11–4.—The "closing volume," expressed as a percent of vital capacity, increases with advanc- ing age in the normal adult. *Dashed line* indicates the upper limit of "normal."

likely, of the change in the volume at which airway closure occurs.

As one expires to low lung volumes, terminal airways close, beginning with those in the more dependent regions of the lung. The volume at which airway closure begins is called the closing volume. The age-related changes in lung and airway properties in the elderly result in closure of airways at higher lung volumes, i.e., an increase in closing volume with age (Fig 11–4). When terminal airways close, the lung units served by these airways no longer participate in volume change or contribute to expiratory flow. This may serve to explain the observed decrease in V̇max at low lung volumes. In the very elderly, the volume at which closure occurs in dependent regions may exceed the FRC. All of these factors lead to further ventilation-perfusion inequalities which are, in turn, reflected by the decrease in Pa$_{O_2}$ with advancing age noted earlier.

Ventilatory Function

During childhood, both volumes and expired flows increase as one develops. Because chil- dren develop at varying rates, measurements of ventilatory function correlate, but with height rather than age in younger children. Later in childhood, there is an acceleration in growth and concomitant increase in lung volumes and flows with both age and height. Finally, in the adult, there are changes associated with senescence.

Because lung volume is related to overall body size, height correlates with three-dimensional measurements of volume. Height diminishes very little with age in the adult. The total lung capacity (TLC), once achieved in early life, also decreases very little with advancing age. As a consequence of age-related changes in lung mechanics, however, the vital capacity (VC), functional residual capacity (FRC), residual volume (RV), and the various timed volume measurements commonly derived from spirometric evaluations also change over the years.

The FRC, determined by the balance between lung and chest wall elastic forces, increases with advancing age. The RV, and consequently the RV/TLC ratio, increase with age, and there is a parallel decrease in VC. Inasmuch as V̇max decreases with age, timed volumes representing average flows over portions of the FVC maneuver decrease accordingly.

The forced expiratory volume in the first second of expiration, FEV_1, is, in effect, the average flow during that first second and is the measurement most commonly used to evaluate ventilatory impairment. The determination of abnormality is made by comparing the measurement from a given individual with a predicted reference value, a predicted "normal." As we noted before, age enters into the equation used to determine the expected result. Several "prediction equations" are available based on analyses of data from normal, healthy subjects. Most of these studies suggest that in adults, the FEV_1 declines at the rate of 25–30 ml/year. In reality, it is not likely that ventilatory function declines in a linear fashion at a fixed rate even in normal, healthy people. Rather, it appears that there is very little decline in FEV_1 in young adults, after

which the decline begins gradually, accelerating in middle age in a nonlinear fashion. The linear prediction equations may not reflect accurately the real changes which occur over time, though they do offer useful approximations to use in interpreting test results.

In conclusion, the overall effect of aging on lung function is the sum of various interrelating factors. The lung, however, has considerable reserve, and the changes observed with aging are subtle and have little impact on health in general, even when extrapolated to the maximum extreme of potential life span. Advancing age alone will not result in impairment of function. The decrease in certain measurements of lung function which are part of the normal aging process must be distinguished from those which are produced by disease, insult, or injury, changes which may be sufficient to produce impairment.

READING LIST

Murray J.F.: *The Normal Lung*. Philadelphia, London, Toronto, W. B. Saunders Co., 1976, pp. 315–316.

The chapter on aging in this book, in addition to a general discussion of the subject, describes the effect of age on arterial oxygen tension.

Bode R., Dosman J., Martin R.R., et al.: Age and sex differences in lung elasticity and in closing capacity in nonsmokers. *J. Appl. Physiol.* 41:129–135, 1976.

Gibson G.J., Pride N.B., O'Cain C., et al.: Sex and age differences in pulmonary mechanics of normal nonsmoking subjects. *J. Appl. Physiol.* 41:20–25, 1976.

Knudson R.J., Clark D.F., Kennedy T.C., et al.: Effect of aging alone on mechanical properties of the normal adult human lung. *J. Appl. Physiol.* 43:1054–1062, 1977.

Turner J.M., Mead J., Wohl M.E.: Elasticity of human lungs in relation to age. *J. Appl. Physiol.* 25:664–671, 1968.

The effects of age on lung mechanics are described in these articles.

Knudson R.J., Slatin R.C., Lebowitz M.D., et al.: The maximal expiratory flow-volume curve: normal standards, variability, and effects of age. *Am. Rev. Respir. Dis.* 113:587–600, 1976.

The effect of age on ventilatory function is discussed in this article.

Anthonisen N.R., Danson J., Robertson P.C., et al.: Airway closure as a function of age. *Respir. Physiol.* 8:58–65, 1970.

Buist A.S., Ross B.B.: Predicted values for closing volumes using a modified single breath nitrogen test. *Am. Rev. Respir. Dis.* 107:744–752, 1973.

Holland J., Milic-Emili J., Macklem P.T., et al.: Regional distribution of pulmonary ventilation and perfusion in elderly subjects. *J. Clin. Invest.* 47:81–92, 1968.

Knudson R.J., Lebowitz M.D., Burton A.P., et al.: The closing volume test: Evaluation of nitrogen and bolus methods in a random population. *Am. Rev. Respir. Dis.* 115:423–434, 1977.

The effects of age on distribution of ventilation and airway closure are discussed in these articles.

PART II

Pathophysiology

12

Lung Function Testing: General Considerations

TESTS OF LUNG FUNCTION have been mentioned frequently in discussions of the evaluation and management of respiratory insufficiency states. Although it is not the purpose of this volume to describe the techniques of testing or the details of pulmonary function test interpretation, a few general comments are in order.

General Uses of Lung Function Tests

Measurements of functional impairment of the lung have an established role in clinical medicine. In some instances they allow detection of abnormalities prior to the development of symptoms, physical signs, or even radiologic findings. They provide objective or at least semiobjective measurements of the severity of impairment from a known disease. Such measurements are useful in following the course of a patient, assessing the efficacy of therapy, determining prognosis, estimating operative risks, and documenting the severity of disease for medicolegal purposes. Lung function tests also have led to a better understanding of the many disease processes that involve the lung, and they have provided an invaluable clinical research tool.

In addition, as noted frequently throughout this book, these tests are often useful in differentiating various disease states that affect the lung. But it is important to recognize the limi-

tations of measurements of functional impairment in differential diagnosis. Such measurements are rarely diagnostic of a specific disease, since they usually fail to define the exact anatomical location of the abnormality and almost never indicate its etiology. Typical patterns of functional abnormality have been described for many diseases, but such patterns are not pathognomonic and are often absent early in the course of a disorder. Only respiratory disorders defined in physiologic terms can be excluded on the basis of negative pulmonary function test results.

Assessment of Abnormality

Laboratory measurements are used to quantify lung function. The resulting values must be interpreted in terms of "normal." "Normal" or, more properly, "reference" values are based on data from people who have been free of cardiorespiratory disorders and, in most cases, who have never smoked. In interpreting values for lung function measurements obtained on a given patient, one compares those values with those predicted for a healthy person of the same characteristics. Depending on the measurement, those characteristics may include age, body size, sex, and race. A significant departure from a predicted value connotes abnormality.

The definition of abnormality may be based on one of two criteria: either the departure from normal is of physiologic significance or the value departs significantly from a statistical norm. The criterion one uses depends on the measurement. For some measurements, abnormality is said to exist when a value departs sufficiently from normal to be of physiologic significance regardless of age, sex, or body size. Measurements of blood gas tensions or pH are evaluated on the basis of physiologic significance. Normal values for Pa_{O_2} and Pa_{CO_2} may be affected by the altitude at which one resides, and aging will influence the normal value for Pa_{O_2} (see chap. 11). Of importance, however, is not the value itself but the consequences of abnormal values. Thus, significant departure from the normal narrow range for pH is always of physiologic significance. Hypoxemia can be said to exist when the Pa_{O_2} falls below a critical level inasmuch as diminished tissue oxygen supply is always critical, regardless of cause.

Other measurements of lung function, such as lung volumes, expiratory flows, or diffusing capacity, are assessed on the basis of departure from statistically derived reference values. The anticipated or predicted "normal" value is usually derived from the appropriate regression equation in which age and body size are pertinent variables.

Two methods are used when considering variables that are dependent on body size, size correction, and size compensation. Size correction is accomplished by comparing one individual's test results with values obtained in a large group of normal subjects of the same sex, age, and body size. Average data for the normal group allow prediction of a value for the individual and expression of his lung function measurement as a percentage of its predicted value.

Various problems are inherent in the use of such predicted values determined from size correction. Should nonsmokers be compared with "normal" population groups that include both smokers and nonsmokers, or should there be separate normal values for smokers and nonsmokers? Similarly, should physical conditioning be taken into account? How do we rule out the possibility that the individual being examined might belong at the extreme of the normal distribution rather than at its mean if he had no

lung disease? The latter problem is especially troublesome. For example, a patient may have a VC of 5 L, the predicted value for his sex, age, and height. However, before development of a pulmonary disorder, his own VC may have been 7 L, greater than that predicted but within the normal distribution of values for the population. Thus, when tested and considered normal, this patient already may have lost more than one fourth of his VC, even though his test results indicate 100% of predicted function. In fact, the problem may be even more complicated. Because of variability in normal subjects, a VC may not be considered definitely abnormal until it is less than 80% of that predicted. In the instance noted above, the patient's VC would have to fall below 4 L (less than 60% of his initial value) before a definite abnormality would be recognized.

If one can determine a predicted "normal" value for a given measurement on a given patient, how great a departure from that predicted value should one permit before labeling the result abnormal? It is important to remember that the predicted value is the mean of values derived from a large group of healthy people of the same age, sex, height, and race, and that there is between-subject variability within that "normal" population. The "limits of normal" must take this biologic variation into consideration, and that variability may well be different for different measurements. For example, the variability in $\dot{V}max$ values is considerably greater than the variability observed in FVC or FEV_1, and, consequently, the limits of normal must be much greater for $\dot{V}max$ than for FEV_1. One may set the lower limit of normal at 55% of predicted for $\dot{V}max_{75\%}$ but at 75% of predicted for FEV_1. A fixed limit of 80% of predicted clearly is inappropriate for all measurements of lung function.

Whereas size correction compares one individual's performance with that of a large group of supposedly normal subjects, size compensation compares two different measurements made in the same individual, each of which depends on body size. This procedure is useful when two values normally parallel each other in a given individual. For example, if a normal subject has a VC above that predicted, he should also have an FEV_1 above that predicted. In the face of a high VC, an FEV_1 at the lower end of the normal range will give an abnormally low FEV_1/FVC ratio, indicating some obstructive abnormality. In this case, the ratio is more discriminatory than either its numerator or denominator.

But there are serious problems if such ratios are interpreted without regard to the absolute values from which they are derived. For example, the FEV_1/FVC ratio is a poor guide to the severity of an obstructive abnormality. If both the FEV_1 and FVC improve after administration of a bronchodilator, their ratio may be unchanged. In this instance the ratio fails to detect an obvious improvement in overall lung function.

The RV/TLC ratio is elevated when RV is high or when VC is reduced to a greater extent than RV. Although a high ratio is one of the characteristic findings of emphysema, it is also seen in restrictive disorders associated with a small TLC, a severe reduction in VC, and a slight reduction in RV.

In the case of specific compliance and specific conductance measurements, compliance and conductance values are divided by the existing lung volume. Although it is true that this eliminates to a degree the effect of body size on compliance and conductance measurements, it may lead to great confusion in the presence of lung disease. A normally compliant but large, emphysematous lung may have a low specific compliance. This hardly indicates that the lung is excessively stiff. Similarly, it is possible to be misled by a normal specific conductance in an abnormally small lung. In this case the decreased airways conductance may be masked when it is divided by an abnormally small lung volume.

Proper Performance

The results of a test will, of course, be misleading if a test is not performed correctly. It is important, therefore, that the patient be thoroughly instructed in how to perform the test, that performance is monitored as the test is administered, and that the test be repeated so that the results can be examined for consistency and reproducibility.

Proper performance of spirometric tests requires the effective cooperation of the subject. Full inspiration and complete expiration are required to measure accurately the maximum volume excursion or vital capacity. The expiratory effort must be vigorously initiated and the effort sustained to achieve maximum expiratory flow throughout the maneuver. Failure of proper performance can often be detected by inspecting the spirogram but is best revealed by examining the maximum expiratory flow-volume (MEFV) curve. The MEFV curve provides the best index of best performance and effort. Because subtle changes in the slope of the volume-time spirogram are difficult to detect, the MEFV curve contains detail not otherwise revealed. The MEFV curve should exhibit an initial rapid increase in flow followed by a diminishing flow with volume, and the curve should not terminate abruptly with a sudden cessation of flow.

Occasionally, a patient willfully withholds maximum effort. This type of malingering is usually readily detected if the tests are repeated and results are examined. The MEFV curve should be highly reproducible, and it is extremely difficult to reproduce a deliberately falsified test. Fortunately, frank malingering is rare. Unsatisfactory tests more often indicate that the patient does not completely understand what is expected of him or that his performance is hampered by fatigue, chest pain, and so on. In such a case, repeating the tests at a later date will usually produce more satisfactory results.

Other tests place fewer demands on the subject, such as tests of inert gas distribution, measurements of diffusing capacity, and, of course, arterial blood gas determinations. Such tests may be useful in evaluating the suspected malingerer.

Misleading Terminology

The names of tests do not always accurately reflect their significance in an abnormal lung. Examples are dynamic compliance and diffusing capacity. Dynamic compliance values may be as closely related to the airways abnormality as to the elastic properties of the lung when measured in patients with airways obstructive disease. Diffusing capacity tests reflect a conglomeration of abnormalities instead of measuring specifically the capacity for gas exchange at the alveolar-capillary barrier.

The names of some other tests are misleading if we fail to recognize that they are "as if" measurements. For example, the very complex problem of nonuniform distribution of ventilation and perfusion throughout the lung is often quantified in terms of physiologic shunting and alveolar dead space. These terms indicate that the overall effect of maldistribution of blood and gas is similar to that which would occur if some fraction of the blood flow traversed totally unventilated areas and some portion of the ventilation reached totally unperfused alveoli. In fact, no totally bloodless or totally unventilated alveoli need actually exist, and these terms certainly do not indicate that poor ventilation or perfusion is limited to an anatomically definable lung region. The terms "alveolar" and "physiologic dead space" are particularly misleading, since they do not measure a space at all, but only a quantity of wasted ventilation.

The term "anatomical shunting," as used by physiologists, refers to blood that finds its way from the right atrium to the peripheral arteries without reaching air-containing alveoli. This may result from a defect in the intraventricular septum (as in congenital heart disease) or from an abnormal vascular channel in the lung (as in pulmonary AV fistula). But the same physiologic effects will be produced by normal pulmonary vessels that traverse totally atelectatic or completely fluid- or disease-filled alveoli. Such anatomical-like shunting is not distinguishable from a true anatomical vascular abnormality on the basis of lung function tests.

The names of other tests are more applicable to normal than pathologic lungs. For example, it is difficult to interpret an "airways resistance" measurement in obstructive airways disease when there is no constant relationship between applied pressure and air flow. In severe emphysema, inspiratory airway resistance may be normal, while expiratory airway resistance becomes markedly elevated during a forced expiratory effort. Since some airways resistance measurements are taken during inspiration, a normal airways resistance measurement can be obtained in a patient with chronic obstructive pulmonary emphysema.

Considerable confusion may occur with the terms "hyper-" and "hypoventilation." In the presence of a large physiologic dead space, overall minute volume must be elevated to maintain a normal effective alveolar ventilation and normal Pa_{CO_2}. If the wasted ventilation is great enough, a patient may even have alveolar hypoventilation despite overall hyperventilation. The adequacy of alveolar ventilation is indicated by Pa_{CO_2}. The presence of overall hyperventilation can be determined only by measurements of minute volume.

Finally, care must be taken in interpreting terms used to describe patterns of functional abnormality. A "restrictive" abnormality on spirometry indicates only a decrease in the volume excursion of the lung. It may result from a wide variety of disorders, including weakness of the respiratory muscles, and does not necessarily relate to a specific type of lung pathology. An "obstructive" pattern simply indicates that there is expiratory slowing. This may result from excessive collapse of airways during forced expiration owing to loss of lung elastic recoil. It does not necessarily indicate an intrinsic airways disease with a physical obstruction to air flow.

Testing for Asymptomatic Respiratory Impairment

In certain situations evidence of a respiratory insufficiency state is sought in a patient who exhibits no signs or symptoms of cardiopulmonary disease. Any complete clinical evaluation that includes a chest roentgenogram and ECG should include spirometry as a basic lung function test. Lung function tests also have been used in mass screening for pulmonary disorders. Evidence indicates, however, that case detection in mass surveys rarely leads to effective therapy. Unless such surveys are combined with effective followup procedures, they are useful only as part of carefully planned and controlled research studies.

Subjects who are exposed to potentially harmful inhalants should be followed up with serial lung function tests as well as chest roentgenograms. Functional abnormalities may precede obvious radiologic change. The type of lung function testing needed varies with the type of dysfunction characteristically produced by the inhalant. Exposure to such substances as asbestos, beryllium, ozone, or the allergens that cause farmer's lung may produce reduction of diffusing capacity before there is ventilatory impairment. With other inhalants a ''bronchospastic'' reaction is expected rather than an effect on parenchymal tissues, as in byssinosis, acute exposure to sulfur dioxide, or atopic asthma. In such cases, slight degrees of airways obstruction may be detected by direct measurements of airways resistance before there are clinical findings and occasionally even before there are discernible changes in the spirogram. In some of the fibrosing pneumoconioses (e.g., silicosis), changes in lung compliance may precede spirometric abnormalities.

It may be advisable to determine whether there is pulmonary involvement from a suspected or known systemic disease before there are clinical or radiologic signs of a pulmonary disorder. Diffusing capacity and even spirometric abnormalities sometimes precede definite radiologic changes in disorders that are widely distributed throughout the lung, including scleroderma, other collagen-vascular diseases, acute miliary tuberculosis, and sarcoidosis.

Spirometric tests are the most widely used for detection of otherwise unsuspected pulmonary dysfunction. In combination with chest roentgenograms, these simple tests detect most clinically significant respiratory disorders. They are highly suitable for routine screening. As noted above, early functional changes resulting from involvement of the lung by a systemic disease or from exposure to certain inhaled noxious agents may be detected only if diffusing capacity is included in the screening tests.

Screening tests of lung function are important for preoperative evaluation even when cardiopulmonary disease is not suspected. This use will be considered later in this chapter.

Testing to Evaluate Questionable Radiologic Abnormalities

In several instances the radiologist may have difficulty in determining the significance of a suggestive abnormality on chest roentgenogram. The most frequent is an appearance of pulmonary hyperinflation with low diaphragms and generalized increased radiolucency. Although suggesting pulmonary emphysema, this type of roentgenogram may be seen in otherwise normal individuals. Before a patient is told that he has emphysema, a diagnostic term that implies a progressive, disabling disorder, irreversible airways obstruction should be demonstrated. A normal forced expiratory flow raises doubt as to the significance of a radiologic suspicion of emphysema.

It must be admitted that the problem is more complicated than indicated above. Some anatomical emphysema may exist without significant ventilatory abnormality. A syndrome of dyspnea and pulmonary hyperinflation without expiratory slowing is thought by some to precede the classic disabling airways obstructive syndrome generally ascribed to emphysema. It may be possible to confirm a radiologic suspicion of emphysema with diffusing capacity and pressure-volume measurements even before expiratory slowing is demonstrable. But in ordinary clinical practice, a diagnosis of emphysema implies a progressive, disabling obstructive lung disease. Before this diagnosis is given to a patient, the radiologic impression should be confirmed by demonstration of expiratory slowing on spirometric tests.

Another type of roentgenogram that is difficult to interpret is one with a very fine reticular appearance. Without physiologic tests, it may be difficult to decide whether this represents an early diffuse interstitial disease or is only a normal variant. Demonstration of reduced VC or diffusing capacity indicates that the radiologic abnormality is significant, requiring further diagnostic study.

Testing to Evaluate Disability

It is essential to distinguish impairment from disability. Impairment refers to a reduction in specific body or organ function, whereas disability is an inability to perform a specific task or activity. A physiologic test may provide a precise estimate of the impairment of specific lung function. But its implications in terms of disability depend on other factors, including the demands of the activity, environmental and social circumstances, psychologic considerations, and motivation. For these reasons there is an imperfect relationship between impairment and disability.

Medical incapacity is defined still differently. It takes into account both the level of impairment and the potential harm to the patient if he performs certain activities. Even if not physiologically impaired, a patient with a recent myocardial infarction is ''incapacitated'' by his disease. A patient also may be incapacitated as a result of emotional factors.

The pulmonary function laboratory is concerned primarily with determining impairment. The chest physician uses this determination of impairment in his overall assessment of medical incapacity. Determination of occupational disability depends on various additional factors, including availability of a job suited to the patient's abilities. In practice, ''disability'' is usually determined in relationship to eligibility for benefits from some social agency. Criteria are

then quite arbitrary, often depending as much on availability of funds as on medical indications.

Various pulmonary function measurements, considered in relationship to occupational demands, have been shown to be related to work status in patients with chronic airways obstruction who are not applying for disability benefits. In such patients the likelihood of occupational disability can be determined from the degree of ventilatory impairment, physical exertion demanded by the occupation, and presence or absence of ECG abnormality, as indicated in Table 12–1. A minority of patients continue to work at active jobs once the FEV_1 falls below 800 ml, but the majority of patients continue to work if the FEV_1 is above 1.1 L, unless they are engaged in a very strenuous occupation. Other pulmonary function tests do not significantly improve the overall prediction of work status, but more detailed studies may be important in individual patients in whom there is a discrepancy between apparent impairment and ventilatory tests. For example, we have observed an emphysematous patient with an FEV_1 of 1.7 L who had a very insensitive respiratory center and severe hypercapnia, hypoxemia, and cor pulmonale. This patient was incapacitated for almost any type of gainful employment, although his likelihood of working was good according to the guidelines of Table 12–1. In general, patients should not continue to work if they have definite clinical signs of cor pulmonale.

There is much less information relating the severity of restrictive disorders to work status. Various factors used to grade the severity of impairment are indicated in Table 12–2. The severity of cor pulmonale also must be considered.

TABLE 12–1.—DISABILITY SCORES FOR PATIENTS WITH CHRONIC
BRONCHITIS AND EMPHYSEMA*

FEV_1, L	SCORE	ECG	SCORE	OCCUPATION	SCORE
>1.3	0	Normal	0	Light work	0
1.1–1.3	10	Suspicious	10	Moderate work	20
0.9–1.1	20	Abnormal	20	Heavy work	40
0.7–0.8	30				
<0.7	40				

*The sum of scores roughly estimates the percentage probability that a patient will no longer be working full time.

TABLE 12–2.—SEVERITY OF IMPAIRMENT IN A RESTRICTIVE TYPE OF DISEASE*

VENTILATORY IMPAIRMENT (% PREDICTED VC)	DIFFUSION LIMITATION (% PREDICTED D_L)	HYPOXEMIA ON EXERCISE (% Sa_{O_2})	ALVEOLAR HYPERVENTILATION (Pa_{CO_2})	SEVERITY
>90	>80	>94	34 torr	None
70–90	65–80	90–94	32–34 torr	Mild
50–70	50–65	85–90	28–32 torr	Moderate
35–50	35–50	75–85	25–28 torr	Severe
<35	<35	<75	<25 torr	Very severe

*The table does not imply consistent relationships among VC, D_L and blood gas abnormalities. The severity of each type of abnormality should be graded independently. D_L = diffusing capacity: Sa_{O_2} = arterial oxygen saturation.

When all of the abnormalities are mild and there is no evidence of myocardial insufficiency, patients are generally able to work at any but the most demanding job. Indeed, in the absence of blood gas abnormalities, patients with restrictive lung diseases may feel able to work until VC is markedly reduced.

In view of the paucity of data and the poor correlation between exercise tolerance and physiologic tests (especially in the restrictive disorders), final assessment of impairment should take into account the history of dyspnea and observations of the patient's breathing during a standardized exercise test. The latter should be a routine procedure in any disability evaluation.

Preoperative Evaluation

PREOPERATIVE SCREENING.—Patients without obvious pulmonary disease are often referred to the pulmonary function laboratory preoperatively to exclude subclinical respiratory dysfunction, especially of the obstructive type. In view of the difficulty in early clinical diagnosis of obstructive lung diseases, such preoperative screening is justifiable, especially in older patients. Detection of an obstructive defect allows institution of therapeutic procedures to improve the patient's tolerance for surgery, allows a rational choice of anesthetic agents, and indicates a program of postoperative care to lower the probability of complications. The requirements for preoperative screening are similar to those for routine examinations discussed earlier in this chapter. Observing the patient during exercise is

not a satisfactory substitute for a well performed physiologic test.

EVALUATING OPERATIVE RISK.—Severe airways obstruction is associated with an increased operative mortality. A maximum voluntary ventilation below 50% of that predicted, maximum expiratory flow rate below 220 L/min, or very low FEV_1 indicates an increased risk. Operative mortality is especially high when airways obstruction is associated with hypercapnia or ECG abnormalities. Severity of restrictive ventilatory impairment is less closely related to postoperative survival, and there have been no adequate studies relating diffusing capacity to operative risk. However, since diffusing capacity shows a marked decline after thoracotomy (generally falling more than does VC with wedge resection or lobectomy), it is logical to regard a very low diffusing capacity as a relative contraindication to pulmonary resection.

In view of the paucity and variability of reported data and their uncertain applicability to current surgical techniques, it is not possible to determine the precise risk of an operative procedure in a patient with pulmonary dysfunction. Surgical mortality depends on cardiovascular as well as pulmonary status. Guidelines for preoperative assessment of surgical risk are presented in Table 12–3; interpretations are deliberately vague.

The resistance and distensibility of the pulmonary vascular bed may be more important than the VC in determining the risks of pulmonary resection, and frank pulmonary hypertension is an important contraindication to surgery. Cardiac catheterization for measurement of pul-

TABLE 12–3.—EVALUATING OPERATIVE RISK FROM PULMONARY FUNCTION TESTS

FINDINGS	INTERPRETATION
Normal tests	No increased risk demonstrated
Obstructive disorders	
*MVV > 50%, FEV_1 > 1.5 L; normal blood gases	Little increased risk if special precautions taken in management
MVV 35–50%, FEV_1 1–1.5 L; normal Pa_{CO_2}; no more than slight hypoxemia; normal ECG	Definitely increased risk even with proper management. A relative contraindication to surgery
MVV 35–50%, FEV_1 1–1.5 L; normal Pa_{CO_2}; slight hypoxemia; abnormal ECG	Greatly increased operative risk. A contraindication to major elective surgical procedures
MVV < 35%, FEV_1 < 1 L; normal Pa_{CO_2}; mild hypoxemia; normal ECG	Greatly increased operative risk. A contraindication to major elective surgical procedures. Probably precludes extensive lung resection
MVV < 35%, FEV_1 <1 L; elevated Pa_{CO_2}; severe hypoxemia or abnormal ECG	Extremely high operative risk. Only mandatory surgery justifiable. Probably precludes any pulmonary resection
Restrictive disorders	
VC > 50%, D_L > 50%; normal blood gases	Little increased operative risk
VC 35–50%, D_L > 50%; slight hypoxemia on exertion	Some increase in operative risk, but not a serious contraindication to surgery, except extensive lung resection
VC < 35%, D_L < 50% or frank hypoxemia	Greatly increased operative risk, especially contraindicating extensive lung resection

*MVV = maximum voluntary ventilation.

monary hemodynamics is indicated when extensive lung resection is contemplated in a patient with poor pulmonary function.

DETERMINING THE FUNCTIONAL IMPORTANCE OF THE PORTION OF LUNG TO BE RESECTED.—If overall lung function is normal or only slightly impaired, removal of a diseased area will not lead to disabling physiologic impairment. But when tests are already markedly abnormal, extensive lung disease must exist. It is then essential to demonstrate that the planned resection will not lead to an intolerable degree of pulmonary insufficiency. This problem is common in surgery for tuberculosis, extensive bronchiectasis, or lung neoplasm associated with diffuse obstructive emphysema.

The fraction of the total ventilation and the fraction of the total perfusion being performed by the lung to be resected may be measured to determine the expected functional loss. Regional ventilation may be estimated by fluoroscopy, and the differential function of the two lungs may be measured precisely with bronchospirometry. In addition to estimates of fractional ven-

tilation and blood flow, differential RV and diffusing capacities can be studied by bronchiospirometry, but the clinical importance of these latter measurements is uncertain.

The hemodynamic effect of removing a portion of the vascular bed may be predicted by observing the effect of balloon occlusion of the vessel to be transected or of temporary occlusion of that vessel at the time of surgery. A sharp rise in PAP contraindicates so extensive a resection. Balloon occlusion of a portion of the pulmonary vascular bed has been combined with differential bronchospirometry to provide the ultimate preoperative assessment of the effects of pneumonectomy.

Newer techniques provide accurate and relatively simple means for assessing regional lung function. Regional blood flow may be estimated by lung perfusion scanning; together with fluoroscopy, this provides sufficient information for preoperative evaluation of most patients. Radioactive gas techniques using ^{133}Xe can provide quite precise estimates of ventilation as well as blood flow to relatively small areas of the lung.

When these methods are available, they are supplanting most other techniques.

In summary, when extensive lung resection is contemplated in a patient with considerably reduced lung function, it may be necessary to perform elaborate studies to determine the feasibility of surgery. But most often, the physician only needs assurance that the portion of lung to be removed is not responsible for a disproportionately large fraction of the overall ventilation and lung perfusion. Fluoroscopic examination combined with radioactive lung scanning and standard pulmonary function tests suffices for preoperative evaluation of such patients.

ASSESSMENT OF PROGNOSIS.—To determine the advisability of any type of elective surgery in a patient with known chronic respiratory insufficiency, it is necessary to know the level of the patient's pulmonary dysfunction. Measurements of functional impairment are essential for estimating survival of patients with chronic airways obstruction.

DETERMINING FUNCTIONAL INDICATIONS FOR SURGERY.—With fibrothorax, decortication may be indicated if blood flow and ventilation to the affected side are markedly impaired. Indication for surgery may be clarified by bronchospirometry or other studies of regional lung function, especially in patients with bilateral lung disease.

Indications for resection of bullae in patients without diffuse lung disease generally depend on observations other than pulmonary function tests. Progressive enlargement on roentgenogram, recurrent or persistent pneumothorax, recurrent infection, or compression of surrounding lung tissue may be reasons for surgical intervention. Studies of regional ventilation and perfusion may be helpful in determining the functional importance of bullous lesions. Thorough evaluation requires angiography to assess the extent of the bullous disease and its effect on surrounding lung.

It is considerably more difficult to evaluate possible benefits of lung resection in a patient with chronic generalized airways obstruction who appears to have especially severe disease in one lung region. Resection of emphysematous areas of lung has been recommended to remove major sites of physiologic shunting or alveolar dead space or to reduce lung volume. The desirability of reducing lung volume has not yet been demonstrated, nor can it be determined by preoperative testing. In considering resection of a site of shunting or alveolar dead space, radioactive gas studies can confirm that ventilation and perfusion are especially disproportionate in some lung region. Even with such studies, however, it is difficult to determine the importance of this region in the overall functional disturbance. Removal of any portion of lung will produce some increase in overall vascular and airways resistances and will reduce diffusing surface. The physician must decide if the theoretical gain from resection is worth the inevitable overall loss of function. To justify removal of a portion of the lung in an attempt to reduce shunting, it should be demonstrated that occlusion of the blood supply to the region significantly improves Sa_{O_2} without raising PAP. Resection for the purpose of reducing alveolar dead space requires demonstration that occlusion of the regional bronchi and blood vessels improves arterial Pa_{CO_2}. These criteria for surgery are rarely fulfilled. The major indication for lung resection in patients with emphysema is compression of relatively normal appearing lung by an expanding bulla. Angiography provides the best assessment of both the severity of compression and the apparent normalcy of the compressed lung.

READING LIST

ATS Statement—Snowbird Workshop on Standardization of Spirometry. *Am. Rev. Respir. Dis.* 119:831–838, 1979.

Epidemiology Standardization Project. III. Recommended Standardization Procedures for Pulmonary Function Testing. *Am. Rev. Respir. Dis.* 118 (no. 6, pt. 2):55–88, 1978.

These two papers present guidelines for instrumentation and methodology of lung function testing.

Tisi G.M.: Preoperative evaluation of pulmonary function. *Am. Rev. Respir. Dis.* 119:293–310, 1979.

This is a recent "state of the art" review.

Lung Function Testing:
Practical Applications

RESPIRATORY DISORDERS are commonly described in clinical terms according to their signs, symptoms, and physical findings. In actuality, they are problems resulting from altered lung function. The understanding and subsequent management of a disorder are facilitated by concentrating on the underlying pathophysiologic abnormality rather than only on the overt clinical manifestation of dysfunction. Once the problem is stated in functional terms, tests may be performed to define and clarify the problem. The physician's perception of the problem serves as a guide to selection of the tests. From the data provided by test results, one can detect the presence of altered function, determine the type of dysfunction, and assess the severity of the abnormality. Lung function tests seldom provide a definitive diagnosis, however. The definition of a specific disease is often couched in morphological terms, requiring knowledge of altered structure. Lung function tests are essentially noninvasive, for they must not appreciably affect the phenomena they are intended to measure. Thus, structural abnormalities can only be inferred from measurements of function, such inference being often based on imperfect knowledge of the correlation between structure and function.

Elsewhere we have discussed the basic mechanisms and principles on which the various measurements of lung function are based. By selecting the appropriate tests, derangements in these mechanisms can be revealed. Derangements often fall into patterns which in turn appear to be characteristics of various types of disease states. Respiratory impairment may be classified on the basis of lung function tests, a physiologic classification describing the functional consequences of underlying cardiorespiratory disease.

Arterial blood gas measurements assess the overall function of the respiratory system and are consequently nonspecific. Spirometric or related tests of ventilatory function, on the other hand, offer some degree of specificity. Such tests are carried out almost routinely, often as the only test performed, and are generally used as a primary basis for a physiologic classification of respiratory disorders. If spirometry alone does not fully characterize the disorder, however, other tests may be required until all features of the dysfunction are revealed. It is not cost-effective to require a complete battery of tests for every patient. Decisions regarding tests and their selection should be made sequentially and according to need.

It is not within the purview of this book to describe pulmonary function testing in technical detail. What follows is simply a description of how tests can be used to characterize respiratory disorders.

Distinguishing Obstructive From Restrictive Ventilatory Disorders

From measurements of the maximum volume excursion and of maximum expiratory flow from

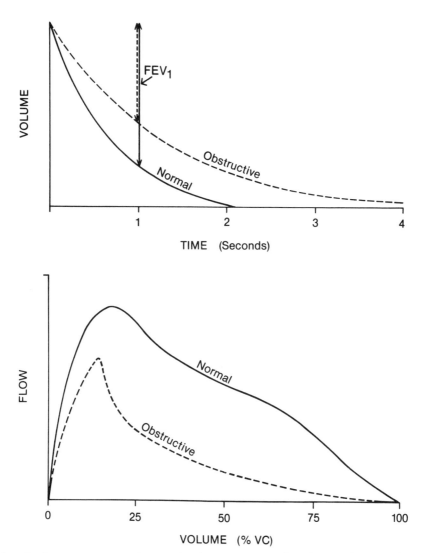

Fig 13–1.—At the top is a typical normal volume-time spirogram *(solid line)* contrasted with the spirogram of a patient with obstructive airways disease *(dashed line).* Below are shown the comparable maximum expiratory flow-volume curves.

the forced expiratory vital capacity (FVC) maneuver, differentiation is possible between obstructive and restrictive ventilatory abnormalities. In this context, "obstructive" refers to airways obstruction characterized by reduced maximum expiratory flow. Although this term is commonly used, it could be considered a misnomer inasmuch as it does not imply the presence of obstruction in the sense of actual occlusion of conducting airways. The proposed alternative, "airflow limitation," is also inexact inasmuch as flow-limiting mechanisms always operate in determining the maximum limit of expiratory flow, Vmax. While "airflow" or "ventilatory impairment" may be more appropriate terms, we will retain the term "airways obstruction" in this discussion. The term "restrictive" implies only diminished volume, but it is important to define the volume described.

A purely *obstructive* ventilatory abnormality is, by definition, distinguished by decreased forced expiratory flow. This is revealed by a decreased forced expiratory volume in the first second (FEV_1) of the FVC maneuver and a characteristic abnormal shape of the maximum expiratory flow-volume (MEFV) curve (Fig 13–1). The volume excursion, or FVC, should be well preserved but in reality, with increasing severity of obstruction, the FVC may be reduced as the residual volume (RV) becomes increased with "air trapping." In such cases, the slow inspiratory vital capacity (IVC) may be greater than the FVC. Not only should the size corrected FEV_1, expressed as a percent of predicted, be diminished, but also the size compensated FEV_1/VC ratio should reveal a disproportionate reduction in flow. While most normal healthy individuals can expire 80% to 85% of their FVC in the first second, an obstructive abnormality is indicated when this value falls below 75% in young individuals, 70% in middle-aged persons, or 65% in the elderly. As a consequence of "air trapping," some reduction of the FVC may be expected when the FEV_1/VC ratio is very low. As a rule, however, the VC as a percentage of predicted should be reduced less than half as much as the FEV_1 in an uncomplicated airways obstructive disorder. Thus, a VC as low as 70% of the predicted level might be expected from an airways obstruction that reduces the FEV_1 to 40% of its predicted level (reductions of 30% and 60%, respectively). With greater degrees of VC impairment in the presence of a low FEV_1/VC ratio, the physician should suspect that some factor other than airways obstruction is limiting thoracic excursion. "Mixed" patterns of this type are often seen with congestive heart failure or with pneumonia complicating the obstructive airways disease.

A *restrictive* ventilatory disorder is distinguished by a reduced VC. A restrictive ventilatory abnormality may be said to exist if the value falls below approximately 80% of predicted in young adults, below 75% in the middle-aged, or below about 65% of predicted in the very elderly. With restrictive ventilatory impairment, absolute values for FEV_1 are often reduced as well, and forced expiratory flow measurements may fall below the normal range. However, flows will be reduced only in propor-

TABLE 13–1.—OBSTRUCTIVE VS. RESTRICTIVE VENTILATORY ABNORMALITY

	VC	FEV_1	$100 \times FEV_1/VC$
Normal	Normal	Normal	Normal
Restrictive	Reduced	Normal or slightly reduced	Normal
Obstructive	Normal or slightly reduced	Reduced	Reduced

tion to the volume excursion, and the FEV_1/VC ratio should be normal unless there is complicating airways obstruction.

Some guidelines for differentiating obstructive and restrictive ventilatory abnormalities are given in Table 13–1. Ideal examples of obstructive and restrictive abnormalities are found in textbooks more often than in the clinical laboratory. Some reduction in VC is common when there is severe airways obstruction, the result of air trapping and an increase in RV. Mild reduction in forced expiratory flow is common when there is restriction of lung volume owing to incomplete expansion of the lung with loss of the earliest, most rapid portions of the forced expiration. In practice, the distinction between obstructive and restrictive ventilatory impairment is based on a disproportionate reduction in either forced expiratory flow rates or maximum volume excursion.

It should be noted that a reduction in VC with normal expiratory flow allows one to say only that a restrictive *ventilatory* abnormality exists. This should be distinguished from pulmonary restriction or so-called restrictive disease. To be accurate, in many laboratories the term "restrictive disease" is used only when both VC and TLC are reduced. When used this way, the term is synonymous with the "small lung pattern." It involves additional measurement of RV and therefore differs from restrictive *ventilatory* abnormality based on spirometric findings alone. In fact, the term "restrictive disease" is best avoided because it implies a diagnostic category, whereas in fact it simply indicates a type of functional change that occurs in many different lung diseases.

TABLE 13–2.—VENTILATORY ABNORMALITIES

Typically Obstructive (see chap. 27)
  Bronchial asthma
  Reversible obstructive bronchitis
  Chronic obstructive lung disease (emphysema-chronic bronchitis syndrome)
  Upper airways tumor or stenosis
  Mucoviscidosis
Mixed or variable
  Congestive heart failure
  Exposure to chemical irritants
  Coal workers' pneumoconiosis, silicosis, etc.
  Carcinoma involving a main bronchus
  Bronchiectasis
  Asthma, bronchitis, or emphysema complicating a restrictive disorder (especially tuberculosis and kyphoscoliosis)
  Noncommunicating bullae, lung fibrosis, or heart failure complicating an obstructive disorder
Typically restrictive
  Neuromuscular disease (see chap. 21)
  Chest wall diseases (see chap. 22)
  Pleural diseases (see chap. 23)
  Parenchymal lung diseases (see chaps. 24, 25)

Some disorders that typically produce obstructive, restrictive, and mixed ventilatory abnormalities are listed in Table 13–2. There is more overlap of findings than can be shown in Table 13–2, and mixed patterns may be encountered in most of the disorders listed as obstructive or restrictive. Except with syndromes defined in physiologic terms, we cannot exclude a diagnosis solely because of its failure to produce a supposedly typical pattern of ventilatory abnormality.

Testing for Obstructive Disorders

The pattern of airways obstruction discussed above and illustrated in Figure 13–1 is characteristic of the diffuse airways involvement of the asthma-obstructive bronchitis-emphysema type of disease. A disproportionate reduction in FEV_1 distinguishes this type of obstruction. Other measurements or tests may be employed to further physiologically characterize the disorder.

BRONCHIAL LABILITY

It is common practice to determine the reversible component of obstructive airways disease by spirometric testing before and after the administration of a bronchodilator aerosol. When diminished expiratory flows become normal after bronchodilator administration, one can state with confidence that the obstructive abnormality results from a form of reversible bronchospasm such as asthma. However, even in an acute attack of bronchial asthma, it is unusual to find immediate reversion to normal after one administration of a bronchodilator. Any significant response is meaningful. Failure of test results to revert to normal may indicate only an incomplete immediate response to one type of therapy at the time of testing. The airways obstruction may still show a gradual improvement over days, weeks, or even months. Airways obstruction should not be considered irreversible until abnormalities persist despite prolonged and intensive medical therapy. Results in a patient who showed a slow response to therapy are summarized in Table 13–3.

When a patient improves after bronchodilator use, both expiratory flow rates and VC increase. The increased volume excursion results from opening of previously occluded airways. The result may be a stable or even worsening $FEV_1/$ VC ratio and $FEF_{25\%-75\%}$ despite the obvious improvement in ventilatory function demonstrated by increase in the absolute values of the FEV_1 and VC. Improvement with bronchodilators should always be assessed from the change in absolute FEV_1 and VC and not by the change

TABLE 13–3.—EFFECT OF TREATMENT ON THE COURSE OF PULMONARY FUNCTION TESTS IN A
PATIENT WITH REVERSIBLE AIRWAYS OBSTRUCTION

	INITIAL TESTS				
	Before Isoproterenol	After Isoproterenol	10 Days	3 Mos	12 Mos
VC (as % predicted)	67.0	72.0	101.0	108.0	110.0
FEV_1 (L)	1.0	1.3	1.5	2.4	3.0
FEV_1/VC (as %)	38.0	47.0	38.0	58.0	70.0
$FEF_{25\%-75\%}$ (as L/sec)	0.4	0.4	0.8	1.3	2.5
MVV* (as % predicted)	33.0	35.0	73.0	93.0	118.0

*MVV = maximum voluntary ventilation.

in the FEV_1/VC ratio alone. (Ideally, flow rates should be compared at identical lung volumes before and after treatment, as is done with an "isovolume" $FEF_{25\%-75\%}$ or with carefully analyzed flow-volume curves.)

In some instances, the FEV_1 may fall within the range of normal before the administration of bronchodilator and then show a significant increase afterward. Such a result is highly suggestive of a very mild form of bronchospasm.

Spirometry is also used to test for bronchial reactivity to a challenge. Many patients with asthma report that exercise may bring on an attack. This can be verified in the laboratory by repeating spirometric measurements following vigorous exercise. Often ventilatory function may appear to improve immediately on cessation of exercise, but subsequent deterioration over a matter of minutes is confirmatory of exercise-induced bronchospasm. In some laboratories, inhalation of frigid air has been used as an airway challenge.

In other cases, one may wish to determine whether a patient has abnormally reactive airways and would be more likely to respond adversely to something in the environment. Patients with airway hyperreactivity will respond more readily than normal subjects to low doses of an aerosolized bronchoconstrictor agent such as methacholine or histamine. Serial spirometric testing with sequential administration of increasing concentrations of the challenge drug can be used to assess airway sensitivity. Under special circumstances, specific environmental or industrial irritants or antigenic substances have been used in a similar fashion in bronchial challenge

studies when it is important to determine the exact cause of a patient's paroxysmal airways obstruction.

In some persons with very reactive airways, the performance of the FVC maneuver may itself induce bronchospasm. In the attempt to obtain reproducible results by repeated testing, the FEV_1 may be observed to fall with successive maneuvers. Such results are quite significant and should not be discarded because they appear inconsistent.

EMPHYSEMATOUS VS. BRONCHIAL TYPE OF OBSTRUCTION

Slowing of forced expiratory flow may be the result of primary intrinsic airways disease or secondary to the loss of lung elastic recoil characteristic of emphysema. Intrapulmonary airways are embedded in lung parenchyma and depend on parenchymal recoil for their external support. With loss of lung recoil, therefore, not only is the pertinent driving pressure producing maximum expiratory flow decreased, but the caliber of the airways is also diminished. Although one might like to distinguish primary airways dysfunction from an emphysematous disorder, rarely does one find chronic irreversible airways obstruction of the "pure" emphysematous type. Once diseases of specific etiology, such as pneumoconioses, have been excluded, most patients with chronic ventilatory impairments will be found to have varying degrees of chronic bronchitis or emphysema. The most one can expect from lung function tests is to try to quantify the severity of emphysema or bronchial disease rather than to distinguish one from the other. Thus, when one has detected the presence of significant airways obstruction from spirometric testing, other tests may be indicated to characterize the disorders further.

Measurements of airway resistance during quiet breathing reflect primarily the function of the more central airways. When used in bronchial challenge studies, such measurements are often sensitive indicators of airway reactivity. It is not uncommon, however, to find patients whose measurements of resistance appear normal in the presence of an abnormal FEV_1. In such cases, one can assume that the airway dysfunction resides in more peripheral airways. An increase in resistance or, conversely, a decreased specific conductance, is suggestive of intrinsic airway disease.

Persistent loss of lung elastic recoil is considered to be the physiologic hallmark of emphysema. Such measurements are not available in most laboratories, however, and when available, they may detect only marked abnormality. The shape factor derived from exponential analysis of pressure-volume data has proved valuable in this context, but has yet to be proved useful in other than research studies.

Insofar as the diffusing capacity is affected by ventilation-perfusion relationships, some abnormality may be observed in the presence of intrinsic airways disease. In emphysema, however, a decrease in diffusing capacity accompanies the enlargement of airspaces, alveolar destruction, and loss of gas-exchanging surface area characteristic of the disease. Thus, the degree of abnormality of diffusing capacity correlates reasonably well with the amount of emphysema. Because hyperinflation with an increase in TLC is a feature of emphysema, expressing the results as diffusing capacity per liter of lung volume enhances the sensitivity of the test.

Although additional lung function tests help further to characterize an obstructive disorder in terms of its parenchymal and airway components, the results of such tests only provide approximations and should not be viewed as precise. They only augment clinical and roentgenographic data.

OCCLUSIVE OBSTRUCTION

Although most airway obstructive disorders are diffuse and characterized by expiratory slowing, total or partial occlusion of large airways may occur, presenting a different pattern of dysfunction. Measurements other than spirometry alone may be helpful in such cases.

With complete obstruction of a major bronchus, atelectasis results. If the lung is otherwise normal, the ventilatory abnormality will be restrictive rather than obstructive. But an incomplete obstruction may produce a check-valve effect, with overdistention of the involved portion of the lung. If a major airway is affected, the physiologic abnormalities may resemble those seen in the emphysema-bronchitis syndrome. A localized wheeze or unilateral hyperinflation on chest roentgenogram often provides a clue to the diagnosis, which must then be confirmed by bronchoscopy or bronchography. Ventilation scans can also reveal the localized nature of the airways abnormality.

When a smaller airway is involved or when there is a less high-grade obstruction, there may be little effect on either expiratory flow rates or volume excursion. Hypoxemia owing to shunting of blood through the obstructed area and abnormal inert gas distribution may be noted.

UPPER OR CENTRAL AIRWAY OBSTRUCTION

As noted in chapter 26, obstruction to airways above the carina may mimic diffuse obstructive airways disease, although such obstructions are often long unrecognized. Measurements of arterial blood gases, diffusing capacity, and inert gas distribution are usually normal. Even when ventilatory impairment is present, the abnormalities are often difficult to discern from the volume-time spirogram. The maximum voluntary ventilation, which requires both inspiratory and expiratory effort and adequate flows in both directions, is usually reduced.

Although heretofore we have dealt primarily with measurements derived from the forced expiratory vital capacity maneuver, abnormalities

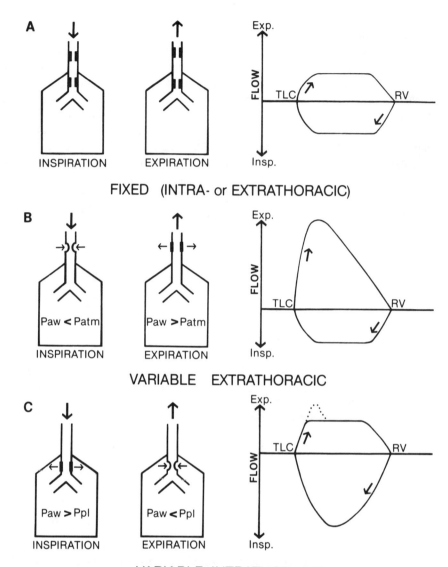

Fig 13–2.—Supracarinal upper airways obstruction may produce characteristic flow-volume abnormalities depending on the type and site of obstruction. **A,** if the obstruction is fixed, both inspiratory and expiratory flows will be decreased whether the obstruction is intrathoracic or extrathoracic (for purposes of illustration, obstruction is shown in both locations). **B,** when a variable obstruction is extra-thoracic in location, the airway narrows during inspiration when airway pressure is less than atmospheric and only inspiratory flow is diminished. **C,** when a variable obstruction is intrathoracic in location, airway pressure is less than pleural pressure during expiration, and only expiratory flow is diminished.

resulting from obstruction to upper airways are most clearly demonstrated by examining complete inspiratory and expiratory flow-volume loops. One of three principal patterns of abnormality may be revealed by the flow-volume loop, the pattern depending on the characteristic and location of the obstructing lesion. These patterns are illustrated in Figure 13–2.

When the airway obstruction is "fixed," the cross-sectional area at the point of obstruction will not change in response to changing transmural pressure. Under such circumstances, both inspiratory and expiratory flows are reduced, much as if a flow-limiting orifice were inserted in the airway, as shown in Figure 13–2,A. This bidirectional reduction in flow occurs whether the site of obstruction is intrathoracic or extrathoracic.

When the airway cross-sectional area at the point of the obstruction can change in response to transmural pressure changes, however, the obstruction is considered variable, and one of two flow-volume patterns is possible, depending on whether the site of obstruction is extrathoracic (Fig 13–2,B) or intrathoracic (Fig 13–2,C). The influence of transmural pressure on the obstruction is also illustrated in Figure 13–2. When the site of obstruction is in extrathoracic airways, during inspiration the pressure within the airway will be negative with respect to the exterior atmospheric pressure, the airway will further narrow, and inspiratory flow will be diminished. During expiration, however, the pressure within the airway will be positive with respect to atmospheric pressure, and the airway will tend to dilate, permitting near-normal expiratory flow. These relationships are reversed when the site of obstruction is in intrathoracic airways. In the latter case, during inspiration, the pressure within the airways will be positive with respect to the negative pleural pressure outside the airways. Airways would tend to dilate during inspiration but then narrow during expiration, when pleural pressure becomes positive. As a consequence, expiratory flow but not inspiratory flow would be reduced.

Whereas flow-volume loops provide a useful physiologic classification of supracarinal obstruction, final determination of the site and nature of the obstructing lesion can be made endoscopically.

PERIPHERAL AIRWAYS DYSFUNCTION

When an obstructive disorder is confined to very peripheral airways, the dysfunction is often difficult to detect. Because disabling chronic obstructive airways disease has been thought to have its origins in these small airways, there has been interest in detecting abnormality at the level of these airways. For purposes of definition, small airways are those 2 mm or less in diameter. Abnormalities in tests purported to detect dysfunction in peripheral airways have been said to characterize "small airways disease." Unfortunately, the term "small airways disease" is unwarranted in that, while used to describe results of tests, it implies a diagnostic category.

Even a moderate degree of obstruction in peripheral airways may have little effect on common spirometric measurements of flow, such as FEV_1. Inasmuch as the total cross-sectional area of peripheral airways is much greater than the summed cross-sectional area of the larger central airways, peripheral airways contribute a very small percentage of the total resistance to airflow. Consequently, a doubling in resistance to flow through a significant proportion of small peripheral airways would have an undetectable effect on total airway resistance. The problem, therefore, is one of detecting the presence of peripheral airway abnormality when standard spirometric measurements appear normal.

FREQUENCY DEPENDENCE OF DYNAMIC COMPLIANCES.—If flow through a given airway is slowed, the lung units served by that airway would respond less quickly by changing volume in response to a change in pressure. When a significant number of airways are thus affected, it will appear that the overall pressure-volume response of the lung will diminish with increasing frequency of breathing, the phenomenon of frequency dependence of dynamic compliance. Based on this principle, the observation of frequency dependent compliance has been attributed to narrowing of small peripheral airways. However, measurements of dynamic compliance at different breathing frequencies are technically difficult, causing some discomfort and requiring considerable subject cooperation. Such measurements are generally confined to research laboratories and very seldom performed in the clinical pulmonary laboratory.

DIMINISHED $\dot{V}max_{75\%}$.—As described in chapter 6, during forced expiration, $\dot{V}$max is determined largely by the resistance of airways upstream of points at which lateral airway pressure is equal to pleural pressure, the equal pressure points (EPP). In a normal subject, during the first 70%–75% of the maneuver, the EPP are located in central airways, but during expiration of the last 25% of the FVC, the EPP move alveolarward. Near the end of the maneuver, therefore, $\dot{V}$max is determined primarily by resistance of more peripheral airways and consequently should be diminished if there were obstruction in smaller airways. Based on these theoretical considerations, flow measurements near the end of the MEFV curve have been examined and "predicted normal" values determined for measurements such as $\dot{V}$max after 50% or 75% of the FVC has been expired ($\dot{V}$max$_{50\%}$ and $\dot{V}$max$_{75\%}$, respectively).

The clinical interpretation of a reduced $\dot{V}$max$_{75\%}$ in the presence of a normal FEV_1 and FEV_1/VC ratio is uncertain. The measurement itself requires that the subject has completely expired to residual volume. Though the flow may be effort-independent, complete expiration does require effort and determines the volume scale from which flow measurements are made. Values for $\dot{V}$max$_{75\%}$ exhibit great within-subject and between-subject variability, and the range of "normal" is quite large. Any disease causing a region of the lung to empty slowly would result in a reduced $\dot{V}$max$_{75\%}$. Thus, in interpreting the isolated occurrence of a reduced $\dot{V}$max$_{75\%}$ one should note it, but not attach clinical significance to it.

"CLOSING VOLUME".—During complete expiration, at low lung volumes, airway closure occurs, beginning in the most dependent regions of the lung. The lung volume at which closure begins to occur is thought to correspond with the beginning of the terminal rise in nitrogen concentration recorded during the single-breath nitrogen washout, or "closing volume," test described in chapter 10. There are data indicating that the airways that close are about 0.6 mm in diameter, the most peripheral of the conducting airways. It has been postulated that if an abnormality exists in small airways, closure will occur prematurely, and the closing volume will be greater than normal. Many smokers have been found to have increased closing volumes despite normal spirometric test results.

Several measurements can be derived from the single-breath nitrogen test (Fig 13–3). Whereas the closing volume, expressed as the CV/VC ratio, and the closing capacity, expressed as CC/TLC ratio, are presumably measurements related to airway closure, when applied to population studies, the slope of the phase III alveolar plateau was the most sensitive measurement in that it detected as abnormal a larger proportion of a subpopulation defined as

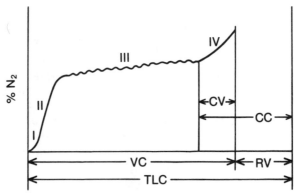

Fig 13–3.—Several measurements can be derived from the single-breath nitrogen test as expired volume is plotted against percent nitrogen; the "closing volume" (CV) expressed as CV/VC, the "closing capacity" (CC or the sum CV + RV), expressed as CC/TLC, or the slope of phase III, expressed as % N_2/L.

other than "normal." As we have noted in chapter 10, however, the slope of phase III is primarily an index of distribution, and many factors can influence it. Because many disease processes result in abnormal distribution of function, it is perhaps not surprising that the slope of phase III is the most sensitive of the measurements derived from this test. Indeed, patients with obvious obstructive airways disease in whom maldistribution of function would be expected very often exhibit an increase in the nitrogen slope of phase III.

Nevertheless, the meaning of an abnormality detected by the single-breath nitrogen test, particularly in the absence of any other abnormality, is uncertain. There is poor concordance between measurements from this test and spirometric or MEFV measurements. Although the single-breath nitrogen test may reveal abnormalities in subjects with normal spiromtery, the opposite is also true. It is not at all certain that this test is specific for small airways dysfunction. Although the test has been employed in many studies, the clinical or prognostic significance of an abnormality detected only by this test is as yet unknown.

DENSITY-DEPENDENT $\dot{V}$max.—The various factors which determine or limit maximum expiratory flow were reviewed in chapter 6. In addition to these factors, which include driving pressures, airway geometry, and airway behavior, flow is also partly a function of the physical properties of the expired gas, i.e., gas density (ρ) and viscocity (μ). In an attempt to determine the site of airways obstruction within the tracheobronchial tree, MEFV curves have been compared breathing air and after breathing a mixture of 80% helium and 20% oxygen (HeO_2). Helium, and therefore the HeO_2 mixture, is considerably less dense but more viscous than air. As a consequence, the $\dot{V}$max breathing HeO_2 will differ from the $\dot{V}$max breathing air, the difference and the magnitude of the difference depending, in turn, on the flow patterns and airway geometry. It was postulated that a failure to increase $\dot{V}$max appropriately in the mid-VC after breathing HeO_2 was indicative of obstruction to flow in small peripheral airways.

When flows are measured at the same lung volume, it can be assumed that the driving pressure is the same regardless of the gas expired. According to the EPP concept, therefore, $\dot{V}$max is then determined by the resistance of airways upstream of the EPP. The test for density dependence of $\dot{V}$max was based on several assumptions; namely, that the EPP were in the same location breathing air and HeO_2 and that the flow patterns were also identical. Normally, in the mid-VC, the EPP are located in central airways. Under these circumstances, the upstream segment is, in effect, a summed conduit the cross-sectional area of which diminishes from terminal airways toward central airways (see Fig 13–5). A major portion of the pressure fall down this conduit represents the energy expended to accelerate gas molecules from the region of large total cross section to the central airways of smaller cross section. This convective accelerative resistance is dependent only on gas density and is independent of gas viscosity. Therefore, compared with air, one would observe a substantial increase in flow breathing the

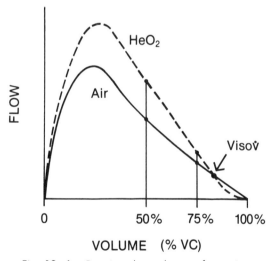

Fig 13–4.—Density dependence of maximum expiratory flow is measured by comparing the MEFV curve breathing air *(solid curve)* with that breathing 80% helium-20% oxygen *(dashed curve)*. Measurements include the increase in flow at 50% or 75% of the expired VC and the volume at which the two curves converge, the volume of isoflow (Viso$\dot{v}$).

less dense HeO_2 gas. At low lung volumes, however, the EPP move alveolarward, and the upstream airways, considered in terms of the summed cross-sectional area of sequential generations of branching, represent a conduit which narrows to a lesser degree down its length. In very peripheral airways where the total cross-sectional area is extremely large, flow velocities are very low, and it is presumed that pure laminar flow may occur. Laminar flow resistance is independent of gas density and depends only on gas viscosity. If upstream segment resistance is primarily laminar, or viscous, then one would observe a lesser increase in flow breathing HeO_2 and, indeed, flow may even be lower breathing the more viscous but less dense mixture. A com-

parison of air and HeO_2 MEFV curves in a normal subject is shown in Figure 13–4.

As we have noted, abnormality confined to small peripheral airways may be difficult to detect and have little effect on the MEFV curve breathing air. To preserve V̇max in the presence of peripheral airway obstruction, the upstream resistance must also be preserved. For this to occur, the upstream segment, it is reasoned, must be made shorter by a more peripheral location of the EPP to compensate for the peripheral airway abnormality as illustrated in Figure 13–5. It would follow that phenomena normally observed at low lung volumes would occur at higher lung volumes, convective accelerative resistance would be lower, and the increase in

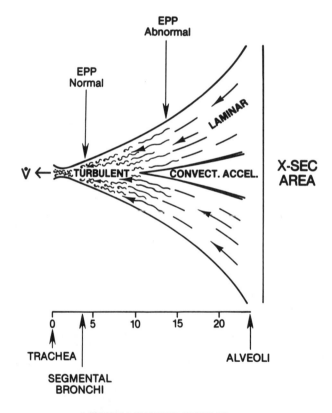

AIRWAY GENERATIONS

Fig 13–5.—The test of density dependence was based on the concept of flow patterns through airways when the airways are considered to be a summed conduit which narrows from alveoli to central airways. Normally, EPP are located in central airways and flow is determined by the sum of laminar flow resistance, turbulent flow resistance, and convective accelerative resistance down the upstream segment. If EPP are located peripherally, flow is determined primarily by laminar flow resistance, and convective acceleration is of less significance.

flow normally observed in the mid-VC would be diminished. Also the point at which the air and HeO_2 MEFV curves converge, the volume of isoflow, or Visov̇, would occur at a higher lung volume. Based on this reasoning, peripheral or small airway obstruction will be revealed by diminished response of increased flow breathing HeO_2. Measurements which have been made include the percent increase in flow (Δ V̇max) or HeO_2/air flow ratio at 50% or 75% of the expired vital capacity or the Visov̇ as a percent of VC.

Although the test for density dependence seems simple as described, its application is less simple. Comparison of V̇max values must be made at the same lung volume. Consequently, the volumes expired breathing the two gases must be identical. Measurements of V̇max from MEFV curves show within-subject and between-subject variability, a variability which is compounded when two V̇max values are compared. This variability further complicates the determination of the volume of isoflow, the precise point at which two converging curves actually cross.

When the test of density dependence of V̇max has been applied, the results have often been disappointing. It has not proved to be a "more sensitive" test and has been found to yield "normal" results in a large proportion of patients who have obstructive airways disease demonstrated spirometrically.

Because of disappointing results, the basis for the test has come under closer examination. The original concept on which the test of density dependence was based involved certain simplifying assumptions which may not be justified. There is evidence to suggest that the EPP may not be in the same location when breathing different gases. It was also assumed that the classic laws of fluid mechanics could be applied and that the flow regimens would be identical. The latter is particularly unlikely. The flow regimen is, in part, determined by the Reynolds number:

$$Re = \frac{\rho u d}{\mu}$$

where u = velocity and d = tube diameter. When flows are identical, and consequently u

and d are also identical, inasmuch as the density, ρ, and viscosity, μ, of the two gases are quite different, the Reynolds number and, hence, flow pattern would be quite different for the two gases. In a branched system, pure laminar flow, completely independent of density, is unlikely to exist. Gas density begins to assume an ever-increasing role in determining flow as the flow pattern becomes disturbed, and ultimately turbulent until convective accelerative resistance becomes dominant. No single flow regimen can describe the entire tracheobronchial tree. Rather, all regimens exist as a continuum throughout the tracheobronchial tree, density and viscosity contributing in varying degrees to pressure-flow relationships in the various airway generations.

In the description of flow limiting mechanisms in chapter 6, it was apparent in the equation for flow at wave speed

$$\dot{V}max = \left(\frac{1}{\rho}\right)^{0.5} \left(\frac{dPtm}{dA}\right)^{0.5} A^{1.5}$$

that flow would be greater if the gas was less dense. On this basis, knowing the density of air and HeO_2, one could predict difference in V̇max if the other factors in the equation were held constant. If the increase in V̇max breathing HeO_2 were anything other than predicted on the basis of density difference alone, it follows that the other factors, which describe airway properties, must be different for the two gases, and that therefore the choke point is not in the same location for both gases.

Tests purported to be specific for peripheral airways dysfunction have thus far proved disappointing. Although the tests discussed here may well reveal something abnormal, the significance of the abnormalities has yet to be demonstrated, and the usefulness of the tests themselves is uncertain. They do not have a role in the clinical pulmonary laboratory.

Testing for Restrictive Disorders

A restrictive disorder is one in which lung volumes are reduced for whatever reason. When the VC, measured during spirometry, is less than the lower limit of normal for one's age, a restrictive ventilatory disorder may be suspected. As noted earlier, some diminution of VC may occur in obstructive disorders as a result of air-trapping. Forced expiratory flows and FEV_1 may be less than predicted when lung volumes are reduced but, in the absence of obstruction, flows should be reduced in proportion to volume and the FEV_1/VC ratio should be normal. When spirometry reveals such a restrictive ventilatory disorder, additional tests will help further to characterize the disorder. Measurements of total lung capacity (TLC) and diffusing capacity (DL_{CO}) are usually indicated, providing useful adjuncts to clinical observations and roentgenographic data.

Several methods are available for the measurement of TLC. Plethysmographic methods are considered more accurate when there are airways obstruction and abnormal distribution of ventilation. In purely restrictive disorders, however, inert gas equilibration or washout techniques are quite satisfactory. Moreover, the nitrogen washout curves or helium equilibration times are usually quite normal and provide useful information.

The most obvious cause of a purely restrictive disorder is decrease in the amount of available lung tissue, as a result of either a congenital abnormality or, more commonly, surgical resection. The remaining lung will function normally, and overall function will be reduced only in proportion to lung volume. Other restrictive disorders may be divided into two categories, extrapulmonary or intrapulmonary.

EXTRAPULMONARY DISORDERS

Respiratory muscle weakness (discussed in chap. 21) or a stiff chest wall may limit the volume excusion during both inspiration and expiration. As a consequence, TLC will be reduced and the RV slightly elevated. In spite of the reduced VC, there is normal distribution of inspired gas and normal physiologic dead space. Because alveolar volume is reduced, the DL_{CO} may also be reduced, but it will be reduced in

proportion to lung volume and the DL_{CO}/L remains normal. Arterial blood gas values may remain normal, although in severe cases they may reflect alveolar hypoventilation.

A low pressure at the mouth during a maximum inspiratory or expiratory effort against a closed airway is an important finding in respiratory muscle weakness, helping to distinguish it from organic lung disease. Also, intrathoracic pressure (measured by esophageal balloon) fails to become markedly negative on full inspiration when the restrictive pattern results from chest wall disease. This is in contrast to the high pressures in patients with excessively stiff lungs. Differentiating organic muscle weakness from debility, poor cooperation, or malingering is more difficult. Fluoroscopic studies assist in diagnosis of diaphragmatic disorders, and severe generalized neuromuscular disorders are usually clinically obvious.

It seems logical to determine the elastic properties of the thoracic wall in order to distinguish muscle weakness from stiffness of the thoracic cage, but such studies are notoriously unreliable (especially in dyspneic patients) and are usually undertaken only in research laboratories.

More complex disorders are often observed associated with marked kyphoscoliosis or fibrothorax. In addition to reduction of TLC, VC, and RV, the disorder is complicated by nonuniform ventilation and ultimately by pulmonary hypertension. Here, physiologic abnormalities range from simple reduction of VC to severe respiratory insufficiency with alveolar underventilation and venous admixture. The picture may be further complicated if chronic or recurrent infections supervene, leading to superimposed bronchitis or localized fibrotic changes in the lung.

In summary, standard lung function tests suggest the possibility of chest wall disease or respiratory muscle weakness when, despite a restrictive ventilatory impairment, there is a normal distribution of inspired gas; normal physiologic dead space; a normal or near-normal diffusing capacity; somewhat elevated RV; and blood gases that are either normal or indicative only of hypoventilation, especially if the lung fields are radiologically normal. Mouth pressure and esophageal balloon studies may help to confirm the diagnosis. Severity of the physiologic derangement of function closely parallels the severity of the mechanical disorder.

INTRAPULMONARY DISORDERS

Diffuse interstitial lung disease alters the mechanical properties of the lung and can be characterized by a spectrum of pathophysiologic abnormalities. The interstitial parenchymal involvement renders the lung less compliant and should result in a change in the shape of the pressure-volume curve. Such changes, however, are often so subtle that even by exponential analysis of the curve it is difficult to distinguish the "stiff" lung from the normal. Moreover, though diffuse, the disease process is seldom if ever uniform. Abnormalities in lung function may range from relatively slight to severe, and there is quite often poor correlation between lung function and the roentgenographic extent of the disease process.

Typically, VC and RV are both reduced, producing an abnormally small TLC. For this reason, as noted previously, the term "restrictive disease" has been applied to this "small lung pattern" of abnormality. The diffusing capacity may be low but may only be reduced in proportion to the volume restriction with a normal $D_{L_{CO}}/L$ lung volume. Arterial carbon dioxide and oxygen tensions may be normal or low. Often blood gas abnormalities are not severe and, when hypoxemia is present, its pattern is that of a ventilation-perfusion imbalance (i.e., low resting Pa_{O_2}, variable fall in Pa_{O_2} with exertion and incomplete correction with 28% oxygen as discussed in chapter 15).

When little but volume restriction is observed, the pattern of abnormality is not distinctive. It may occur in any extensive disease of the lung not associated with airways obstruction, air trapping, emphysema, or bullae. The pattern also is seen after extensive pulmonary resection and sometimes early in the course of diffuse pa-

renchymal disease. A complete list of causes would encompass most of the parenchymal, interstitial, or infiltrative lung disease, including those involving the lung in a localized or patchy manner. The pattern is found most notably in sarcoidosis, pneumoconiosis, extensive primary or secondary neoplasm, disseminated acute and chronic lung infection, postinflammatory fibrosis, and in some cases of congestive heart failure.

In its more severe and distinctive form, interstitial lung disease is often accompanied by ventilation-perfusion imbalance, impaired diffusing capacity, chronic hypocapnia, and hypoxemia. The combination of these physiologic abnormalities with interstitial parenchymal disease has led to the coining of the term "alveolar-capillary block syndrome." In the fully developed form of this syndrome, lung function tests reveal the following pattern:

1. Ventilatory tests that are normal or restrictive in type.

2. Marked reduction in pulmonary diffusing capacity, with a greater decrease of diffusing capacity than of VC or TLC (a low diffusing capacity/lung volume ratio).

3. Comparable degree of reduction in RV and VC; TLC normal or small; RV/TLC ratio normal or only slightly elevated.

4. Alveolar hyperventilation, or at least the absence of hypoventilation (i.e., Pa_{CO_2} normal or low).

5. Arterial hypoxemia that is mild at rest but increases markedly with exertion and is almost fully corrected by small increments in inspired P_{O_2} (e.g., 28% oxygen or 2 L/min by nasal catheter). This pattern of hypoxemia, typical of a diffusion defect, is the most characteristic feature of the syndrome.

The term "alveolar-capillary block" has been applied to this pattern because the results are those one might expect if there was a physical barrier to transfer of oxygen (or carbon monoxide in the measurement of $D_{L_{CO}}$) from the alveolus to the alveolar capillary due to thickening of the alveolar wall. While conceptually useful, the term itself may be a misnomer. Within the wall separating two alveolar spaces, the capillary endothelium and alveolar epithelium of one of the alveoli are closely applied; interstitial thickening may further separate the capillary only from the other alveolus. Actual limitation to gas diffusion probably contributes little to the blood gas abnormality or reduced DL_{CO}, whereas a reduction in the number of functioning alveoli or increased ventilation-perfusion inequalities secondary to altered mechanics serve to explain most of the derangement in function. A ventilatory-perfusion imbalance is generally present and may be the most important cause of arterial oxygen unsaturation, especially in later stages of disease. In any case, the concept of alveolar-capillary block is useful in delineating a pattern of physiologic abnormalities generally associated with diffuse interstitial lung disease. Such diseases and their classification are considered in chapter 25.

Although we may try to describe restrictive disorders according to the above categories, physiologic abnormalities that accompany a restrictive ventilatory abnormality are quite variable, and there is no pattern that can be regarded as pathognomonic for a specific disease. Many cases of restrictive disorders encountered in the clinical laboratory do not fulfill the criteria for either the "small lung pattern" or the "alveolar-capillary block syndrome." These show a nonspecific reduction of VC accompanied by a normal or slightly elevated RV, a high RV/TLC ratio, a normal or only slightly reduced diffusing capacity, and blood gases which are either within the normal range or indicative of a mild ventilation-perfusion imbalance. Physiologic tests usually do not allow further differential diagnosis of this nondescript restrictive impairment, which can result from debility secondary to any chronic illness or from a great variety of lung diseases, both localized and diffuse.

Lung Function Abnormalities with Normal Spirometry

Although most disorders of respiratory function are accompanied by abnormalities in ordinary spirometric tests, some physiologic alterations occur without apparent ventilatory dysfunction.

ARTERIAL BLOOD GAS ABNORMALITIES

There are many nonrespiratory causes of arterial hypoxemia, many of which are discussed in chapter 29. Anatomical vascular abnormalities (e.g., pulmonary AV fistulas and congenital heart diseases) may produce severe hypoxemia in the absence of ventilatory abnormalities. Right-to-left shunting also is found in hepatic disease and rarely with a localized pulmonary abnormality too small to affect materially other aspects of lung function.

Disorders of ventilatory drive may lead to underventilation of alveoli and hypercapnia without associated spirometric abnormalities. This suggests a primary insensitivity of the respiratory center or a depression of ventilatory drive owing to drug intoxication or a CNS disease.

DIFFUSING CAPACITY ABNORMALITIES

Although a restrictive pattern is usually a feature of interstitial lung disease, the ventilatory defect may be small enough that spirometric studies will be considered normal. Nevertheless, a decreased diffusing capacity may still be present.

The diffusing capacity may be reduced when anemia is present. Hemoglobin concentration should be taken into account before interpreting any reduction of the diffusing capacity.

Conversely, erythrocytosis or increased pulmonary blood flow may cause an abnormally high diffusing capacity. This is occasionally observed in congenital heart disease and early congestive heart failure.

ABNORMAL GAS DISTRIBUTION

Bullae, even of considerable size, may not impair spirometric tests if there is no associated diffuse lung disease. If they communicate with the bronchial system, such bullae can lead to abnormalities of inert gas distribution and elevation of RV. The same findings may occur in a localized incomplete airways obstruction below the carina.

READING LIST

Kryger M., Bode F., Antic R., et al.: Diagnosis of obstruction of the upper and central airways. *Am. J. Med.* 61:85–93, 1976.

Miller R.D., Hyatt R.E.: Obstructing lesions of the larynx and trachea: clinical and physiologic characteristics. *Mayo Clin. Proc.* 44:145–161, 1969.

Miller R.D., Hyatt R.E.: Evaluation of obstructing lesions of the trachea and larynx by flow-volume loops. *Am. Rev. Respir. Dis.* 108:475–481, 1973.

Upper or central airway obstruction is comprehensively discussed in these articles.

Woolcock A.J., Vincent N.J., Macklem P.T.: Frequency dependence of compliance as a test for obstruction in the small airways. *J. Clin. Invest.* 48:1097–1106, 1969.

The basis for frequency dependence of dynamic compliance as a test for peripheral airways dysfunction is described in this article.

Knudson R.J., Burrows B., Lebowitz M.D.: The maximal expiratory flow-volume curve: its use in the detection of ventilatory abnormalities in a population study. *Am. Rev. Respir. Dis.* 114:871–879, 1976.

Sensitivity of diminished $\dot{V}max_{75\%}$ is discussed in this article.

Buist A.S., Ross B.B.: Predicted values for closing volumes using a modified single breath nitrogen test. *Am. Rev. Respir. Dis.* 107:744, 1973.

Buist A.S.: Early detection of airways obstruction by the closing volume technique. *Chest* 64:495, 1973.

Buist A.S.: The single-breath nitrogen test. *N. Engl. J. Med.* 293:438, 1975.

Dollfuss R.E., Milic-Emili J., Bates D.V.: Regional ventilation of the lung, studied with boluses of 133-xenon. *Respir. Physiol.* 2:234, 1967.

Holland J., Milic-Emili J., Macklem P.T., et al.: Regional distribution of pulmonary ventilation and perfusion in elderly subjects. *J. Clin. Invest.* 47:81, 1968.

Knudson R.J., Lebowitz M.D., Burton A.P., et al.: The closing volume test: evaluation of nitrogen and bolus methods in a random population. *Am. Rev. Respir. Dis.* 115:423–434, 1977.

Knudson R.J., Lebowitz M.D.: Comparison of flow-volume and closing volume variables in a random population. *Am. Rev. Respir. Dis.* 115:423–434, 1977.

McCarthy D.S., Spencer R., Greene R., et al.: Measurement of "closing volume" as a simple and sensitive test for early detection of small airway disease. *Am. J. Med.* 52:747, 1972.

Although a great many papers have been published on the "closing volume" test, the preceding are a few useful references on this subject.

Despas P.J., Leroux M., Macklem P.T.: Site of airway obstruction in asthma as determined by measuring maximal expiratory flow breathing air and a helium-oxygen mixture. *J. Clin. Invest.* 51:3235–3243, 1972.

Dosman J., Bode F., Urbanetti J., et al.: The use of a helium-oxygen mixture during maximum expiratory flow to demonstrate obstruction in small airways in smokers. *J. Clin. Invest.* 55:1090–1099, 1975.

Knudson R.J.: Detection of early airways dysfunction, in Loeppky J.A., Riedesel M.L. (eds.): *Oxygen Transport to Human Tissue.* Proceedings of Luft Symposium held on June 25–27, 1981, Albuquerque, New Mexico. New York, Elsevier North-Holland, Inc., Publishers, 1982, pp. 319–333.

Meadows J.A. III, Rodarte J.R., Hyatt R.E.: Density dependence of maximal expiratory flow in chronic obstructive pulmonary disease. *Am. Rev. Respir. Dis.* 121:47–53, 1980.

Mink S., Ziesmann M., Wood L.D.H.: Mechanisms of increased maximum expiratory flow during HeO_2 breathing in dogs. *J. Appl. Physiol.* 47:490–502, 1979.

Mink S.N., Wood L.D.H.: How does HeO_2 increase maximum expiratory flow in human lungs? *J. Clin. Invest.* 66:720–729, 1980.

The use of density dependence of $\dot{V}max$ as a test for early or peripheral airways dysfunction is controversial. Several views are expressed in these articles.

Forster R.E.: Exchange of gases between alveolar air and pulmonary capillary blood: pulmonary diffusing capacity. *Physiol. Rev.* 37:391–452, 1957.

Ogilvie C.M., Forster R.E., Blakemore W.S., et al.: A standardized breath holding technique for the clinical measurement of the diffusing capacity of the lung for carbon monoxide. *J. Clin. Invest.* 36:1–17, 1957.

The measurement of diffusing capacity of the lung has a long history, and many articles have been written on the subject. Therefore, only two classic references are listed, the first of which is an early comprehensive review of the subject.

14

Hypercapnia and Respiratory Acid-Base Abnormalities

Detection of Hypercapnia

WITH MARKED AND RAPID increases in Pa_{CO_2}, the patient may experience headache, somnolence, tremor, or altered mentation. Asterixis is sometimes noted. But clinical symptoms and signs are unreliable, and early diagnosis and evaluation of hypercapnia depend on arterial blood gas analysis with measurements of both pH and Pa_{CO_2}. Arterial blood gases should be measured promptly on exacerbation of symptoms of severe chronic lung disease. Measurements of venous carbon dioxide content or combining power are of little use in determining if there is acute carbon dioxide retention. Normal limits for Pa_{CO_2} range from 34 to 45 torr, at least for altitudes up to 4,000 ft. At higher altitudes, values tend to be slightly lower.

Mechanisms and Differential Diagnosis of Hypercapnia

The determinants of Pa_{CO_2} are easily discussed if we make the following assumptions: (1) under steady-state conditions, all metabolically produced carbon dioxide ($\dot{V}_{CO_2}$) is eliminated through the lung, and (2) there is complete equilibration of carbon dioxide between blood and gas in functioning or "effective" alveoli (effA), insuring that the carbon dioxide tension of blood leaving the lung and reaching peripheral arteries (Pa_{CO_2}) equals the carbon dioxide tension of these effective alveoli ($Peff_{A_{CO_2}}$). According to the first assumption, $\dot{V}_{CO_2}$ equals the fractional concentration of carbon dioxide in effective alveoli times the minute ventilation of these alveoli ($\dot{V}effA$). The fractional concentration of carbon dioxide in these alveoli is the $Peff_{A_{CO_2}}$ divided by the barometric pressure (P_B). Therefore,

$$\dot{V}_{CO_2} = \dot{V}effA \times Peff_{A_{CO_2}}/P_B$$

Since the second assumption indicates that Pa_{CO_2} equals $Peff_{A_{CO_2}}$,

$$\dot{V}_{CO_2} = \dot{V}effA \times Pa_{CO_2}/P_B$$

By rearranging this equation, the determinants of the arterial CO_2 tension (Pa_{CO_2}) are evident:

$$Pa_{CO_2} = P_B \times \dot{V}_{CO_2}/\dot{V}effA_{CO_2}$$

Thus, the Pa_{CO_2} is directly proportional to the carbon dioxide produced by the body and inversely proportional to the effective alveolar ventilation. Since P_B is a constant, no other factors enter into consideration. For Pa_{CO_2} to remain constant, $\dot{V}effA$ must increase or decrease in proportion to the metabolically produced carbon dioxide, at least under steady state conditions. Hypercapnia results when $\dot{V}effA$ is too low for the metabolic conditions. If $\dot{V}effA$ is fixed, the level of Pa_{CO_2} is a function of the $\dot{V}_{CO_2}$.

What factors determine $\dot{V}$effA? Obviously, $\dot{V}$effA must be related to the overall minute ventilation. *The lower the minute ventilation, the higher the* Pa_{CO_2}, *if all other factors are equal.* But not all of the minute ventilation reaches functioning alveoli. Some is wasted on the anatomical dead space. With each breath, approximately 150 ml of fresh air (depending on body size) is required to flush out the upper airway. The anatomical dead space ventilation therefore depends on the respiratory rate. It equals the volume of the upper airways times respiratory frequency. With a minute ventilation of 6 L and an anatomical dead space of 150 ml, the effective alveolar ventilation cannot exceed 1.5 L at a respiratory rate of 30 per minute, but it might be as high as 4.5 L if the respiratory rate were 10 per minute. Thus, *at the same minute ventilation, the more rapid the ventilation, the lower the* $\dot{V}$effA *and the higher the* Pa_{CO_2}. An increase in respiratory rate must be accompanied by an increase in minute ventilation if the Pa_{CO_2} is to be held constant.

One additional factor enters into the determination of $\dot{V}$effA. Some alveoli are well ventilated but poorly perfused with blood. That is, they have a high ventilation/perfusion ($\dot{V}A/\dot{Q}$) ratio. The ventilation to such alveoli is largely wasted. Despite their high ventilation, little carbon dioxide exchange can occur. Carbon dioxide exchange is also limited in alveoli with low $\dot{V}/\dot{Q}$ ratios. Blood perfusing such underventilated alveoli is inadequately cleared of carbon dioxide. The total defect in carbon dioxide excretion resulting from $\dot{V}A/\dot{Q}$ inequalities may be expressed in terms of an alveolar dead space ventilation. A small amount of alveolar dead space ventilation occurs at the apices of normal lungs, where perfusion is more limited than ventilation. The effect is much more important in diseased lungs in which localized perfusion abnormalities are present. Though it occurs in almost all types of pulmonary diseases, the mechanism is most obvious in pulmonary embolism where the perfusion of a portion of the lung is blocked. Any ventilation to the affected area will be wasted in terms of carbon dioxide exchange. Thus, *if all other factors are equal, the greater the alveolar dead space ventilation, the lower the* $\dot{V}$effA *and the higher the* Pa_{CO_2}.

In summary, the determinants of Pa_{CO_2} include: (1) carbon dioxide production, (2) minute ventilation, (3) anatomical dead space ventilation, and (4) alveolar dead space ventilation. (The combination of anatomical and alveolar dead space has been called the physiologic dead space, but it is preferable to separate them when considering the determinants of hypercapnia.) The differential diagnosis of hypercapnia may be considered under the above headings.

Carbon dioxide production may be increased by exercise, high work of breathing, a systemic infection, or even by anxiety. An increase in $\dot{V}_{CO_2}$ will result in hypercapnia if there is no concomitant increase in minute ventilation.

Minute ventilation depends on the balance between ventilatory drive and the ability of the respiratory apparatus to respond to that drive. An individual's respiratory drive is a function of the inherent sensitivity of his respiratory center but may be reduced by certain drugs (especially sedatives and narcotics), by alkalosis, or by excessive oxygen tensions. The hypoxic stimulus of altitude increases the drive to breathe. Thus, normal Pa_{CO_2}'s tend to be somewhat lower at high altitude than the normal sea level range of 34–45 torr.

The ability of the respiratory apparatus to respond depends on several factors. Neuromuscular disorders (e.g., myasthenia gravis, Guillain-Barré syndrome, and bulbar poliomyelitis) may lead to hypercapnia if the respiratory muscles become involved. Even without a frank neurologic disease, respiratory muscle function may be affected by fatigue. Thus, after struggling for a prolonged period to maintain an adequate minute ventilation, a patient in status asthmaticus may ultimately begin to underventilate. Pain on respiration may lead the patient to limit his breathing voluntarily. Muscle splinting or spasm accompanying pleurisy or rib fracture or discomfort following thoracic or upper abdominal surgery may contribute to diminished ventilation as well as lead to other complications. Finally, the ability of the respiratory system to respond to increased drive depends on the inherent mechanical properties of the lungs and chest wall themselves. Although any severe thoracic disease may lead to hypoventilation, restrictive disorders are much less likely to limit total minute ventilation than are obstructive abnormalities.

Ventilation of the conducting airways constitutes *anatomical dead space ventilation*. In modern medical practice it is not uncommon for an external dead space to be added inadvertently, thereby aggravating hypercapnia. The added dead space may be in the form of a face mask that is not continuously flushed with fresh air, a respiratory valve with a large internal dead space, or a tube connecting the patient with a respiratory valve. When tracheostomy or endotracheal intubation is done in an attempt to reduce anatomical dead space (a procedure of dubious value), the apparatus attached to the patient may have a larger dead space than the upper airway.

Many factors may contribute to increased respiratory frequency, thereby increasing anatomical dead space ventilation per minute. Anxiety, stiffening of the lung (as with pulmonary vascular congestion, atelectasis, or pneumonia), and chest wall pain all may lead to a rapid, shallow breathing pattern.

Increased *alveolar dead space ventilation* may result from almost any disorder of the lung parenchyma that leads to increased nonuniformity of ventilation/perfusion ratios. If overall ventilation is not limited, this can be compensated by an increased minute volume. But increased dead space ventilation is apt to lead to increased Pa_{CO_2} if the patient has a limited ventilatory capacity, as in severe airways obstruction.

In evaluating hypercapnia, the physician should consider the possible contributions of all of the factors mentioned above. Failure to deal with all of them may lead to ineffective management. For example, the Pa_{CO_2} of a patient with severe airways obstruction in exacerbation may be related in large part to anxiety with excessive tachypnea and an unnecessarily elevated metabolic rate. Simple reassurance may help a great deal in controlling hypercapnia while measures designed to improve lung function are being instituted.

Effects of Hypercapnia

An elevation of Pa_{CO_2} must be accompanied by a decrease in Pa_{O_2}. In a patient with a normal lung at sea level, dangerous hypoxemia does not result until the Pa_{CO_2} reaches quite high levels (over 75 torr). But if the patient is already hypoxemic as a result of physiologic shunting from an associated lung disease, even a slight increase in Pa_{CO_2} and a fall in Pa_{O_2} may result in a dangerous level of hypoxemia. The amount of fall in Pa_{O_2} accompanying an increase in Pa_{CO_2} is discussed in chapter 15.

Acid-base changes also accompany hypercapnia. An acute increase in Pa_{CO_2} results in a predictable decrease in arterial pH, the blood being an imperfect buffer. With persistence of hypercapnia, renal retention of bicarbonate and amelioration of the pH change occur. The usual pH changes in acute and chronic hypercapnia are shown in Figure 14–1. This figure has proved of great value in interpretation of pH changes that develop in the course of an episode of carbon dioxide retention. It allows differentiation of acute from chronic hypercapnia on the basis of the observed pH abnormality. It also indicates the amount of pH compensation generally achieved with varying degrees of carbon dioxide retention. With severe hypercapnia, renal mechanisms are incapable of maintaining the pH within normal range. Finally, Figure 14–1 indicates the degree of respiratory compensation (alteration in Pa_{CO_2}) that can be expected in metabolic acidosis and alkalosis.

Development of acidosis secondary to hypercapnia (respiratory acidosis) is associated with a shift of potassium out of the cells, resulting in increased renal excretion and depletion of body K^+ despite relatively normal or even high serum K^+ levels. With correction of acidosis, potassium reenters the cells, and low serum levels result unless exogenous K^+ is provided. Thus, hypokalemia is likely to develop during the recovery phase from acute hypercapnia.

Respiratory acidosis appears to potentiate the hypertensive effect of hypoxemia on the pulmonary circulation. It may also contribute to CNS symptoms. Certainly, headache, tremor, aste-

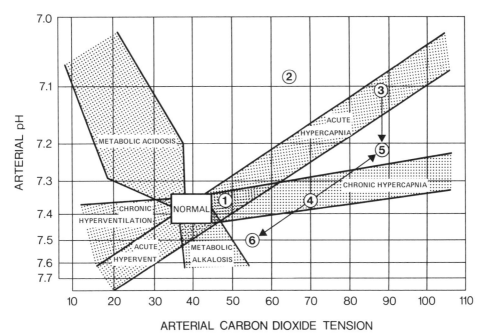

Fig 14–1.—Blood gas interpretation. Graph presenting a summary of reported data from patients with the various acid-base disturbances noted. In a patient with metabolic defects, the graph indicates the expected degree of respiratory compensation (Pa_{CO_2} change from increase or decrease in ventilation). In a patient with ventilatory problems, it shows the expected range of pH response to changes in Pa_{CO_2}. The six points indicated on the graph exemplify possible values in a hypercapneic subject: **(1)** Mild hypercapnia. In this range acute cannot be distinguished from chronic carbon dioxide retention unless the patient's usual Pa_{CO_2} is known. **(2)** A combination of hypercapnia and metabolic acidosis. Often noted in severe acute ventilatory failure as a result of lactic acidosis from severe hypoxemia. **(3)** Acute respiratory acidosis. Seen with rapid development of underventilation in a patient with a previously normal Pa_{CO_2}. **(4)** Chronic carbon dioxide retention. Fully compensated chronic hypoventilation may be noted persis-

tently in patients with severe chronic lung disease or may be seen after a day or two in patients with acute ventilatory failure. **(5)** A mixture of acute and chronic hypercapnia. This may indicate partial compensation of acute hypercapnia (see *arrow* from point *3*) or acute worsening of chronic hypercapnia (see *arrow* from point *4*). **(6)** A combination of metabolic alkalosis and hypercapnia of respiratory origin. This may result from too rapid correction of chronic hypercapnia by an artificial respirator (see *arrow* from point *4*). In this case, the bicarbonate retained to compensate for the more severe hypercapnia is now metabolically inappropriate, resulting in metabolic alkalosis. Also, a value of this type commonly occurs from potassium chloride deficiency complicating improving ventilatory failure. Note that the slopes of the arrows connecting points *4, 5,* and *6* follow the slope of the acute hypercapnia band. Abrupt changes in Pa_{CO_2} result in pH changes along this slope regardless of the starting point on the graph.

rixis, somnolence, and even coma are common in this clinical situation. But these signs and symptoms appear to relate more closely to the hypoxemia, rapidity of change in the Pa_{CO_2}, and acidosis that accompany hypercapnia than they do to the Pa_{CO_2} level itself.

READING LIST

McCurdy D.K.: Mixed metabolic and respiratory acid-base disturbances: diagnosis and treatment. *Chest* 62 (suppl.):35–43, 1972.

A good overall discussion of the interpretation of acid-base disturbances.

Rastegar A., Thier S.O.: Physiologic consequences

and bodily adaptations to hyper- and hypocapnia. *Chest* 62 (Suppl.):28–34, 1972.

A good discussion of the body's compensation for changes in Pa_{CO_2}.

Schwartz W.B., Relman A.S.: A critique of the pa-rameters used in the evaluation of acid-base disorders. *N. Engl. J. Med.* 268:1382–1388, 1963.

This article clearly describes the difference between in vitro and in vivo interrelationships of pH, Pa_{CO_2}, and HCO_3^-.

15

Hypoxemia and Erythrocytosis

HYPOXEMIA is defined as a reduction in Pa_{O_2} or arterial oxygen saturation (Sa_{O_2}). This is not the only determinant of the adequacy of tissue oxygenation. Delivery of oxygen to tissues also depends on other factors (see chap. 9), such as hemoglobin concentration, which determines the total quantity of oxygen that can be carried in arterial blood, and the rate of blood flow to the tissues, which determines the total oxygen supplied to the tissues per minute.

Detection of Hypoxemia

The clinical diagnosis of hypoxemia is notoriously unreliable. Cyanosis is noted regularly only when hypoxemia is very severe, and most clinical cyanosis results from impaired blood flow rather than from low Pa_{O_2}. Arterial blood gas analysis is essential for accurate diagnosis.

In most modern laboratories Pa_{O_2} is measured directly by an oxygen electrode system. Some type of oximetric or manometric measurement may provide a direct estimate of Sa_{O_2}. It is desirable to make *both* Pa_{O_2} and Sa_{O_2} measurements routinely. This provides an in-laboratory check on the validity of each determination. Also, there are ranges of Pa_{O_2} and Sa_{O_2} on the steep portion of the oxyhemoglobin dissociation curve in which small changes in tension reflect large and highly significant changes in saturation. Furthermore, in clinical conditions such as carbon monoxide poisoning (see chap. 30), use of the Pa_{O_2} will be misleading as an indicator of arterial oxygenation. Under these circumstances,

the Sa_{O_2} will more precisely reflect the clinical status of the patient.

Some laboratories make a practice of reporting an Sa_{O_2} calculated from the Pa_{O_2}, using a standard oxygen dissociation curve. This practice cannot be condoned. The oxygen dissociation curve is not fixed. Not only does it vary among individuals, but it also may change with time in the same subject. For example, a shift to the right may occur with chronic hypoxemia, a result of increase in red cell 2,3-DPG. Although the hemoglobin is normally 50% saturated at a Pa_{O_2} of 26 torr, this same degree of saturation may occur at 35 torr or higher in a chronically hypoxemic individual, facilitating unloading of oxygen in peripheral tissues. In such instances, calculated Sa_{O_2} values are misleading.

Mechanisms and Differential Diagnosis of Hypoxemia

A reduction in Sa_{O_2} may occur for several reasons. Differentiation of the mechanism is important in differential diagnosis. The mechanism can be determined by relatively simple procedures available in most institutions. The mechanisms of hypoxemia are summarized in Figure 15–1, and the means of differentiating them are outlined in Table 15–1.

ALVEOLAR HYPOVENTILATION.—Alveolar hypoventilation is reflected by hypercapnia and must result in a decrease in Pa_{O_2}. For ordinary clinical purposes, the fall in Pa_{O_2} resulting from hypoventilation may be estimated to be equal to

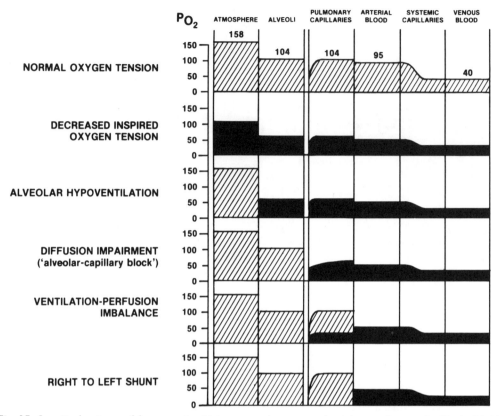

Fig 15–1.—Mechanisms of hypoxemia. (Adapted from Gaensler E.A., Constantine H.: Applied pulmonary physiology. *Postgrad. Med.* 36:431, 1964.)

the rise in Pa_{CO_2}. When the respiratory gas exchange ratio (CO_2 excretion/O_2 consumption) is less than 1, as it is in most individuals, the fall in Pa_{O_2} will actually be slightly greater. Conversely, a rise in Pa_{O_2} will be observed with hypocapnia or hyperventilation.

The effect of changes in alveolar ventilation on Pa_{O_2} is shown in Figure 15–2, where the relationship between Pa_{O_2} and Pa_{CO_2} is illustrated assuming a normal respiratory gas exchange ratio of 0.8 and an environmental oxygen tension of 160 torr. Greater reduction of Pa_{O_2} than shown in Figure 15–2 indicates that there is an additional cause for hypoxemia, most often a concomitant ventilation-perfusion imbalance as described below.

The effects of exertion on the hypoxemia of underventilation are unpredictable and depend on the ventilatory response to exercise. In some

patients with primary alveolar hypoventilation, for example, exercise results in improvement in both Pa_{CO_2} and Pa_{O_2}. In most patients with hypoventilation secondary to chronic lung disease, however, exertion increases both hypercapnia and hypoxemia.

If ventilation is not further depressed, supplemental oxygen would be expected to increase Pa_{O_2} by the same amount as inspired oxygen tension is increased. Thus, it is easy to increase the Pa_{O_2} to normal in a pure hypoventilation problem. Inspiration of 28% oxygen enriches the inspired oxygen tension by approximately 50 torr. This would fully correct any significant hypoxemia that might be due to underventilation.

DECREASED INSPIRED OXYGEN TENSION.—This occurs with high altitude, rebreathing expired air, and excessive rates of external combustion of oxygen. Rebreathing is associated

TABLE 15–1.—MECHANISMS OF HYPOXEMIA

			ARTERIAL O_2 TENSION			
			Air Breathing		28% O_2 Breathing	100% O_2 Breathing
MECHANISM	COMMON CAUSES	ARTERIAL CO_2 TENSION	Rest	Exercise		
Decreased inspired oxygen tension	Altitude	Decreased	Decrease predictable from altitude	No significant change	Increases approx 50 torr	Increases to within 250 torr of barometric pressure >400 torr
Alveolar hypoventilation	Depressed respiratory center Obesity syndrome Neuromuscular diseases Severe obstructive lung diseases	Increased	Decrease predictable from increase in Pa_{CO_2}	Variable (depends on effect on Pa_{CO_2})	Increases approx 50 torr minus the increase in Pa_{CO_2}	>400 torr
Diffusion limitation (alveolar-capillary block)	Diffuse parenchymal lung diseases	Normal or decreased	Little decrease, except terminally	Marked decrease	Increases more than 50 torr	>400 torr
Ventilation-perfusion imbalance (physiologic shunting)	All types of pulmonary diseases	Normal or decreased (unless also hypoventilating)	Variable amount of decrease	Usually decreases	Increases less than 50 torr	>400 torr
Right-to-left shunts anatomical	Congenital heart disease Pulmonary AV fistula	Normal or decreased	Variable amount of decrease	Usually decreases	Increases less than 50 torr	<400 torr (<200 torr if Pa_{O_2} is <55 torr on room air)
anatomical-like	Atelectasis Various severe lung diseases	Normal or decreased (unless also hypoventilating)	Variable amount of decrease	Usually decreases	Increases less than 50 torr	<400 torr

with a high Pa_{CO_2} and may be considered a form of hypoventilation. The diagnosis of altitude hypoxemia presents no diagnostic problem as long as the clinician is aware of the expected fall in Pa_{O_2} with increasing altitude. Surprisingly, there are minimal data concerning limits of Pa_{O_2} at various elevations, particularly for older individuals. Table 15–2 provides a rough guideline, although as a general rule, the Pa_{O_2} will change approximately 2.24 torr for each 1,000-ft increase or decrease in altitude (see chap. 11).

Values at the lower end of the normal range are unusual in vigorous young adults. Lower normal values for young children and older individuals reflect a larger amount of ventilation-perfusion imbalance at these ages. Obviously, the Pa_{O_2} at altitude depends on the degree of hyperventilation. This is somewhat variable, in part relating to the degree of acclimatization to altitude. Even at sea level the normalcy of a Pa_{O_2} value must be considered in light of the accompanying Pa_{CO_2}. If a patient is hyperventilating, as reflected by a low Pa_{CO_2}, the Pa_{O_2} should normally be near the upper limit of normal range. Figure 15–2 indicates the expected relationship between Pa_{O_2} and Pa_{CO_2} in normal individuals at sea level.

There is normally little fall in Pa_{O_2} on exercise at the altitudes usually encountered in the United States. With altitude hypoxemia, supple-

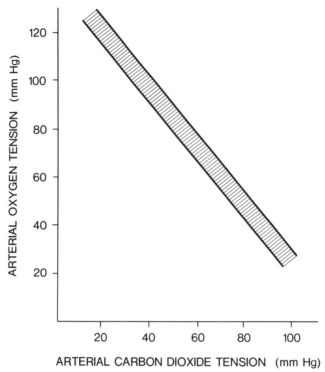

Fig 15–2.—Expected relationship of Pa_{CO_2} and Pa_{O_2} in normal individuals with respiratory exchange ratio of 0.8 at sea level, when Pa_{CO_2} is varied by increasing or decreasing effective alveolar ventilation. (Modern terminology would express gas tension in terms of torr rather than mm Hg.)

mental oxygen tends to raise Pa_{O_2} by the same amount as the oxygen tension is increased in the inspired gas.

DIFFUSION IMPAIRMENT.—Localized impairment of alveolar gas exchange may lead to a pattern of ventilation-perfusion imbalance (see below). An overall problem with gas diffusion, however, leads to a different pattern of hypoxemia. This has been described as an alveolar-capillary block (see chap. 13). This type of hypoxemia is rarely encountered in its pure form. More often some degree of alveolar-capillary

block may complicate the more fundamental problem of ventilation-perfusion imbalance, but this is difficult to diagnose with certainty. In any case, the following pattern suggests an overall diffusion impairment and, when noted, is most likely a result of a diffuse parenchymal lung disease: (1) relatively mild hypoxemia at rest, (2) very marked fall in Pa_{O_2} on mild exercise, (3) normal or low Pa_{CO_2} (carbon dioxide is a much more diffusible gas than oxygen), and (4) a greater than expected increase in Pa_{O_2} with small increments in inspired oxygen tension. There is no pure diffusion defect compatible with life during air breathing that will result in a Pa_{O_2} tension below 80 torr while the patient inspires 28% oxygen.

VENTILATION-PERFUSION IMBALANCE.—The most common mechanism for hypoxemia is ventilation-perfusion imbalance. It simply indicates that some of the pulmonary blood flow does not become normally oxygenated despite traversing

TABLE 15–2.—RANGE OF NORMAL Pa_{O_2}

ALTITUDE	AGE 10 TO 60 YR	UNDER AGE 10 AND OVER AGE 60 YR
Sea level	84–110 torr	>70
2,000 ft	78–104 torr	>67
4,000 ft	72–98 torr	>64
6,000 ft	66–92 torr	>61
8,000 ft	60–86 torr	>58

air-containing alveoli. Most commonly, this results from localized areas of hypoventilation. If some perfused alveoli do not receive their fair share of ventilation (i.e., they have a low ventilation/perfusion ratio), the blood perfusing them will be inadequately oxygenated. Similar problems may result from localized areas of diffusion impairment; e.g., when the local rate of diffusion of oxygen from alveolus to capillary is insufficient to fully oxygenate the capillary blood flow in some of the alveoli. A small amount of ventilation-perfusion imbalance is always present, since ventilation and blood flow are not perfectly matched even in normal individuals (see chap. 10)

Ventilation-perfusion imbalances should produce some carbon dioxide retention as well as hypoxemia. However, this can be readily compensated by an increase in overall ventilation, and carbon dioxide retention is usually equated with alveolar hypoventilation rather than ventilation-perfusion imbalances. Similar compensation for hypoxemia cannot occur by increased ventilation, since blood leaving normally ventilated alveoli is already almost fully saturated with oxygen.

The most extreme example of a ventilation-perfusion imbalance occurs when mixed venous blood perfuses nonventilated areas of lung, thereby acting as a right-to-left shunt (see below).

Exercise produces a variable effect on the hypoxemia resulting from ventilation-perfusion imbalances, although Pa_{O_2} usually falls to some extent. Supplemental oxygen produces less increase in Pa_{O_2} than would be predicted from the increase in inspired oxygen tension, but the administration of 100% oxygen induces a Pa_{O_2} greater than 400 torr.

RIGHT-TO-LEFT SHUNTS.—Right-to-left shunts are vascular communications occurring whenever unoxygenated venous blood fails to participate in gas exchange within the lungs, and eventually mixes with oxygenated blood. A small amount of right-to-left shunting is normally present as a result of blood flow through the cardiac thebesian veins and the bronchial circulation. Pathologic extrapulmonary right-to-left shunts are also observed in many congenital heart disorders. Since the respiratory system is normal, hyperventilation can occur in response to blood gas changes, and Pa_{CO_2} is maintained at normal or even low levels. Exercise generally causes a further fall in Pa_{O_2}, but the amount of change varies depending on hemodynamic alterations.

Within the lungs, right-to-left shunts may result from pulmonary arterial-venous fistulas or, more commonly, from perfusion of nonventilated areas of the lung. The latter may occur as a consequence of atelectasis, severe emphysema, bronchiectasis, or extensive parenchymal consolidation. In these conditions, however, right-to-left shunts may only contribute a small fraction to the observed hypoxemia. The larger portion is usually a result of ventilation-perfusion imbalances.

Right-to-left shunting is very resistant to correction by supplemental oxygen. A right-to-left shunt that leads to a Pa_{O_2} of 50 torr during air breathing will not allow the Pa_{O_2} to rise above 100 torr even during inhalation of pure oxygen. For clinical purposes, the presence of pathologic right-to-left shunting can be detected by the failure of the Pa_{O_2} to exceed 400 torr during pure oxygen breathing.

Effects of Hypoxemia

Minor degrees of hypoxemia produce few obvious physiologic changes. Slight hyperventilation, minor impairment of intellectual performance and subtle visual changes may be noted, but most of the clinically significant effects of hypoxemia are not seen until the Pa_{O_2} falls below 45 torr. The following may then be noted:

1. Pulmonary hypertension, aggravated by any coexisting respiratory acidosis. This is an important mechanism in the development of cor pulmonale.

2. Increase in cardiac output, representing a further strain on cardiac function.

3. Deleterious effects on myocardial function, especially when there is associated coronary artery disease.

4. Impaired renal function with a tendency to retain sodium.

5. Altered CNS function, usually characterized by headache, lethargy, or somnolence. With severe acute hypoxemia, convulsions and permanent brain damage may result.

6. A tendency to anaerobic metabolism with lactic acidosis. This may lead to a severe reduction in pH in patients with concomitant respiratory acidosis.

Evaluation of Cyanosis

Cyanosis is a bluish discoloration of skin, nailbeds, or mucous membranes attributed to excessive hemoglobin unsaturation. Reduced hemoglobin is purple, in contrast to the bright red of oxyhemoglobin. Ostensibly, cyanosis occurs when superficial capillaries contain more than 5 gm of reduced hemoglobin per 100 ml of blood. However, the presence or absence of cyanosis is determined by the subjective impression of the observer. This may be influenced by the thickness or pigmentation of the skin, the state of the superficial capillary bed, and even the ambient light. As a result, cyanosis is not a sensitive indicator of oxygen supply to tissues. Plethora associated with erythrocytosis may mimic cyanosis, whereas severe hypoxemia in the presence of anemia will not produce cyanosis.

A differential diagnosis of the discoloration suggestive of cyanosis is given in Table 15–3. Included for consideration are arterial hypoxemia, circulatory changes, and abnormal pigmentation, which may give a bluish cast to the skin. Localized cyanosis reflects a circulatory disorder involving reduced blood flow or distention of venules in the affected area. Diffuse "peripheral" cyanosis, not involving central areas such as the tongue and conjunctiva, usually reflects a low cardiac output state, such as heart failure or shock, but may be difficult to distinguish clinically from the "central" cyanosis seen with arterial hypoxemia.

Arterial oxygen should always be measured whenever generalized cyanosis is observed. Because severe hypoxemia may exist before cyanosis is recognized clinically, the absence of

TABLE 15–3.—CAUSE OF CYANOTIC APPEARANCE

Arterial hypoxemia
  Low inspired oxygen tension
  Alveolar hypoventilation
  Diffusion impairment
  Ventilation-perfusion imbalance
  Right-to-left shunting
Circulatory abnormality
  Low cardiac output
  Local reduction of blood flow
  Increased venous pressure
  Other causes of venous engorgement
Abnormal blood or skin pigments
  Argyria
  Met- or sulfhemoglobinemia
  Exogenous pigment
Erythrocytosis

this physical finding should never be taken as an indication of adequate arterial oxygenation.

Some relatively rare conditions may produce a superficial discoloration suggestive of cyanosis. Argyria resulting from silver ingestion may lead to a bluish gray discoloration of the skin. Unlike true cyanosis, the discoloration of argyria does not blanch on pressure.

Methemoglobin cannot combine reversibly with oxygen, is dark in color, and produces the appearance of cyanosis. Methemoglobinemia should be suspected if the oxygen capacity of the blood is low in the presence of a normal total hemoglobin or if oximetric measurements indicate unsaturation in spite of a normal oxygen tension. Spectroscopic analysis of the blood will confirm the diagnosis.

Evaluation of Erythrocytosis

Chronic severe oxygen deficiency stimulates the output of erythropoietin, which, in turn, stimulates the bone marrow to produce red blood cells. Any situation characterized by chronic hypoxemia may be associated with secondary erythrocytosis. In patients with chronic respiratory disorders, there is often an associated increase in plasma volume, minimizing the increase in hematocrit. In these patients measurements of hemoglobin or hematocrit do not reflect accurately the actual increase in red cell mass.

When a hemoglobin in excess of 16.5 gm or

a hematocrit above 55 is encountered, it must be determined if this is associated with hypoxemia. Although slight reduction in oxygen saturation has been reported with polycythemia rubra vera, an Sa_{O_2} below 92% or a Pa_{O_2} below 60 torr at sea level strongly suggests that the erythrocytosis results from an abnormality in oxygenation. Unfortunately, arterial oxygenation may be variable in hypoxemic patients, and a single normal blood gas value does not exclude secondary erythrocytosis. Arterial samples should be obtained on exercise as well as when the patient is reclining and close to a basal state (at least 5 to 10 minutes of rest should be allowed between inserting the arterial needle and withdrawing blood). Arterial carbon dioxide and bicarbonate should be measured as well as oxygen levels, and spirometric and diffusing capacity measurements should be made. Any significant abnormality raises serious doubt about a diagnosis of polycythemia rubra vera. Although some pulmonary dysfunction may occur in late stages of this disease, in earlier stages lung function tests are normal except for an unusually high diffusing capacity.

Secondary erythrocytosis may also occur as a result of hypoxemia from primary alveolar hypoventilation or from disturbances of ventilation during sleep. These problems are discussed in chapter 20. In addition, nonpulmonary causes of secondary erythrocytosis, such as neoplasms, renal cysts, and abnormal hemoglobins with an increased affinity for oxygen (left-shifted curve), may also need to be considered.

READING LIST

Berlin N.I.: Diagnosis and classification of the polycythemias. *Semin. Hematol.* 12:339–347, 1975.

A review of the diagnosis and evaluation of the various polycythemias.

Comroe J.R., Botelho S.: Unreliability of cyanosis in recognition of arterial anoxemia. *Am. J. Med. Sci.* 214:1–6, 1947.

The classic article demonstrating the failure of cyanosis to correlate with arterial oxygenation.

Davidson F.F., Glazier J.B., Murray J.F.: The components of the alveolar arterial oxygen tension difference in normal subjects and in patients with pneumonia and obstructive lung disease. *Am. J. Med.* 52:754–762, 1972.

Illustrates the mechanisms contributing to hypoxemia in patients with pneumonia and airways obstructive diseases.

Harris E.A., Kenyon A.M., Nisbet H.D., et al.: The normal alveolar-arterial oxygen tension gradient in man. *Clin. Sci.* 46:89–104, 1974.

This article demonstrates the variability observed in the normal alveolar-arterial oxygen tension gradient and shows how it changes with age.

Lundsgaard C., Van Slyke D.D.: Cyanosis. *Medicine* (Baltimore) 2:1–76, 1923.

The classic monograph reviewing the subject of cyanosis.

Make B.: Diagnosis and management of hypoxemia. *Compr. Ther.* 4:42–49, 1978.

A brief review of the evaluation and treatment of hypoxemia.

Quan S.F., Kronberg G.M., Schlobohm R.M., et al.: Changes in venous admixture with alterations of inspired oxygen concentration. *Anesthesiology* 52:477–482, 1980.

Demonstrates how venous admixture changes as inspired oxygen is altered in patients with acute lung disease.

Raven M.S., Epstein R. M., Malm J.R.: Contribution of thebesian veins to the physiologic shunt in anesthetized man. *J. Appl. Physiol.* 20:1148–1156, 1965.

Documents the contribution of intracardiac veins to the normal venous admixture in man.

Riley R.L., Cournand A.: 'Ideal' alveolar air and analysis of ventilation perfusion relationships in the lungs. *J. Appl. Physiol.* 1:825–847, 1949.

The classic article proposing the concept of the "ideal alveolar gas composition" and the influence on blood gases of imbalances of ventilation and perfusion.

16

Cardiovascular Responses to Respiratory Disorders

Pulmonary Hypertension

The lesser circulation is a low-pressure system with low resistance and marked distensibility. Under normal circumstances, cardiac output can increase two to three times without leading to a significant increase in pulmonary artery pressure (PAP). Thus, the pulmonary vasculature is able to decrease its resistance markedly in response to an increase in blood flow. As the pulmonary vascular bed becomes attenuated by disease, however, it becomes increasingly unable to accommodate increments in flow without an increase in PAP, and when two thirds to three fourths of the vascular bed has been lost, pulmonary arterial hypertension is noted even at rest.

Anatomical alterations in the pulmonary vascular bed are only one cause of hemodynamic alterations in patients with respiratory disorders. Of at least equal importance is the hypoxemia that often accompanies these diseases. Hypoxemia has a twofold effect. It increases the cardiac output and, at the same time, increases the tone of the vascular bed. With this increase in tone, resistance cannot fall to accommodate the increased flow and PAP rises, as shown in Figure 16–1.

When the pulmonary vascular bed is progressively attenuated without concomitant hypoxemia, as in primary pulmonary vascular disease

and certain types of emphysema, cardiac output decreases. The low cardiac output minimizes the pulmonary artery hypertension that would otherwise occur as a consequence of the elevated pulmonary vascular resistance. In early stages PAP may be normal at rest, and PAP elevations only occur when cardiac output is increased with exercise. As the disease progresses, some resting pulmonary hypertension develops despite the low cardiac output. The low cardiac output of these patients leads to tissue hypoxia even though the Pa_{O_2} is near normal. This may account in part for such symptoms as weakness, easy fatigue, and coldness of the extremities. Definite diagnosis of this low cardiac output state requires actual measurement of cardiac output.

In the presence of hypoxemia cardiac output is well maintained despite attenuation of the vascular bed. As a consequence, resting pulmonary hypertension is an early development. It is aggravated by any accompanying respiratory acidosis, which potentiates the pulmonary hypertensive effects of hypoxemia. In fact, hypoxemia and hypercapnia may lead to severe pulmonary hypertension even in the absence of anatomical changes in the vascular bed, as in the primary alveolar hypoventilation syndromes. A brief period of oxygen breathing produces only

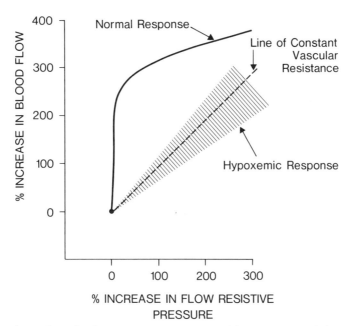

Fig 16–1.—The relationship of pulmonary artery pressure to pulmonary blood flow during exercise in a normal individual showing little increase in pressure with increases in flow up to two to three times resting levels. This is due to a marked fall in resistance of the normal vascular bed when flow is increased by exertion. With hypoxemia the tone of the vascular bed is increased, and a normal fall in vascular resistance does not occur in response to an induced increase in blood flow, resulting in pulmonary hypertension.

slight reduction in PAP, but more marked reduction occurs over several weeks of oxygen supplementation. This suggests that chronic hypoxemia leads to muscular hypertrophy as well as to increased tone of pulmonary vessels.

Signs suggestive or indicative of pulmonary hypertension include dilatation of the main pulmonary arteries and fullness of the apical vessels on ordinary chest radiology; loss of the normal apex to base gradient of blood flow on lung scans made in the sitting or standing position; an increase in the second pulmonic sound; ECG evidence of right ventricular hypertrophy (RVH), and, most definitively, direct demonstration of high PAP values on cardiac catheterization.

In a few patients development of pulmonary hypertension causes right-to-left flow through a patent foramen ovale that was of no functional consequence when right ventricular pressures were normal. The superimposition of anatomical shunting from this mechanism on the physiologic shunting resulting from the underlying lung disease may lead to severe, refractory hypoxemia.

Cor Pulmonale

Cor pulmonale is defined as an "alteration in structure or function of the right ventricle resulting from disease affecting the structure or function of the lung or its vasculature, except when this alteration results from disease of the left side of the heart or congenital heart disease."[*]

Remarkably little is known about the development of right ventricular dysfunction as a consequence of chronic pulmonary diseases. As already mentioned, in the absence of hypoxemia, a low cardiac output state with relatively normal

_____

*Inter-Society Commission: Pulmonary Heart Disease Study Group. *Circulation* 41:A–17–23, 1970.

resting PAP may develop. According to the above definition, this might be regarded as a "low output type" of cor pulmonale. It is accompanied by few clinical signs of right ventricular disease and is not usually associated with congestive heart failure.

Once frank resting pulmonary hypertension has developed, some clinical evidence of right ventricular disease can usually be found. Earliest evidences are usually electrocardiographic. Later, physical and radiologic signs of RVH are found. Congestive heart failure may develop insidiously or first occur abruptly during an acute exacerbation of the underlying lung disorder.

Many factors contribute to the development of congestive heart failure in patients with cor pulmonale. Increasing hypoxemia leads to increased PAP and further right ventricular strain. It also directly impairs myocardial function and contributes to fluid retention. Congestive heart failure may also develop secondary to an increased demand for cardiac output consequent to increased work of breathing, fever, or anxiety in patients with chronic lung diseases. Once congestive heart failure develops, a vicious circle is initiated, as depicted in Figure 16–2. Hypervolemia from congestive heart failure results in pulmonary vascular congestion and further deterioration of lung function. A resulting worsening of blood gases further aggravates the pul-

monary hypertension, causing additional deterioration of lung function. With appropriate therapy, the circle is interrupted, and both cardiac and pulmonary function improve.

There are several problems in the diagnosis of cor pulmonale. The diagnosis is easily missed if the patient is first seen in an episode of frank heart failure. The underlying pulmonary disorder may not be obvious, and all signs may be ascribed erroneously to intrinsic heart disease. The presence of severe, persistent blood gas abnormalities or of RVH should suggest the possibility of underlying lung disease.

It is also easy to overdiagnose cor pulmonale in patients with chronic respiratory disorders. Chronic dependent edema is common in these patients, even in the absence of cardiac dysfunction. This is probably related to the tendency to fluid retention from blood gas changes, impaired venous return to the chest, and venous stasis from prolonged inactivity. Also, tachycardia may be marked in patients with respiratory insufficiency even in the absence of heart disease. Finally, certain ECG changes occur in these patients that do not necessarily indicate cor pulmonale. Examples include delayed transition of the QRS complexes in the precordial leads (clockwise rotation), slight right axis deviation, and prominent P waves. The most reliable ECG indicator of RVH in these patients is a dominant

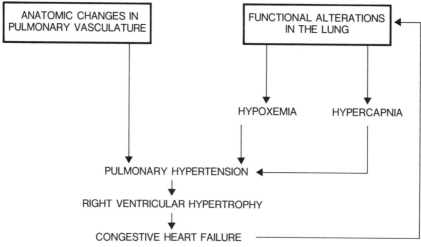

Fig 16–2.—Mechanisms of pulmonary hypertension and congestive heart failure from cor pulmonale.

R wave in the right precordial leads. Another reliable indicator of cardiac disease is increasing heart size and, particularly, a fluctuation in heart size in association with symptoms suggesting congestive heart failure. Physical signs of RVH are notoriously unreliable in patients with chronic lung diseases. Newer methods of assessing cardiac function using radioisotopic techniques and echocardiograms should lead to improved diagnostic precision.

Optimum management of chronic cor pulmonale requires improvement of the underlying respiratory disorder and control of hypoxemia. In many patients prolonged oxygen therapy can lead to relief of pulmonary hypertension and regression of RVH. Successful treatment of acute congestive heart failure secondary to cor pulmonale also requires prompt relief of hypoxemia. While this alone may result in marked improvement, small phlebotomies, diuretics, and vigorous attempts to relieve the underlying respiratory problem are also of importance. Digitalis should not be used in the treatment of acute congestive heart failure secondary to cor pulmonale. It is of questionable efficacy and is very likely to result in intoxication in these patients, who have fluctuating blood gas and serum electrolyte values and in whom there is already a tendency for cardiac arrhythmias to develop.

Differential Diagnosis of Right Ventricular Hypertrophy

Neither pulmonary hypertension nor RVH necessarily indicates an underlying respiratory disorder. PAP may be elevated as a consequence of a high pulmonary venous pressure resulting from a left atrial or left ventricular disease. In this case pulmonary wedge pressure (PWP) measurements made at cardiac catheterization will be elevated, and calculations of pulmonary arteriolar resistance (cardiac output/[PAP − PWP]) will be normal, indicating that abnormalities in the pulmonary vessels themselves do not explain the pulmonary hypertension.

Pathogenic mechanisms for RVH are summarized in Table 16–1. Most cases result from congenital or rheumatic heart disease or are associ-

TABLE 16–1.—MECHANISMS OF RIGHT VENTRICULAR HYPERTROPHY

Diseases of right ventricular outflow tract
  Pulmonary valvular or infundibular stenosis
  Obstructing lesions of main pulmonary arteries
  Persistent ductus arteriosus
Diseases of lung or pulmonary vessels (cor pulmonale)
  Obstructive lung diseases
  Restrictive lung diseases
  Recurrent pulmonary emboli
  Primary pulmonary vascular diseases
Diseases affecting pulmonary venous pressure
  Obstructive abnormalities of pulmonary veins
  Obstructive abnormalities in left atrium or mitral valve
  Chronic left ventricular failure of any cause
Diseases leading to persistent high pulmonary blood flow
  (especially congenital heart diseases with left-to-right shunting of blood)
Persistent hypoxemia
  Altitude
  Right-to-left shunts
  Secondary to pulmonary disease (cor pulmonale)
  Chronic hypoventilation (cor pulmonale)

ated with a severe lung disease that is clinically obvious. Any diffuse disease of the lung parenchyma may result in cor pulmonale with RVH, but chronic obstructive lung diseases are the most common causes. Frank RVH usually occurs with airways obstructive problems only when there is concomitant severe hypoxemia and marked ventilatory impairment (FEV$_1$ below 1 L). In patients with relatively normal blood gases or with mild ventilatory impairment, a contributing cause of the RVH should be suspected.

When the cause of RVH is not evident after considering the history, physical findings, chest x-ray, ECG, and simple lung function tests, the following types of disorders must be considered:

1. "Silent" mitral valve disease, atrial septal defect or one of the rarer diseases of the left atrium or pulmonary veins.

2. Primary vascular disease of the lungs, recurrent pulmonary emboli, or diffuse interstitial lung disease that is difficult to visualize on chest roentgenogram and produces little ventilatory impairment.

3. Defect in the right ventricle itself, pulmonary stenosis, or an abnormality of the main pulmonary arteries.

Cardiac fluoroscopy and echocardiography are

helpful in determining whether left atrial enlargement exists, as would be expected with mitral valve disease. Additional lung function studies such as diffusing capacity, physiologic dead space, and arterial blood gas measurements may provide evidence of a pulmonary vascular disorder or primary alveolar underventilation problem. A lung scan may help in diagnosis of pulmonary emboli. If the diagnosis remains uncertain, cardiac catheterization and angiographic studies are necessary. Even if the specific underlying disease remains obscure, these studies should at least allow localization of the defect to the right ventricle, pulmonary valve area, pulmonary vessels, or left atrium and indicate the direction of further evaluation.

READING LIST

Fishman A.P.: Hypoxia on the pulmonary circulation: how and where it acts. *Circ. Res.* 38:221–331, 1976.

A still current review of the mechanism of effects of hypoxemia on the pulmonary circulation.

Fishman A.P.: Chronic cor pulmonale. *Am. Rev. Respir. Dis.* 114:775–784, 1976.

A state of the art review with an extensive reference list.

Matthay R.A., Berger H.J.: Cardiovascular performance in chronic obstructive pulmonary diseases. *Med. Clin. North. Am.* 65:489–524, 1981.

A more up-to-date review of hemodynamic changes in airways obstructive diseases, with 254 references.

Respiratory Failure

General Considerations

Respiratory failure exists when respiratory dysfunction is of such a degree that gas exchange is no longer adequate to maintain normal arterial blood gas levels. The term may be applied to any patient who is hypoxemic or hypercapnic from a respiratory disease. Respiratory failure is usually observed under three different clinical circumstances. First, it may occur acutely in a patient with no preexisting respiratory disease. Second, its onset may be insidious, produced by a form of chronic respiratory dysfunction. Last, in patients with chronic respiratory failure, there may be sudden exacerbations of their illness, resulting in acute respiratory failure superimposed on chronic respiratory failure. Therapeutic modalities for these forms of respiratory failure frequently differ.

Acute Respiratory Failure

Conditions that produce respiratory failure can be placed into two categories as shown in Table 17–1—those whose primary physiologic consequence is to impair oxygenation, and those whose primary consequence is a depression of ventilation with resultant hypercapnia. Symptoms and signs of hypoxemia and hypercapnia are shown in Table 17–2. They are nonspecific and can be observed in many medical conditions. Furthermore, they are unreliable guides to the severity of blood gas changes. Therefore,

the diagnosis of acute respiratory failure requires arterial blood gas analysis. In patients without a history or clinical findings consistent with a chronic respiratory disorder, an elevation of the Pa_{CO2} is diagnostic of an acute impairment in ventilation. However, the acute development of hypoxemia does not necessarily result from an impairment in oxygenation. Hypoventilation by itself can produce hypoxemia (see chap. 15). Determination of whether there is a primary defect in oxygen gas exchange can be made by calculation of the alveolar-arterial oxygen tension difference: $P(A-a)O_2 = PA_{O2} - Pa_{O2}$. The alveolar PO_2 can be estimated using a simplified version of the alveolar gas equation:

$$PA_{O2} = \left(P_B - P_{H2O}\right)FI_{O2} - \frac{Pa_{CO2}}{0.8}$$

where PA_{O2} = alveolar PO_2, P_B = barometric pressure, and P_{H2O} = partial pressure of water vapor at body temperature assuming full saturation. If this difference is less than 6 torr breathing room air, there is no impairment in oxygenation. Breathing pure oxygen, the $P(A - a)O_2$ may be as high as 30 torr without a defect in oxygen gas exchange being present.

Treatment for acute respiratory failure depends on whether the respiratory disorder has caused primarily an impairment in oxygenation, ventilation, or, rarely, both. In cases where there is only relatively mild hypoxemia, supplemental oxygen using a nasal cannula or a simple mask may correct the hypoxemia. Using these

TABLE 17–1.—TREATMENT OF ACUTE
RESPIRATORY FAILURE

Impairment of ventilation: Hypercarbia with a normal
    $P(A - a)O_2$
Depression of respiratory drive—drugs, CNS
    disease
Neurologic disorders—poliomyelitis, Guillain-
    Barré syndrome
Chest wall abnormalities—myopathies,
    kyphoscoliosis

Impairment of oxygenation: Increased $P(A - a)O_2$
                                with usually a
                                normal Pa_{CO_2}
    Pneumonia
    Pulmonary edema
    Asthma

TABLE 17–3.—GUIDELINES FOR VENTILATORY
SUPPORT IN ACUTE RESPIRATORY FAILURE

Respiratory rate	>35 min^{-1}
Vital capacity	<15 ml/kg body weight
Inspiratory force	<25 cm H_2O
Pa_{O_2}	<60 torr (high flow mask with 100% O_2)
P_{CO_2}	>55 torr

devices, it generally is not possible to provide an inspired oxygen concentration greater than 50%. When higher concentrations are required, a tight-fitting reservoir mask can usually deliver up to 90% inspired oxygen. However, need for a reservoir mask generally denotes respiratory failure of such severity that endotracheal intubation and mechanical ventilation with PEEP are indicated. Therapy under these circumstances is similar to that described for adult respiratory distress syndrome (see chap. 28). When the primary abnormality is a severe impairment in ventilation which cannot be immediately reversed, mechanical ventilation should be employed. Oxygen therapy is not required unless there is persistent hypoxemia after hypercapnia is corrected. General criteria for initiating ventilatory support in both forms of acute respiratory failure are listed in Table 17–3. Whether the primary manifestation is hypoxemia or hypercapnia, the specific cause of respiratory failure should be identified and treated in all cases.

TABLE 17–2.—SIGNS AND SYMPTOMS OF
HYPOXEMIA AND HYPERCARBIA

RESPIRATORY	CEREBRAL	CARDIAC
Tachypnea	Restlessness	Bradycardia
Apnea	Irritability	Tachycardia
Chest wall retractions	Headaches	Hypotension
Cyanosis	Seizures	Hypertension
Grunting	Coma	
	Papilledema	
	Asterixis	

Chronic Respiratory Failure

Patients with progressive respiratory disorders such as chronic obstructive airways diseases may eventually have hypoxemia and hypercapnia as their pulmonary function worsens. When mild, these chronic blood gas abnormalities are often remarkably well tolerated, partly as a result of the numerous mechanisms available to compensate for alterations in gas exchange. Renal retention of bicarbonate helps maintain pH at normal levels in the face of carbon dioxide retention. Shifts in the oxyhemoglobin dissociation curves with changes in arterial pH and P_{CO_2}, changes in erythrocyte 2,3-DPG, increased erythropoiesis, and increase in cardiac output all help maintain tissue oxygenation despite blood gas abnormalities. As a result, severe progressive hypoxemia and hypercapnia may develop insidiously without obvious clinical signs.

In general, a Pa_{CO_2} above 50 torr or a Pa_{O_2} below 60 torr at sea level has been accepted as indicative of respiratory failure. Since patients with chronic lung disease are able to tolerate some hypoxemia without clinical impairment, it is perhaps misleading to designate such mild chronic hypoxemia as respiratory failure. However, in view of our definition, it must be appreciated that many stable, ambulant patients with chronic lung disease are in a continuous state of mild chronic respiratory failure that requires no specific therapy. It is necessary to treat chronic hypoxemia only if it is severe or is associated with problems resulting from cor pulmonale. Well-compensated chronic hypercapnia requires no specific therapy and is not associated with specific symptoms. Use of oxygen therapy in chronic obstructive airways disease is discussed in further detail in chapter 27.

Acute Respiratory Failure in Chronic Lung Disease

The clinical course of patients with chronic lung disease may be punctuated by periodic exacerbations which produce an acute deterioration in gas exchange superimposed on a preexisting chronic process. If baseline blood gas values are unknown, acute respiratory failure is assumed to exist when hypoxemia or hypercapnia is associated with an acute symptomatic exacerbation or when arterial pH is lower than expected for a chronic, well-compensated hypercapnia. The relationship of pH to P_{CO_2} in acute vs. chronic hypercapnia, as well as in other acid-base disturbances, is shown in Figure 17–1. (This figure was explained in some detail in chapter 14.)

Before initiating therapy, arterial blood gas analysis should be obtained, except in the most extreme emergencies, both to document the presence of superimposed acute respiratory fail-

ure and to determine its severity. Initial attempts to correct hypoxemia should be made using low flow oxygen via nasal cannula at 1–2 L/min or a 24%–28% Venturi-type mask. Extreme caution should be exercised to prevent giving more oxygen than required to correct the hypoxemia. Many patients with chronic carbon dioxide retention have a diminished hypercapnic drive to breathe and a reduced sensitivity to hydrogen ion. Hypoxemia is often the major remaining stimulus to respiration. Too rapid correction or overcorrection of hypoxemia may lead to respiratory depression, with a further increase in carbon dioxide retention and acidosis. Very high inspired oxygen tensions may cause respiratory arrest.

The danger in intermittent oxygen therapy must be stressed. If a patient's ventilation is depressed by oxygen treatment, he becomes more dependent than ever on oxygen supplementation. If oxygen is suddenly discontinued, fatal levels of hypoxemia may develop. This results from the difference in body stores of carbon dioxide and oxygen. During a period of oxygen-

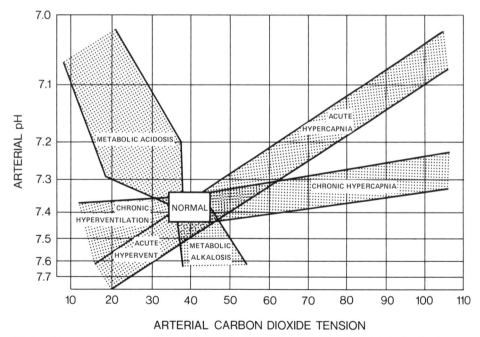

Fig 17–1.—Blood gas interpretations. Observed pH-P_{CO_2} relationships in various types of acid-base disturbances. (See Fig 14–1 for further explanation.)

induced hypoventilation, considerable storage of carbon dioxide occurs, but the high inspired oxygen cannot produce much increase in body oxygen stores. When oxygen treatment is discontinued, it will take some time to "unload" the accumulated carbon dioxide, especially if ventilation does not increase promptly. As a result, Pa_{CO_2} remains elevated while inspired Po_2 is lowered abruptly, leading to severe hypoxemia.

Most patients with chronic obstructive airways diseases in whom acute respiratory failure develops during an exacerbation of their disease do not require mechanical ventilation, even if they show a moderate increase in Pa_{CO_2}. As a result of the sigmoid shape of the oxyhemoglobin dissociation curve, administration of small amounts of supplemental oxygen usually raises the Pa_{O_2} to between 50 and 60 torr or near a saturation of 90% without totally removing the hypoxic ventilatory stimulus. Furthermore, in these patients, vigorous therapy of the underlying disorder and of any cardiac complications, and avoidance of all sedative and narcotic therapy, usually results in sufficient improvement in ventilation to lower the arterial carbon dioxide to the patient's chronic level. Specific management of exacerbations of airways obstructive diseases is provided in chapter 27. Unfortunately, in some clinical situations, any attempt to improve arterial oxygenation results in only worse hypercapnia and respiratory acidosis. In this situation, mechanical ventilation is indicated in selected cases where there is an obvious reversible precipitating cause for the superimposed acute respiratory failure. The decision of whether to initiate mechanical ventilation in patients with chronic lung disease is a difficult ethical problem, and is best made in consultation with the patient's primary care physician, family, and the patient personally. During the chronic management of these patients, it is often possible to discuss the question of eventual ventilatory assistance with the patient before the need arises. In contrast to the patient whose medical history is documented, some patients with chronic airways obstruction develop acute respiratory failure but little is known of their previous medical history. These patients proba-

bly should be given the benefit of the doubt and receive mechanical ventilation.

Other therapeutic considerations include the use of aminophylline, which appears to have a mild respiratory stimulant action that helps to avoid the need for mechanical ventilation in patients with chronic obstructive airways disease. Recent data suggest that it acts by improving respiratory muscle fatigue. In contrast, analeptic agents are rarely indicated as respiratory stimulants in treatment of hypercapnia. Most of these agents increase metabolic oxygen consumption as much as they improve ventilation. Use of intermittent positive-pressure breathing treatments should be avoided, since they may worsen underlying bronchospasm and decrease ventilatory efficiency in patients not familiar with their use. Furthermore, their possible beneficial effects on ventilation are not sustained beyond their actual use.

Ancillary Methods of Treatment

When respiratory failure is complicated by metabolic acidosis, intravenous (IV) administration of sodium bicarbonate is indicated to control the excessively low pH. All patients who have acute respiratory failure during cardiac arrest will have increased levels of lactic acid and require bicarbonate therapy. Repeated measurements of arterial pH should be used to determine the dosage of bicarbonate needed to maintain pH above 7.2.

Hypokalemic hypochloremic alkalosis frequently appears following therapy for acute respiratory failure. Supplemental potassium chloride given IV or orally corrects the defect. Uncorrected, this form of metabolic alkalosis sets the stage for dangerous superimposed respiratory alkalosis due to the increased alveolar ventilation from ventilators. Deaths from severe alkalosis have been described in this setting. If the patient is receiving cardiac glycosides, hypokalemia may also lead to digitalis intoxication.

While the episode of respiratory failure is being treated, a search for its cause should be instituted. Remaining therapeutic measures are then directed primarily at the underlying causes of the respiratory insufficiency. In this regard, it is important to remember that anxiety (especially with excessive tachypnea), intercurrent infection, and a variety of remediable pulmonary complications (e.g., pneumothorax or massive atelectasis from mucus plugging) may precipitate acute respiratory failure in patients with underlying respiratory insufficiency states.

READING LIST

Kettel L.J., Diener C.F., Morse J.O., et al.: Treatment of acute respiratory acidosis in chronic obstructive lung disease. *J.A.M.A.* 217:1503–1508, 1971.

This study demonstrates that most patients with chronic obstructive lung disease and acute respiratory failure can be treated conservatively without mechanical ventilation.

Martin L.: Respiratory failure. *Med. Clin. North Am.* 61:1369–1396, 1977.

This is a general review of the pathophysiology and treatment of all types of respiratory failure.

Martin L.V., Marshall R.L.: Survival of chronic bronchitics after intermittent positive pressure ventilation. *Anaesthesia* 28:10–16, 1973.

In this article the outcome of patients with chronic bronchitis requiring mechanical ventilation is documented.

Mechanical Ventilation and Positive End-Expiratory Pressure

MECHANICAL VENTILATORS are devices that artificially enable gas to move into and out of the lungs. The major indications for use of mechanical ventilation are severe acute impairments in oxygen and carbon dioxide gas exchange as discussed in chapter 17. In addition, mechanical ventilators are employed prophylactically after major surgical procedures in which there is a high probability of immediate postoperative respiratory dysfunction. Mechanical ventilation is sometimes used to hyperventilate patients artificially to lower intracranial pressure and to increase respiratory compensation in the presence of severe metabolic acidosis. Last, in patients with a limited vital capacity due to muscle weakness or neurologic disease, mechanical ventilation is used to avoid atelectasis and retention of secretions even before the development of frank respiratory failure (see chaps. 17 and 21). Overall criteria for institution of mechanical ventilation are shown in Table 18–1 and discussed further in chapters 17, 20, 21, 27, 28, and 30.

Types of Mechanical Ventilators

There are two general categories of mechanical ventilators as outlined in Table 18–2. The most common class of ventilators are those which act by generating positive pressure in the lungs (positive-pressure ventilators). Positive-pressure ventilators can be further divided into those which cycle from inspiration to expiration on the basis of delivering a preset tidal volume (volume-constant ventilators) and those which cycle from inspiration to expiration after a preset positive pressure has been reached within the airway (pressure-limited ventilators). With pressure-limited ventilators, it is difficult to insure a constant tidal volume, since any event such as coughing, bronchospasm, or even production of viscid secretions will increase impedance to inspiration and cause the ventilator to cycle into expiration before the desired tidal volume has been delivered. This can be a severe disadvantage in ventilating the majority of patients with parenchymal lung disease. Currently, pressure-limited ventilators are generally used only in neonatal ventilation and for intermittent positive-pressure breathing treatments (IPPB). Volume-constant ventilators are used in most other clinical situations.

The second major class of ventilators are negative-pressure ventilators, which generally act by producing a subambient pressure outside the lungs. In this class are tank ventilators (iron lung), cuirass ventilators (chest shell), and the rocking bed. The last is a bed with a fulcrum in the middle which pivots up and down, thereby displacing the diaphragm by gravity. All of these devices present major problems in expediting the nursing care of severely ill patients; also,

TABLE 18–1.—CRITERIA FOR INITIATING
MECHANICAL VENTILATION

Respiratory rate	>35 min^{-1}
Vital capacity	<10–15 ml/kg
Maximum inspiratory force	<-25 cm H_2O
Pa_{O_2}	<60 torr using a mask delivering 100% O_2
Pa_{CO_2}	>55 torr

they are relatively inefficient ventilators. They are primarily used for long-term ventilation in patients with neuromuscular disease.

Recently, it has been demonstrated that adequate gas exchange can be maintained using positive-pressure ventilation at rates between 60 and 5,000 breaths per minute. This radical form of ventilation has been termed high-frequency ventilation (HFV). Since delivered tidal volumes are generally less than the anatomical dead space, conventional assumptions regarding the movement of gas into and out of the lungs (see chaps. 6 and 8) do not seem applicable. Adequate gas exchange most likely occurs because of enhanced diffusivity of both O_2 and CO_2 within conducting airways. Theoretical advantages of HFV over conventional ventilation include adequate ventilation at lower airway pressures and therefore less barotrauma, less depression of cardiac output, and more efficient gas exchange. Although its role in clinical medicine remains to be completely defined and its use still investigational, HFV may be more efficacious than conventional mechanical ventilation in the treatment of the respiratory distress syndromes, especially when a large bronchopleural fistula is present, and may provide some advantages during ventilation for certain surgical procedures.

TABLE 18–2.—CLASSIFICATION OF
MECHANICAL VENTILATORS

POSITIVE-PRESSURE
Volume-constant
Pressure-limited
NEGATIVE-PRESSURE
Tank (iron lung)
Cuirass
Rocking bed
HIGH-FREQUENCY

Physiologic Aspects of Positive-Pressure Ventilation

LUNG MECHANICS.—With spontaneous inspiration, the respiratory muscles pull the chest wall out, causing the intrapleural pressure to become more negative. This produces a larger pressure gradient between the mouth and the pleural space, resulting in gas flow down this gradient into the lungs. If airways resistance does not change, the volume of gas which enters the lungs is determined by the compliance of the lungs and the change in pleural pressure. Tidal volume will be larger if the change in pleural pressure is greater or if lung compliance is increased. By generating positive pressure at the mouth, mechanical ventilation also creates a pressure gradient between the mouth and pleural space, resulting in gas flow into the lungs. The changes in pleural pressure and the determinants of tidal volume, however, are different than those noted with spontaneous ventilation. Since the increase in airway pressure with mechanical ventilation must provide the energy to increase not only the volume of the lungs but also the thoracic cavity, assuming no change in airways resistance, tidal volume at a given airway pressure is determined by the compliances of the lung and chest wall together. Therefore, a decrease in either lung or chest wall compliance will result in a smaller tidal volume for any given airway pressure increment. As a result of transmission of airway pressure to the pleural space, pleural pressure becomes more positive with mechanical ventilation. The degree to which positive pressure in the airway is transmitted to the pleural space is determined by the relative compliances of the lung and chest wall. An increase in lung compliance and a decrease in chest wall compliance will allow a large proportion of the positive airway pressure to be transmitted to the pleural space. An example of this latter concept is seen in patients with severe chronic airways obstruction who receive mechanical ventilation. These patients have very compliant lungs, which allow a large proportion of the positive pressure in the airway to be transmitted to the pleural space. Although in normal individuals the chest wall tends to recoil outward at FRC (see chap. 6), in patients with airways obstruction who are hyperinflated, the chest wall may tend to recoil inward. This will magnify the increase in pressure transmitted to the pleural space during positive-pressure ventilation.

CARDIOVASCULAR EFFECTS.—Mechanical ventilation sometimes causes a reduction in cardiac output by impairing venous return to the heart. During spontaneous inspiration, intrapleural and therefore intrathoracic pressure becomes more negative with respect to ambient pressure. This facilitates return of blood to the heart by creating a pressure gradient between the peripheral venous system and the central veins during inspiration. With a positive-pressure inspiration, intrapleural pressure becomes positive with respect to ambient pressure, leading to a reversal of this gradient and impairment of venous return. Usually a reflex increase in peripheral venous tone restores the pressure gradient to normal and prevents any significant fall in blood pressure or cardiac output. However, in patients with intravascular volume depletion, very compliant lungs (as in emphysema), or an impairment of peripheral vascular reflexes, initiation of mechanical ventilation may result in hypotension. This can be counteracted by elevation of the lower extremities or infusion of IV fluids.

DISTRIBUTION OF VENTILATION AND GAS EXCHANGE.—During spontaneous breathing, inspired gas is distributed primarily to the more dependent areas of the lung corresponding generally to lung areas receiving the most perfusion. During positive-pressure ventilation, nondependent areas of the lung receive proportionally more ventilation than they do with spontaneous breathing. This results in less efficient matching of ventilation to perfusion. No clinically significant abnormality is usually observed in patients without parenchymal lung disease, but this may be an important factor in patients with a severe impairment of gas exchange.

WORK OF BREATHING.—In normal individuals the work of breathing contributes a small frac-

tion of the body's oxygen consumption. Alteration of the lung's mechanical properties, such as exists in many disease states, can markedly increase the work of breathing. Initiation of mechanical ventilation in these clinical situations may significantly decrease the work of breathing, leading to a reduction in overall oxygen consumption and an increase in the mixed venous P_{O_2}. Since a concomitant impairment in oxygenation due to right-to-left shunting or ventilation-perfusion imbalance is usually present, this may improve the Pa_{O_2}.

FLUID BALANCE.—Mechanical ventilation often results in fluid retention. This may be due to the effects of increased secretion of antidiuretic hormone. The positive fluid balance is not usually clinically significant and requires no specific treatment, unless positive end-expiratory pressure (PEEP) is also being applied.

Positive End-Expiratory Pressure

Positive end-expiratory pressure is produced by having the patient expire against an above-ambient airway pressure. This generally results in an increase in FRC. In the respiratory distress syndromes (see chap. 28), hypoxemia is produced by atelectasis and regions of the lung with low ventilation relative to perfusion. By increasing FRC, PEEP may open atelectatic alveoli, prevent unstable alveoli from closing during expiration, and improve ventilation in areas with low ventilation/perfusion ($\dot{V}A/\dot{Q}$) ratios. Some data suggest that it may also improve collateral ventilation within the lung. These effects usually result in an increase in the Pa_{O_2}. Although use of PEEP corrects many of the physiologic abnormalities in the respiratory distress syndromes, there is no evidence that it favorably alters the ultimate course of the underlying disease. It is therefore only a technique of providing respiratory support and not a specific therapy.

PEEP also has major detrimental effects. First, the increase in airway pressure produced by PEEP is preferentially transmitted to normal lung areas. This can result in overdistention of normal alveoli and an increase in the dead space/tidal volume (V_D/V_T) ratio. Overdistention of normal alveoli can also divert blood flow away from normal lung areas toward atelectatic areas, resulting in worse hypoxemia. Second, increases in mean airway pressure produced by PEEP are attended by a high incidence of lung barotrauma. Therefore, pneumothorax, pneumomediastinum, and subcutaneous emphysema are frequently observed during PEEP therapy. Third, PEEP often causes a decrease in cardiac output and blood pressure. Several mechanisms have been suggested to explain the detrimental hemodynamic effects of PEEP. Since intrathoracic pressure is increased with PEEP, it may impair venous return and therefore decrease cardiac output. It has also been proposed that PEEP adversely influences myocardial contractility directly or that it causes release of vasoactive mediators, which may cause peripheral systemic vasodilation. Most recently, data have been presented to demonstrate that PEEP produces right ventricular dilation by a marked increase in pulmonary vascular resistance or right ventricular afterload. This leads to a shift of the interventricular septum so that it encroaches on the left ventricular cavity. Left ventricular compliance and left ventricular end-diastolic volume are reduced, producing a decrease in stroke volume and cardiac output. Irrespective of the specific mechanism, hemodynamic compromise secondary to PEEP therapy can often be attenuated by volume expansion and use of vasopressors. In addition, since the degree of airway pressure transmission to the pleural space is lower when lung compliance is reduced, the hemodynamic effects of PEEP may be less evident in the patients who require PEEP the most.

PEEP can be applied during both spontaneous breathing and mechanical ventilation. It can be used during spontaneous breathing when the primary abnormality is hypoxemia without hypercarbia, and when decreasing the work of breathing is not an important consideration. There are two methods used to apply PEEP during spontaneous breathing (Fig 18–1), expiratory positive airway pressure (EPAP) and continuous positive airway pressure (CPAP). With EPAP, the patient inspires at ambient airway pressure, but expires against positive pressure. During CPAP, airway pressure is positive throughout both inspiration and expiration. Although the apparatus for EPAP is less complicated and its effect on cardiovascular function is not as great, it is not as efficient in improving arterial oxygenation and increasing FRC as CPAP. In addition, work of breathing is greater with EPAP. In general, CPAP or EPAP can be used up to an end-expiratory pressure of 15 cm H_2O. Thereafter, the work of breathing becomes excessive, and mechanical ventilation usually is required.

In spite of its detrimental effects, PEEP is one of the major therapeutic modalities in the treatment of the respiratory distress syndromes. PEEP is indicated when the Pa_{O_2} is less than 60 torr and the inspired O_2 concentration (F_{IO_2}) is greater than 0.40–0.50. As shown in Figure 18–2, progressive increments in PEEP can produce a steady improvement in the Pa_{O_2} and intrapulmonary shunt fraction ($\dot{Q}_S/\dot{Q}_T$) in spite of a decrease in oxygen transport ($Ca_{O_2} \times \dot{Q}_T$), which is an indicator of oxygen delivery to the tissues. Therefore, monitoring of arterial blood gases alone cannot adequately determine the best level of PEEP. It is generally agreed that the best method of adjusting PEEP is to maximize oxygen transport. This requires placement of a thermodilution pulmonary artery catheter and repeated measurements of cardiac output after each increase in PEEP level. PEEP is increased in 3–5 cm H_2O increments until oxygen transport is maximized. If the Pa_{O_2} is still inadequate after these maneuvers, and the F_{IO_2} is greater than 0.50, use of volume expansion or vasopressors can be considered to increase the cardiac output so that more PEEP can be added.

Figure 18–2 also shows that the highest lung thorax compliance appears to coincide with the maximum level of oxygen transport with PEEP. If a pulmonary artery catheter cannot be used, measurement of compliance may provide a rough guide for the adjustment of PEEP therapy. However, this relationship is not precise, and

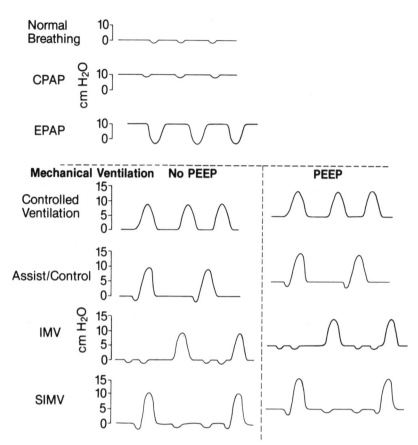

Fig 18–1.—Techniques of mechanical ventilation and methods of applying PEEP. The differences among various techniques of mechanical ventilation and methods of applying PEEP are illustrated according to their effects on airway pressure. Spontaneous inspiration is depicted as negative deflections from the baseline airway pressure at end-expiration, whereas mechanical inspiration is shown as positive deflections.

significant deviations may be present in individual patients.

It has also been suggested that PEEP should be increased to lower the $\dot{Q}s/\dot{Q}_T$ at an F_{IO_2} of 1.0 to less than 0.10. Volume expansion and vasopressors are used to compensate for the hemodynamic impairment produced by PEEP. This method of PEEP adjustment assumes that minimizing the $\dot{Q}s/\dot{Q}_T$ itself favorably alters the course of the underlying lung disease. There is little evidence to support this contention, and this method of PEEP therapy has little to recommend it.

Airway Management During Mechanical Ventilation

When endotracheal intubation is required to institute mechanical ventilation or to apply end-expiratory pressure, a tube with a high-compliance, low-pressure cuff should always be used. This will prevent the occurrence of tracheomalacia resulting from transmission of high-cuff pressures, which previously was frequently observed with low-compliance, high-pressure cuffed tubes. For several reasons, nasotracheal intubation is preferred over the oral route if in-

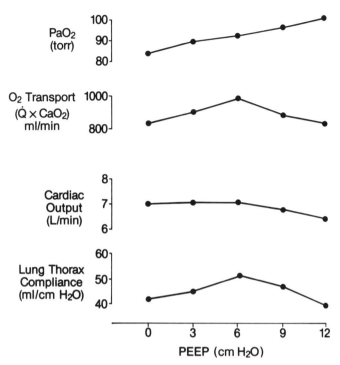

Fig 18–2.—Effects of increasing levels of PEEP on cardiac output, Pa_{O_2}, oxygen transport, and lung thorax compliance. Increasing increments of PEEP produce progressive improvement in the Pa_{O_2} in spite of an eventual reduction in cardiac output and oxygen transport. Lung thorax compliance parallels the changes in oxygen transport and may provide a noninvasive indicator of the effects of PEEP.

tubation is required for longer than one to two days. First, it is generally more comfortable for the patient. Second, nasal tubes are easier to maintain in the correct position, and thus inadvertent dislocation or extubation is less frequent. Last, nasal tubes produce less pressure damage in the larynx.

A source of some controversy is the question of when tracheostomy should be performed on patients who require prolonged mechanical ventilation. Although the use of high-pressure cuffs and consequent tracheal damage previously dictated tracheostomy after a few days of intubation, the advent of low-pressure cuffs has virtually eliminated this complication. Injury to the larynx however, is still produced by prolonged intubation, and has been suggested as an indication for continued early tracheostomy. Unfortunately, tracheostomy is not without its complications, such as late tracheal stenosis, erosion into the innominate artery, and infection at the stoma. Recent studies suggest that the complications from tracheostomy are much more frequent than those from prolonged intubation, especially since the complications from the latter usually spontaneously resolve after extubation. Therefore, in many intensive care units, endotracheal intubation is used for four to six weeks or longer before tracheostomy is considered.

Modes of Ventilation

Positive-pressure ventilation can be administered so that the level of ventilation is determined solely by the minute ventilation provided by the ventilator, or so that part or all of the minute ventilation is initiated by the patient. Schematic representation of the four major modes of ventilation is shown in Figure 18–1.

The patient is in the control mode when the

ventilator delivers breaths at a preset tidal volume and rate regardless of the patient's arterial blood gas levels or his own spontaneous respiratory efforts. Generally, patients are ventilated in this mode only by default, when their own respiratory efforts are lacking.

The assist mode is being used when the patient is allowed to initiate a ventilator breath by generating a fall drop in airway pressure with a spontaneous respiratory effort. The ventilator senses this fall in airway pressure and delivers a mechanical breath. This mode of ventilation allows the patient to set the level of ventilation without having to assume the work of breathing. In most circumstances, a backup ventilatory rate is preset so that if the patient's own respiratory efforts cease, the backup rate will be delivered. When a backup rate is utilized, this mode is referred to as assist/control.

Intermittent mandatory ventilation (IMV) and synchronized intermittent mandatory ventilation (SIMV) are two modes of ventilation in which spontaneous and mechanical ventilation are combined. With IMV the number of ventilator breaths per minute is preset, and the patient is allowed to breathe spontaneously between them. Therefore, total minute ventilation is divided between the patient's and the ventilator's contributions. SIMV is a blend of assist/control and spontaneous ventilation. The only difference between SIMV and IMV is that with the former the patient initiates each of the preset number of ventilator breaths. If there is no respiratory effort within a certain time interval, a ventilator breath is delivered automatically. It does not appear, however, that there is any clinical advantage to using SIMV instead of IMV.

Each of these modes of ventilation can be combined with PEEP. When the assist/control mode is combined with PEEP, the term "continuous positive-pressure ventilation" (CPPV) is used. IMV combined with PEEP is usually referred to as IMV with PEEP or IMV with CPAP.

A source of continuing controversy is whether it is preferable to ventilate using assist/control or one of the IMV modes. There are three major advantages to using assist/control ventilation. First, since the patient is able to control the ventilatory frequency, this mode of ventilation can compensate for changes in the patient's ventilatory requirements. Second, by almost eliminating spontaneous respiratory effort by the patient, respiratory oxygen consumption is minimized. This may be important in sepsis or cardiogenic shock, where oxygen consumption and the work of breathing should be reduced as much as possible. Third, the respiratory muscles are placed at nearly complete rest. The latter potential advantage may be important when respiratory muscle fatigue is a major contributing factor to acute respiratory failure. Several advantages have also been suggested for using IMV. First, since a major portion of the total minute ventilation is a result of spontaneous breathing, the mean intrathoracic pressure will be lower than with assist/control. Therefore, the hemodynamic impairment often observed with mechanical ventilation and PEEP may be less. Second, since the respiratory muscles are being continuously used with IMV, respiratory muscle function may be better maintained. Therefore, the duration of mechanical ventilation and the time required for weaning may be shorter than with assist/control. Third, the ability to breathe spontaneously may prevent the occurrence of asynchronous breathing and decrease the need for sedative agents. Last, by adjusting the relative contributions of the ventilator and the patient to total minute ventilation, it may be easier to maintain normocarbia. In spite of the theoretical advantages proposed for each mode of ventilation, there is little conclusive evidence to suggest that one mode is definitely superior in all cases. When choosing a ventilation mode for an individual patient, the following guidelines are suggested. Assist/control is preferable in cases where oxygen consumption and the work of breathing should be minimized and where fluctuations in neurologic status or respiratory drive, and hence the need for mechanical ventilation, are anticipated. IMV is preferable in patients with severe hemodynamic compromise, and in those who are markedly asynchronous with the ventilator, or have a severe respiratory alkalosis. In most other cases, the mode of ventilation used is probably not important.

Weaning from Mechanical Ventilation

Withdrawal from mechanical ventilatory support is one of the major therapeutic objectives in the treatment of respiratory failure. This process is referred to as weaning. Weaning cannot be considered until the patient is clinically and hemodynamically stable, and the underlying disease process responsible for acute respiratory failure is improving. If these general criteria are met, physiologic data are obtained to demonstrate adequacy of neuromuscular strength, oxygenation, and ventilation (Table 18–3). Weaning can generally proceed if a patient has a Pa_{O_2} of >70 torr while breathing a $F_{I_{O_2}}$ of <0.4 at a PEEP of ≤ 5 cm H_2O; a Pa_{CO_2} of <45 torr; a maximum inspiratory force (MIF) more negative than -25 cm H_2O, and a VC of >10–15 ml/kg.

A PEEP of ≤ 5 cm H_2O is not a contraindication to weaning; however, higher levels must be reduced in increments of 3–5 cm H_2O before weaning can commence. A PEEP reduction can usually be made safely when arterial oxygenation improves at a stable PEEP level, if the lung thorax compliance is unchanged or improving. Premature lowering of PEEP can cause significant hypoxemia, which may require a higher level of PEEP to correct than had been needed before.

There are two methods of ventilator weaning, IMV and the use of short periods of spontaneous breathing. With IMV, the ventilator rate is gradually reduced, allowing the patient to contribute an increasingly greater proportion of the minute ventilation as long as the arterial blood gas values do not deteriorate. Alternatively, a device known as a T-piece is placed at the proximal end of the patient's endotracheal tube to administer a known concentration of oxygen. The patient is then asked to breathe spontaneously for increasingly longer periods of time. These periods are interspersed between periods of mechanical ventilation. This method is known as the T-piece technique. Although IMV has been proposed as being extremely useful in weaning patients who have difficulty using a T-piece, there is little evidence that one method is superior to the other. If patients have difficulty weaning, attention should be directed at determining the reason for their problem. Poor nutrition and weakness, respiratory depressant medications, excessive secretions, and bronchospasm are examples of factors which prevent a patient from weaning.

After a patient has demonstrated that he can breathe spontaneously for 4–24 hours, his endotracheal or tracheostomy tube can be removed. Even so, such patients require close observation, since mechanical ventilation sometimes needs to be reinstituted.

TABLE 18–3.—PHYSIOLOGIC CRITERIA FOR WEANING

Mechanics	
Vital capacity	>10–15 ml/kg
Maximum negative inspiratory force	>25 cm H_2O
Work of breathing	<2.5 kg-m/min
Tidal volume	>5 ml/kg
Maximum minute ventilation	$>$Twice the minute ventilation
Oxygenation	
Pa_{O_2}	>70 torr (PEEP ≤ 5 cm H_2O and $F_{I_{O_2}} \leq 0.4$)
$P(A - a)O_2$ at $F_{I_{O_2}} = 1.0$	<300–350 torr
$\dot{Q}s/\dot{Q}T$ at $F_{I_{O_2}} = 1.0$	<0.1–0.2
Ventilation	
Pa_{CO_2}	35–45 torr
V_D/V_T	<0.6
Minute ventilation	<10 L/min

124   PATHOPHYSIOLOGY

READING LIST

Fairley H.B.: Physiologic effects of mechanical ventilatory support, in Merin R.G. (ed.): *28th Annual Refresher Course Lectures*. Chicago, American Society of Anesthesiologists, 1977, p. 133B.

In this article the physiologic consequences of mechanical ventilation on gas exchange and the pulmonary circulation is discussed with reference to normal individuals and specific disease states.

Froese A.B., Bryan C.A.: High frequency ventilation. *Am. Rev. Respir. Dis.* 123:249–250, 1981.

In this short editorial, the current status of high-frequency ventilation is briefly reviewed.

Hemmer M., Viquerat C.E., Suter P.M., et al.: Urinary antidiuretic hormone secretion during mechanical ventilation and weaning in man. *Anesthesiology* 52:395–400, 1980.

This study documents the increased secretion of ADH and negative free water clearance which occurs during mechanical ventilation.

Luce J.M., Pierson D.J., Hudson L.D.: Intermittent mandatory ventilation. *Chest* 79:678–685, 1981.

This is a good discussion of the indications for use of IMV.

Quan S.F., Hasan F.M.: Difficulties in weaning from mechanical ventilation. *Ariz. Med.* 37:622–625, 1980.

This is a concise review of the problems encountered in weaning patients from mechanical ventilation.

Stauffer J.L., Olson D.E., Petty T.L.: Complications and consequences of endotracheal intubation and tracheostomy: A prospective study of 150 critically ill adult patients. *Am. J. Med.* 70:65–76, 1981.

This is the only long-term prospective study of the complications of endotracheal intubation vs. tracheostomy. It demonstrates that tracheostomy is associated with a higher complication rate.

Stevens P.M.: Positive end-expiratory pressure breathing. *Basics RD* 5:1–6, 1977.

The physiology and indications for the use of PEEP are discussed.

Suter P.M., Fairley H.B., Isenberg M.D.: Optimum end-expiratory airway pressure in patients with acute pulmonary failure. *N. Engl. J. Med.* 242:284–289, 1975.

This is the classic article demonstrating the relationship between improvement in gas exchange with PEEP therapy and adverse consequences in cardiac output. It demonstrates the need for calculating oxygen transport during adjustments of PEEP.

Dyspnea

Mechanisms of Dyspnea

Dyspnea is the subjective sensation of uncomfortable, disordered, or difficult breathing. It is similar to fatigue, apprehension, pain, or malaise in that, like the communication of any experience, it involves both the perception of sensation and the patient's own interpretation of that sensation. Although we can measure objectively various indexes of pulmonary dysfunction, we cannot quantitate the patient's subjective perception of his respiratory discomfort. As would be expected, the correlation between measurements of dysfunction and degree of dyspnea is imperfect. Some patients with apparently satisfactory lung function complain of dyspnea; others, whose poor function should indicate a degree of dyspnea, deny it. Thus, the factors associated with dyspnea must include the patient's subjective sensitivity as well as functional factors such as increased respiratory work or decreased ventilatory capacity.

Virtually nothing is known at present concerning the neural pathways mediating the sensation of dyspnea. Various theories have been proposed, most of which involve perception of an imbalance between two or more of the following: (1) apparent need to breathe, (2) ventilatory drive, (3) work of breathing, (4) ventilation achieved, and (5) neural discharges to the respiratory muscles. No single factor can explain the occurrence of dyspnea in such diverse situations as paralysis of the respiratory muscles, exposure to high altitude, psychogenic disorders, and a variety of bronchopulmonary dis-

eases. In congestive heart failure there is a reasonably good correlation between dyspnea and loss of lung compliance. A correlation between dyspnea and severity of expiratory slowing is noted in chronic obstructive lung diseases. Indeed, in most respiratory disorders, the severity of dyspnea is more closely related to mechanical abnormalities than to blood gas disturbances.

Evaluation of the Dyspneic Patient

The patient usually describes his feelings as "shortness of breath." To determine the roots of this complaint, the physician must first seek answers to the following questions: What factors provoke the sensation? Considering those factors, is the sensation abnormal for an individual of this age and physical condition? Is the sensation one of fatigue, weakness, or chest discomfort rather than difficult, disordered breathing?

Having ascertained that the patient's sensation of shortness of breath is not confused with chest discomfort or explained by age or poor physical condition, the physician then should seek information concerning the objective phenomena that accompany the sensation of dyspnea. The abnormality of breathing should be described in detail, demonstrated by the patient or induced in the physician's presence. If the breathing at the time that dyspnea is noted would not be described as abnormal by an objective observer, the patient may be equating a variant of anginal pain, globus hystericus, or depressive reaction with shortness of breath.

The hyperventilation syndrome, which sometimes masquerades as an organic disorder, is characterized by repetitive deep, sighing respirations, a sensation of inability to expand the chest sufficiently, and a feeling of "not being able to take in enough air." The syndrome is often accompanied by numbness of extremities or lips, carpopedal spasm, light-headedness, or even loss of consciousness. These are all manifestations of acute hypocapnia and respiratory alkalosis.

It is sometimes difficult to distinguish episodic asthma from episodes of hyperventilation. Both may occur at rest, be associated with emotional upsets, and leave no evidence of disease between attacks. If the distinction is not clear from the history, it may be necessary to provoke an attack, testing the patient's ventilatory function and blood gases during the episode. But even between attacks, lung function studies may be helpful. Patients with the hyperventilation syndrome generally have completely normal spirometric tests. They may show frequent sighs during quiet breathing even when asymptomatic, and they frequently have a mild chronic reduction in Pa_{CO_2}. During an episode of dyspnea, Pa_{CO_2} falls markedly and is associated with marked alkalosis. In contrast, asthmatic patients frequently show spirometric evidence of mild airways obstruction that improves with bronchodilator use even between attacks, often have increased airways obstruction induced by exercise, and may be unusually susceptible to the bronchoconstrictor effects of inhaled methacholine. The possibility of recurrent pulmonary emboli should be kept in mind in evaluating patients with episodic, nonexertional dyspnea, even of an asthmatic type.

Slow, labored respirations, especially when accompanied by wheezes, are characteristic of airways obstructive disorders. Chronic airways obstruction is readily diagnosed or excluded by spirometric tests.

Marked tachypnea, resembling the breathing of a normal individual after heavy exercise, is more suggestive of pulmonary vascular congestion secondary to heart disease or a restrictive type of lung disease. Careful cardiac auscultation, radiologic evaluation of heart size, or electrocardiography will reveal some abnormality in almost all patients with a cardiac disorder. Chest radiology, spirometric tests, or blood gas analyses at rest and exercise will be abnormal in the vast majority of patients with bronchopulmonary disease leading to chronic dyspnea.

When the above-noted diagnostic procedures are normal, the physician must still consider severe anemia, primary pulmonary vascular disease, subtle interstitial lung disease not readily apparent on chest roentgenograms, and nonobstructive pulmonary emphysema. It has been reported that dyspnea may occur even in the absence of airways obstruction in some patients with emphysema, as has been noted in some having homozygous α_1-antitrypsin deficiency. To arrive at a final diagnosis in dyspnea of obscure origin, it may be necessary to undertake extensive studies, including measurements of lung volumes and diffusing capacity, inert gas distribution tests, lung scanning with radioisotopes, exercise tolerance tests, measurements of pressure-volume and flow-volume characteristics, α_1-antitrypsin studies, and even cardiac catheterization and angiographic studies.

There are very few patients with unexplained chronic exertional dyspnea in whom a specific diagnosis cannot be made. While in some the dyspnea may be psychogenic, most patients with shortness of breath of emotional origin can be distinguished as having variants of the hyperventilation syndrome. Unexplained dyspnea reminds us of the remaining areas of ignorance regarding the sensory receptors, afferent pathways, and integrative mechanisms responsible for the subjective sensation of dyspnea.

READING LIST

Campbell E.J.M., Agostoni E., Newsom-Davis J.: *The Respiratory Muscles; Mechanics and Neural* *Control.* Philadelphia and London, W.B. Saunders Co., 1970.

Parts of this book, and chapter 14 in particular, are pertinent to the understanding of the mechanisms of dyspnea.

Ciba Foundation Symposium: Porter R. (ed.): *Breathing: Hering Breuer Centenary Symposium.* London, J & A Churchill, 1970.

Similarly, portions of this symposium deal with the sensation we call dyspnea.

Howell J.B.L., Campbell E.J.M.: *Breathlessness.* Oxford, Blackwell Scientific Publications, 1966.

The sensation of breathlessness is also discussed in the published proceedings of this earlier symposium.

PART III

Bronchopulmonary Diseases

Disorders of Ventilatory Drive

A VARIETY OF clinical disorders may depress or stimulate ventilatory drive or otherwise alter the control of ventilation. Depression of ventilatory drive results in a decrease in alveolar ventilation and consequent hypercapnia, whereas stimulation increases alveolar ventilation and reduces Pa_{CO_2}. In the sleep disorders, there appear to be abnormalities in the coordination of ventilation which occur only during sleep in addition to depression of ventilatory drive. Table 20–1 outlines the general causes of abnormalities in the control of ventilation.

The most common causes of suppression of ventilatory drive are pharmacologic agents. Medications and drugs have different sites of action and affect respiration in a variety of ways, as indicated in Table 20–2. Their effect is influenced by various associated factors, including body temperature, sleep, anxiety, acidosis, alkalosis, exercise, and disease states.

A decreased ventilatory drive is readily diagnosed when overall hypoventilation and hypercapnia occur in a patient having an otherwise normal respiratory system. Before frank hypercapnia occurs, however, insensitivity of the respiratory center may sometimes be demonstrated by a decreased ventilatory response to carbon dioxide, i.e., by obtaining an abnormal carbon dioxide response curve (see chap. 3).

It is much more difficult to assess ventilatory drive in a patient with abnormal lung mechanics. However, it is helpful to remember that, in the presence of a normal ventilatory drive, hypercapnia is unusual in airways obstructive dis-

orders until the FEV_1 falls below 1 L. In patients with restrictive ventilatory impairment, hypercapnia rarely develops until the terminal state of illness as long as the ventilatory drive remains intact.

Demonstration of an abnormally low Pa_{CO_2} always indicates increased ventilatory drive. The degree of concomitant pH change helps to decide if the phenomenon is chronic, as may occur in high-altitude residents, or is the result of acute hyperventilation, often caused by anxiety concerning arterial puncture.

The clinical aspects of a few special cases of disordered ventilatory drive are discussed below. These include drug intoxication, the sleep apnea syndromes, sudden infant death syndrome (SIDS), hyperventilation, and advanced chronic obstructive airways disease.

Drug Intoxication
(Overdose, Poisoning)

Virtually all of the drugs known to depress the CNS have been associated at some time with overdose resulting in decreased alveolar ventilation. Overdoses of barbiturates, hypnotics, antidepressants, and narcotics are frequent causes of admissions to respiratory intensive care units and emergency rooms. Coma proceeds from class 0 (asleep but arousable) to class IV (areflexic with respiratory depression). Occasionally, as in the case of narcotic overdose, a specific antagonist may reverse the effects of the intoxicating drug. However, if rapid reversal is

TABLE 20–1.—ALTERATIONS IN
VENTILATORY CONTROL

Causes of decreased ventilatory drive
  Pharmacologic depression of ventilation
  CNS diseases
    Infections
    Tumors and general increases in intracranial pressure
    Vascular diseases
    Trauma
  Idiopathic (primary) hypoventilation
  Alkalosis and hyperoxia
Causes of increased ventilatory drive
  Psychogenic (including reactions to pain)
  Metabolic (fever, hyperthyroidism, bacteremia)
  CNS lesions (strokes, infections, pontine lesions)
  Hormones and drugs (catecholamines, salicylates,
    analeptics)
  Secondary to hypoxia and acidosis
  Ascent to high altitude
Sleep disorders
  Sleep apnea syndromes
  Sudden infant death syndrome

not possible when carbon dioxide retention and respiratory acidosis occur, indicating marked depression of ventilatory drive, endotracheal intubation with mechanical ventilatory support usually is needed. This allows time for the body to metabolize or excrete the excessive quantity of ingested drug, or for use of such measures as diuresis or charcoal hemoperfusion to accelerate or assist the body's clearance mechanisms.

In patients with preexisting respiratory insufficiency, relatively small doses of sedatives, narcotics, or even tranquilizers may cause sufficient reduction in ventilatory drive to lead to hypercapnia. Agents of this type should be avoided whenever possible in patients with severe bronchopulmonary diseases or respiratory muscle weakness.

Sleep Apnea Syndromes

The occurrence of periods of apnea during sleep was recognized by literary scholars for many years before the description in 1956 of a syndrome consisting of obesity, hypersomnolence, periodic breathing, hypoxemia, and right heart failure. It was termed the ''Pickwickian syndrome'' after the ''fat boy'' in Charles Dickens's *The Posthumous Papers of the Pickwick Club* published in 1837. Subsequently, it has been demonstrated that in many cases apnea during sleep is the primary abnormality producing this symptom complex, and that obesity is not a necessary prerequisite.

Apnea is defined as cessation of airflow past the mouth and nose for at least 10 seconds. The sleep apnea syndrome is present when there is documentation of greater than 30 of these episodes during both REM and non-REM sleep. Apneic episodes can be divided into three classifications: (1) central—absence of airflow and ventilatory efforts; (2) obstructive—absence of airflow despite ventilatory efforts; and (3) mixed—a combination consisting of an initial period of central apnea followed by obstructive apnea. Two factors appear to be important in producing apneic episodes during sleep. First, in obstructive apnea, the site of obstruction is located in the oropharynx. This appears to be related to a sudden loss of tone in the muscles surrounding the oropharynx just before the onset of inspiration. The decrease in intraluminal airway pressure with inspiration then results in airway collapse and obstruction. Second, in both central and obstructive apnea, ventilatory re-

TABLE 20–2.—ACTION SITES OF DRUGS AFFECTING RESPIRATION

SITE	EXAMPLE OF AGENT
Carotid and aortic chemoreceptors	Nicotine, oxygen
Pulmonary and coronary receptors	Veratridine
Respiratory chemocenters	Carbon dioxide, acidosis
CNS	Sedative-hypnotics, narcotics, amphetamines
Spinal nerve roots; intercostal nerves	Procaine
Skeletal neuromuscular junction	Tubocurare, neostigmine
Bronchioles	Atropine, epinephrine, histamine
Kidney (via acid-base changes)	Acetazolamide
Metabolic (via acid-base changes)	Aspirin, diuretics, etc.

sponsiveness to hypercarbia and hypoxia are depressed, suggesting that a decrease in ventilatory drive is also present. It is not understood, however, why either of these factors is present in patients with sleep apnea.

Sleep apnea occurs primarily in middle-aged men between the ages of 40 and 60. Its occurrence in women is almost completely limited to those who are postmenopausal. The clinical features associated with the sleep apnea syndromes are listed in Table 20–3. Repetitive episodes of apnea throughout the night produce a cyclical pattern consisting of apnea followed by arousal which leads to a markedly abnormal sleep pattern. With the obstructive form of apnea, snoring is almost a universal feature and may precede the occurrence of other symptoms for many years. Invariably, the snoring is so loud that the patient's bed partner sleeps in another room. Daytime hypersomnolence is also a frequent symptom with obstructive apnea; it may be so severe that the patient will fall asleep in the middle of a conversation or while driving a car. With central apnea, insomnia and frequent nocturnal awakenings are common symptoms. Although symptoms of a sleep disturbance are present in most cases of sleep apnea, these symptoms may not be the result of sleep deprivation. For example, it has been observed that the duration and number of apneic episodes in a sleep apnea patient with hypersomnolence are no different than in patients without this symptom. An alternative hypothesis is that hypersomnolence is related to the degree of oxygen desaturation. With all forms of sleep apnea, morning

TABLE 20–3.—CLINICAL FEATURES OF SLEEP APNEA

Snoring
Hypersomnolence
Insomnia
Abnormal motor activity during sleep
Morning headaches
Intellectual and personality changes
Sexual impotence
Systemic hypertension
Pulmonary hyptertension and cor pulmonale
Erythrocytosis
Arrhythmias
Possible sudden nocturnal death

headache and nausea may occur, simulating the symptoms of a brain tumor. Abnormal motor activity manifested by limb movement and walking during sleep is not uncommon. Psychological problems such as impotence, depression, intellectual deterioration, and enuresis are also a part of the symptom complex.

In addition to the psychological and sleep disturbances, a number of cardiovascular problems are also associated with the sleep apnea syndromes. Long periods of repetitive apnea produce large declines in oxygen saturation. If the syndrome is severe, this may result in pulmonary hypertension and secondary erythrocytosis. An increase in sympathetic discharge or tone during the periods of apnea may result in systemic hypertension. A variety of tachy- and bradyarrhythmias is also observed, which may be the cause of the sudden nocturnal death occasionally associated with this syndrome. Although these cardiovascular disturbances are initiated by physiologic abnormalities during sleep, they ultimately may continue into wakefulness, as demonstrated by the occurrence of cor pulmonale in severe sleep apnea.

The diagnosis of sleep apnea is usually suspected from the clinical presentation of a sleep disturbance in a middle-aged adult male. Definitive evidence is obtained with polysomnography. This procedure consists of the following clinical recordings: (1) EEG and electro-oculogram to determine sleep stages and abnormal cortical activity; (2) monitoring of respiratory airflow; (3) ECG to detect arrhythmias; (4) impedance pneumography, intercostal electromyography (EMG), or esophageal manometry to assess respiratory effort; and (5) ear oximetry or transcutaneous PO_2 monitoring to detect changes in arterial oxygen saturation. Examples of recordings in patients with obstructive and central apnea are shown in Figure 20–1. In addition to confirming the diagnosis of sleep apnea on polysomnography, it is necessary to determine whether there are associated medical conditions which may produce a secondary sleep apnea syndrome or may exacerbate the idiopathic syndrome. These are listed in Table 20–4.

The treatment for sleep apnea is determined

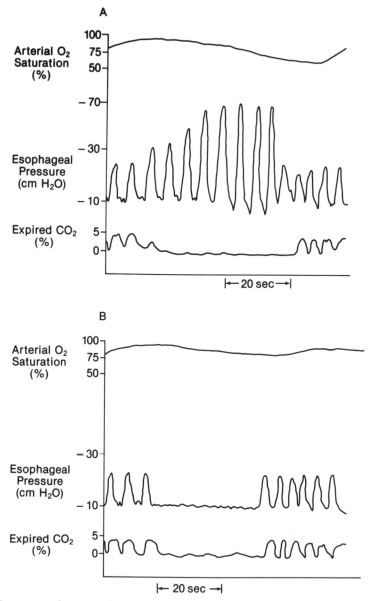

Fig 20–1.—**A,** tracings from a polysomnogram illustrating obstructive apnea. Airflow, as detected by changes in % expired CO_2, ceases for greater than 20 sec, but respiratory effort as measured by esophageal pressures progressively increases. O_2 saturation falls to a nadir of 75%. **B,** tracings from a polysomnogram showing an episode of central apnea. Both airflow and respiratory effort are absent. O_2 saturation decreases to 80%. (Adapted from Coaker L.A. and Quan S.F. Diagnosis and treatment of sleep apnea syndrome in adults. *Ariz. Med.* 38:448, 1981.)

TABLE 20–4.—CONDITIONS PREDISPOSING TO SECONDARY SLEEP APNEA

Upper airway abnormalities (hypertrophied tonsils/adenoids, masses)
Developmental anomalies of the jaw/neck/oropharynx (micrognathia)
Hypothyroidism
Brain stem lesions
Cervical spinal injury
Myotonic dystrophy
Encephalitis
Acromegaly
Shy-Drager syndrome
Goiter

by the type of apnea present and the severity of symptoms. In obstructive apnea, tracheostomy alleviates all of the symptoms, but is associated with significant social and physical debility. It is generally reserved for severe cases. Less severe cases may be helped by use of protriptyline, which appears to act by improving pharyngeal muscle tone during inspiration, or use of nocturnal mask CPAP (see chap. 18). In central apnea, pharmacologically increasing ventilatory drive with medroxyprogesterone or acetazolamide or use of phrenic nerve pacing may be helpful. With mixed apnea, a combination of the above approaches may be necessary. It must be emphasized that there are no firm guidelines in the treatment of sleep apnea, and therapy must be individualized for each patient.

Sudden Infant Death Syndrome

The leading cause of infant mortality between the ages of 1 and 12 months is the sudden infant death syndrome (SIDS), also known as crib death. The usual presentation is one of a previously healthy infant who is found dead after going to sleep for a nap or for the night. In the past, these deaths were attributed to various factors, such as infanticide, occult infection, or suffocation. However, current evidence suggests that these infants suffer from an abnormality of ventilatory control which places them at risk for sudden death.

SIDS appears to be more common in infants between 3 and 18 weeks old and in those who are of low birth weight. There is a slight male preponderance, and a racial predilection in that American Indians and blacks are at greater risk

than whites and Orientals. The incidence in siblings of SIDS infants is 4–7 times the random rate. In addition, two thirds of SIDS infants have been noted to have had a respiratory infection within two weeks of death.

Evidence that an abnormality in ventilatory control is important in the pathophysiology of SIDS has been obtained from a number of studies in "near-miss" SIDS infants (NMSIDS), a population at high risk for eventual death from SIDS. These data suggest that the duration of periodic breathing is greater in NMSIDS than in normal infants. In addition, NMSIDS infants appear to have impaired ventilatory responses to hypoxemia and hypercapnia. The exact role of these factors in producing sudden death, however, is not yet clear.

Clinical management in SIDS has focused on identification and treatment of high-risk infants (NMSIDS and siblings of SIDS victims). Detection of an increased risk is usually done by performing a polysomnogram as previously described or by doing home pneumograms. The latter is a tape recording of ECG, impedance pneumography, and instantaneous heart rate obtained from a home cardiorespiratory monitor. It is then analyzed for cardiorespiratory abnormalities. Infants found to be abnormal by either of these methods are placed on a home apnea monitoring program where their parents are instructed in the purpose of monitoring and in cardiopulmonary resuscitation. Central respiratory stimulants have also been used to decrease the number and duration of apneic episodes. Of these, theophylline has been the most widely used and has shown some efficacy.

Ventilatory Drive and Chronic Obstructive Lung Diseases

Chronic obstructive lung diseases alter lung function through two important mechanisms. First, the efficiency of gas exchange is impaired so that a greater minute ventilation is required to maintain a normal Pa_{CO_2}. Second, airways obstruction imposes an increased mechanical load on the respiratory bellows mechanism so that a greater amount of work is required to maintain an adequate minute ventilation. Therefore, it might be expected that in severe airways obstruction, the impairment in lung function eventually becomes so great that CO_2 retention inevitably occurs. Although it is clear that CO_2 retention in airways obstructive diseases usually is present only when the FEV_1 is less than 1.0 L, mechanical limitation of lung function does not appear to be the sole etiologic factor. It has been demonstrated that among patients with equivalent mechanical lung function, CO_2 retention occurs only in some. In these patients, other factors appear to be important in producing the CO_2 retention. Recent studies demonstrate that patients with chronic airways obstruction and CO_2 retention have a decrease in ventilatory drive and also exhibit a difference in respiratory timing compared with eucapneic subjects. Central ventilatory drive in response to hypercarbia is depressed in patients with chronic hypercapnia. Methods of measuring ventilatory drive were discussed in chapter 3. Many patients with CO_2 retention also are severely hypoxemic. In these latter patients, the peripheral chemoreceptor response to hypoxemia is blunted, a finding similar to that observed in high-altitude residents or children with cyanotic heart disease. This abnormality is not corrected with long-term oxygen administration. Respiratory timing in CO_2 retainers is also different than in eucapneic subjects in that the former exhibit more rapid and shallow tidal breathing. This breathing pattern results in an increase in the V_D/V_T, a decrease in alveolar ventilation, and hence an increase in Pa_{CO_2}.

Sleep disordered breathing has recently been observed to be quite prevalent in chronic obstructive lung diseases. In many patients frequent periods of apnea or hypopnea (decreased, but not complete cessation of airflow associated with arterial oxygen desaturation) produce severe declines in arterial oxygen saturation. Declines in arterial saturation are most severe during REM sleep, and may be related to a decrease in respiratory muscle tone or a decrease in ventilatory drive induced by REM sleep in these patients. In a small subgroup of patients with chronic airways obstruction who have apnea and hypoxemia during sleep, oxygen administration produces a prolongation of the apneic episodes. The clinical implications, however, of the high prevalence of sleep disordered breathing in such patients is not yet clear, and is a subject requiring further investigation.

Hyperventilation Syndrome (Anxiety Syndrome, Anxiety Neurosis)

In its most classic form, this syndrome presents as episodic shortness of breath, as discussed in chapter 19. But the ventilatory change itself is not always noticed by the patient, who may complain instead of other symptoms occurring as a consequence of hyperventilation. These symptoms may be classified as follows:

1. Central nervous system: faintness, dizziness, unsteadiness, impairment of consciousness and memory, feelings of unreality, loss of consciousness.

2. Peripheral nervous system: numbness; tingling; coldness of distal extremities, especially hands and face.

3. Muscular: muscle spasms, myalgias, coarse tremors, twitches, carpalpedal spasms with generalized tetany.

4. Respiratory: shortness of breath, tightness in or about the chest, sighing respirations, excessive yawning.

5. Cardiac: palpitations, tachycardia, "skip beats," atypical chest pains (usually momentarily sharp twinges around or lateral to the nipples, or more persistent dull aching pressure over the lower anterior chest).

6. Gastrointestinal: dryness of the mouth, dysphagia, bloating, belching, flatulence.

7. Psychic: anxiety, tension, apprehension pseudocalmness.

8. Constitutional: fatigue, weakness, insomnia, chronic exhaustion.

Most of these symptoms can be produced in the laboratory with induced chronic hyperventilation.

When patients suspected of having the hyperventilation syndrome perform routine spirometry, they tend to breathe with irregularity. There are frequent changes in the baseline, and the spirographic tracing shows intermittent deep sighs and brief periods of frank hyperventilation. Routine ventilatory tests are usually completely normal, but some individuals have difficulty performing the required ventilatory maneuvers. Measurements of respiratory function independent of voluntary effort, such as compliance, inert gas distribution, and diffusing capacity, are normal. Some patients have an abnormally large increase in ventilation in response to inhaled carbon dioxide. In patients with episodic dyspnea, severe respiratory alkalosis without hypoxemia during an attack is of definite value in confirming the diagnosis. Other patients may have chronic mild alkalosis and persistently low carbon dioxide tension. In the absence of any cause of a metabolic acidosis, an isolated finding of low bicarbonate on a serum sample should suggest this syndrome. Serum electrolytes frequently show low potassium and occasionally a decreased level of serum phosphorus.

READING LIST

Altose M.D., McCauley W.C., Kelson S.G., et al.: Effects of hypercapnia and flow resistive loading on respiratory activity in chronic airways obstruction. *J. Clin. Invest.* 59:500–507, 1977.

Demonstrates that hypercapneic patients with chronic airways obstruction have decreased responses to inhaled carbon dioxide.

Bradley C.A., Fleetham J.A., Anthonisen N.R.: Ventilatory control in patients with hypoxemia due to obstructive lung disease. *Am. Rev. Respir. Dis.* 120:21–30, 1979.

This study demonstrates that hypoxemic patients with chronic airways obstruction have decreased ventilatory responses to hypoxemia and CO_2.

Clark R.W.: Sleep apnea. *Primary Care* 6:653–679, 1979.

A good general review of the diagnosis and treatment of sleep apnea.

Coaker L.A., Quan S.F.: Diagnosis and treatment of sleep apnea syndrome in adults. *Ariz. Med.* 38:446–450, 1981.

A concise review of the pathophysiology, diagnosis, and treatment of sleep apnea.

Guilleminault C., Cummiskey J., Dement W.C.: Sleep apnea syndrome: recent advances. *Adv. Intern. Med.* 26:347–372, 1980.

A comprehensive review of sleep apnea.

Guilleminault C., Cummiskey J., Mott J.: Chronic obstructive airflow disease and sleep. *Am. Rev. Respir. Dis.* 122:397–406, 1980.

This study demonstrates that many patients with chronic airways obstruction have sleep disordered breathing, and in some tracheostomy was beneficial.

Javaheri S., Blum J., Kazemi H.: Pattern of breathing and carbon dioxide retention in chronic obstructive lung disease. *Am. J. Med.* 71:228–234, 1981.

In this study, patients with severe chronic airways obstruction and CO_2 retention were found to have a more rapid respiratory rate and a larger VD/VT than eucapneic subjects.

Kelly D.H., Shannon D.C.: Periodic breathing in infants with near-miss sudden infant death syndrome. *Pediatrics* 63:355–360, 1979.

This study found that the duration of periodic breathing in "near-miss SIDS" infants was greater than in normal subjects.

Littner M.R., McGinty D.H., Arand D.L.: Determinants of oxygen desaturation in the course of ventilation during sleep in chronic obstructive pulmonary disease. *Am. Rev. Respir. Dis.* 122:849–857, 1980.

Demonstrates that patients with chronic airways obstruction develop sleep-related desaturation from impaired ventilatory responses to hypoxia and hypercapnia.

Shannon D.C., Kelly D.H., O'Connell K.: Abnormal regulation of ventilation in infants at risk for sudden infant death syndrome. *N. Engl. J. Med.* 297:747–750, 1977.

In this study, "near-miss SIDS" infants were found to have abnormal ventilatory responses to inhaled carbon dioxide.

Valdes-Dapena M.A.: Sudden infant death syndrome: a review of the medical literature 1974–1979. *Pediatrics* 66:597–614, 1980.

A comprehensive review of the epidemiologic, clinical, and pathologic aspects of SIDS.

Wynne J.W., Block J.A., Hemenway J., et al.: Disordered breathing and oxygen desaturation during sleep in patients with chronic obstructive lung disease. *Am. J. Med.* 66:573–579, 1979.

A study of the frequency and severity of sleep-disordered breathing in chronic airways obstructive diseases.

Neuromuscular Diseases

Respiratory Muscle Weakness or Paralysis

Any neurologic or muscular disease that affects the respiratory muscles may result in alteration of pulmonary function. A list of disorders commonly leading to ventilatory impairment is provided in Table 21–1. When severe, such neuromuscular disorders may cause respiratory failure with frank hypercapnia, but even at an earlier stage there may be sufficient dysfunction to produce dyspnea. When pulmonary function is measured in such patients, there is a loss of VC and often a decrease in maximum voluntary ventilation, but measures of expiratory flow are well preserved. Characteristics that help to distinguish neuromuscular disorders from other causes of a reduced VC are discussed in chapter 13. It should be remembered that patients with impaired respiratory muscle function may show

TABLE 21–1.—NEUROMUSCULAR DISEASES ASSOCIATED WITH VENTILATORY IMPAIRMENT

Muscular
  Dystrophies
  Myotonias
  Polymyositis
Myoneural junction disorders
  Myasthenia gravis
  Botulism
  Tetanus
  Pharmacologic agents (curare-like drugs, anticholinesterases, some antibiotics)
Neurologic
  Guillain-Barré syndrome
  Poliomyelitis
  Amyotrophic lateral sclerosis

extreme sensitivity to respiratory depressant medications and medications which may impair neuromuscular transmission. In such patients narcotics, sedatives, and muscle relaxants should be avoided. Aminoglycoside and polymyxin antibiotics and several cardiovascular agents, such as procainamide, quinidine, and propranolol, must also be used with caution.

Determination of the maximum negative inspiratory pressure or force (MIF) is a useful indicator of respiratory muscle strength. In a less direct way, the VC also provides an index of the progress of a neuromuscular disorder that involves the respiratory muscles. When there is a progressive decline in VC or MIF, the patient must be monitored closely for hypoventilation. Although ventilatory assistance is indicated in the presence of frank hypercapnia, once the VC is less than 15 ml/kg or the MIF is less negative than -25 cm H_2O, some form of ventilatory assistance is required even in the absence of hypercapnia. When respiratory muscle weakness is of this severity, patients are generally unable to generate an effective cough or sigh, which results in retained secretions and atelectasis. Occasionally, ventilatory assistance may be indicated in patients with marginal indices of respiratory muscle strength in order to relieve dyspnea, rest the respiratory muscles, and allow sleep. The type of assistance required depends on the specific clinical state and ranges from a rocking bed to assisted ventilation during sleep to totally controlled ventilation (see chap. 18). When a disease is potentially reversible, as with myasthenia gravis, Guillain-Barré syndrome, or poliomyelitis, it is sometimes better to begin some type of ventilatory assistance as soon as the progressive decline in respiratory muscle function is observed.

Diaphragmatic Paralysis

Hemidiaphragmatic paralysis occurs commonly as a result of interruption of phrenic nerve function. In the past, a common cause was phrenic nerve crush used in treatment of tuberculosis. Diaphragmatic paralysis still results occasionally from surgical procedures in the area of the neck or mediastinum. More commonly, hemidiaphragmatic paralysis results from intrathoracic tumors involving the phrenic nerve. Idiopathic paralysis of the hemidiaphragm also occurs. When unassociated with other disease, it is usually benign.

The diagnosis of unilateral paralysis of the diaphragm usually is first suspected because of an elevated hemidiaphragm on chest roentgenogram or physical examination. Paralysis must be distinguished from a thinning and weakness (eventration) of the diaphragm and from elevations resulting from a subdiaphragmatic lesion, loss of lung volume on that side, or pleural disease that fixes the hemidiaphragm in an elevated position. The various causes of elevation of the hemidiaphragm cannot be reliably differentiated on physical examination. With true paralysis, however, paradoxical motion of the diaphragm is noted on fluoroscopy during rapid ventilatory maneuvers such as sniffing.

Loss of hemidiaphragm function produces a decrease of lung volume and maximum ventilatory capacity, which is accentuated in the supine position. Any preexisting lung function impairment will be increased as a result of loss of diaphragmatic function, but in the absence of underlying lung disease, most patients are asymptomatic.

With the decreasing incidence of diphtheritic polyneuritis and poliomyelitis, bilateral paralysis of the diaphragm is rare. However, it still is observed in severe cases of various polyneuropa-thies and myopathies. It results in a marked reduction in VC and some decrease in expiratory air flow. Arterial hypoxemia has been described in patients with bilateral diaphragmatic paralysis, a consequence of maldistribution of ventilation and perfusion. Both hypoxemia and the ventilatory abnormalities are exaggerated in the supine position and during sleep. Such patients regularly complain of orthopnea.

In the appropriate clinical setting, bilateral diaphragmatic paralysis may be suspected in the presence of otherwise unexplained hypoventilation, and supine paradoxical inspiratory inward movement of the abdomen. The ultimate test to prove the diagnosis is measurement of the maximal change in transdiaphragmatic pressure (P_{di}) gradient from FRC to TLC obtained by simultaneous recording of esophageal and gastric pressures. Change in P_{di} should be greater than 25 cm H_2O in normal individuals, but is generally less than 6 cm H_2O in patients with bilateral diaphragmatic paralysis. Unlike hemidiaphragmatic paralysis, motion of the diaphragms on fluoroscopy may be misleading owing to diaphragmatic movement induced by contraction and relaxation of the abdominal muscles.

Treatment of bilateral diaphragmatic paralysis depends on the severity of ventilatory impairment and the patient's underlying disease. Some form of mechanical ventilatory assistance is frequently required, although in some patients electric pacing of the phrenic nerve or diaphragm has been successfully used. The prognosis for bilateral diaphragmatic paralysis is generally poor, since most of the diseases responsible for the condition are chronic. However, spontaneous remission may occur after paralysis resulting from an infectious polyneuritis.

Respiratory Muscle Fatigue

Fatigue of the respiratory muscles can be produced by excessive ventilatory workloads and may eventually result in hypoventilation. Factors contributing to the development of respiratory muscle fatigue include increased work of breathing, diminished respiratory muscle strength, respiratory muscle insufficiency, and the unavailability of energy-producing substrates for optimal respiratory muscle function.

Examples of clinical situations in which fatigue of the respiratory muscles are thought to contribute to hypoventilation include the adult respiratory distress syndrome (ARDS), neuromuscular diseases, exacerbations of obstructive airways disease, and severe hypoxemia. In ARDS, a decrease in lung compliance and an increase in dead space ventilation both result in an increase in the work of breathing. In addition, hypoxemia may contribute to suboptimal respiratory muscle function. Airways obstructive disorders are characterized by an increase in airways resistance, which increases the work of breathing. There is also hyperinflation of the lungs, which results in a decrease in muscle strength by abnormally lengthening inspiratory muscles so that they are less efficient in developing tension. This is a major problem in status asthmaticus (see chap. 27).

It is important to recognize the significance of respiratory muscle fatigue in patients with neuromuscular disease. Sufficient muscle function may remain to allow maintenance of adequate minute ventilation for a brief period. However, sustaining a normal minute ventilation for a prolonged period may be an excessive load for weak respiratory muscles, and therefore progressive hypoventilation may result from fatigue even without worsening of the underlying disease.

READING LIST

Arzov Z., Mastaglia F.L.: Disorders of neuromuscular transmission caused by drugs. *N. Engl. J. Med.* 301:409–413, 1979.

Discusses the pathophysiology of drug induced disorders of neuromuscular transmission.

Bergofsky E.H.: Respiratory failure in disorders of the thoracic cage. *Am. Rev. Respir. Dis.* 118:581–601, 1978.

A review of the pathophysiology of respiratory failure produced by nonparenchymal lung disease.

Derenne J-Ph., Macklem P.T., Roussos C.: The respiratory muscles: mechanics, control, and pathophysiology (pt. III). *Am. Rev. Respir. Dis.* 118:581–601, 1978.

A review of the role of respiratory muscles in respiratory failure.

Leventhal S.R., Orkin F.K., Hirsch R.A.: Prediction of the need for postoperative mechanical ventilation in myasthenia gravis. *Anesthesiology* 53:26–30, 1980.

A study which identifies the factors predictive of postoperative mechanical ventilation in myastheniagravis.

Luce J.M., Huseby J.S., Marini J.J.: Bilateral diaphragmatic paralysis as a cause of respiratory failure. *West. J. Med.* 132:456–460, 1980.

Demonstrates that diaphragmatic muscle paralysis can present as acute respiratory failure.

Macklem P.T.: Respiratory muscles: the vital pump. *Chest* 78:753–758, 1980.

A discussion of respiratory muscle fatigue.

McMichan J.L., Piepgras D.G., Gracey D.R., et al.: Electrophrenic respiration. *Mayo Clin. Proc.* 54:662–668, 1979.

A discussion of the use of pacing in diaphragmatic paralysis.

Newsom-Davis J., Goldman M., Loh I., et al.: Diaphragmatic function and alveolar hypoventilation. *Quart. J. Med.* 45:87–100, 1976.

A review of the effect of diaphragmatic muscle function in alveolar ventilation.

22

Chest Wall Abnormalities

RESPIRATORY DYSFUNCTION of varying degrees may result from abnormalities or alterations in structure of the chest wall. Temporary alteration in the stability of the chest wall may follow trauma or be the aftermath of a surgical procedure. Fixed chest wall deformities may be congenital, the result of a disease process, or deliberately produced surgically.

Chest Wall Instability

The most common chest wall injury is simple rib fracture. As the result of associated pain and muscle splinting, there is immediate voluntary restriction of tidal volume, compensatory increase in respiratory rate, and voluntary inhibition of the cough reflex. Normal young persons tolerate these changes well. In many elderly persons, and particularly when there is an underlying lung disease, these changes may lead to impaired clearance of secretions, bronchopulmonary infection, worsening of blood gas abnormalities, and even acute respiratory failure. Chest strapping, which further restricts lung volumes, and administration of analgesics, which depress respiration and suppress the cough reflex, only compound the problem. The treatment of choice is relief of pain. When only a few ribs are fractured, judicious use of analgesics may be helpful and will reduce pain and muscle splinting. In more severe cases with multiple fractures, relief of pain by intercostal nerve block may be necessary to produce comfort and allow full chest expansion.

Alterations in function similar to those caused by rib fracture may occur in the immediate postoperative period following simple thoracotomy. A temporary shift of lung perfusion away from the side operated on has also been demonstrated.

A major defect in chest wall continuity with loss of normal thoracic musculoskeletal support results in paradoxical motion of the affected chest wall—"flail chest." Crushed chest injuries with multiple rib fractures, surgical resection of portions of chest wall, or thoracoplasty (decostalization) before skeletal regeneration can produce this phenomenon. As pleural pressure changes during the respiratory cycle, the unsupported chest wall moves in a direction opposite to the normally supported chest wall. This is shown for an abnormality on the right side in Figure 22–1. When intrathoracic pressure is decreased during inspiration, the injured chest wall is pulled inward while the normal chest is expanding. There is also a shift of the mediastinum away from the affected side, with inspiration such that both lungs actually expand and contract synchronously. Overall efficiency of ventilation, however, still is impaired. It has been postulated that the paradoxical chest wall movement would be accompanied by movement of air from one lung to the other, but evidence suggests that this occurs only in the presence of upper airway obstruction.

In spite of the unstable chest wall present in flail chest, in most cases the respiratory disturbance is primarily related to underlying lung contusion, chest wall pain, and decreased cough efficiency. These factors promote retention of

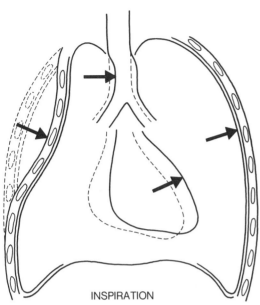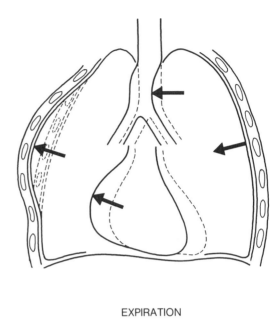

INSPIRATION   EXPIRATION

Fig 22–1.—Mechanical instability of the chest wall (flail chest). *Arrows* indicate direction of motion. Note the paradoxical motion of the unstable portion of chest wall on the right side.

secretions, atelectasis, inflammation, and pneumonitis. Unless there is very severe disruption of the thoracic cage, respiratory insufficiency is poorly related to the degree of chest wall instability. In fact, mortality appears most closely associated with nonrespiratory conditions, such as shock and injuries to other organs.

Treatment of flail chest involves insuring adequate oxygenation and ventilation and appropriate care of injuries sustained by other organ systems. In the patient with a mild to moderate flail chest who is able to maintain adequate ventilation, supplemental oxygen and intercostal or thoracic epidural nerve blocks may be sufficient. In a patient with obvious respiratory insufficiency, mechanical ventilation should be instituted. Surgical stabilization of the chest wall is generally not beneficial.

Fixed Chest Wall Deformities

The type and severity of fixed chest wall deformity determine the degree of cardiorespiratory dysfunction that may result. Four major types of deformity have been well defined: ky-phoscoliosis, ankylosing spondylitis, pectus excavatum and healed thoracoplasty.

Kyphoscoliosis is characterized by angulation of the thoracic spine both laterally and posteroanteriorly. Neurologic and neuromuscular diseases, such as poliomyelitis and tuberculosis of the thoracic spine, are common causes of severe deformities, whereas congenital or idiopathic kyphoscoliosis is usually less severe. Of the four major types of deformity, kyphoscoliosis produces the most severe degree of dysfunction. The deformity and decreased mobility of the bony thorax lead to an increase in the work of breathing. The observed shallow breathing results in a decrease in alveolar ventilation, in spite of an increase in overall ventilation. As a result of the asymmetrical deformity, unequal distribution of ventilation and perfusion occurs, the consequent physiologic shunting leading to hypoxemia. When overall ventilation is severely limited, hypercapnia, respiratory acidosis, and severe hypoxemia may result. Pulmonary arterial hypertension is common, and cor pulmonale is the usual cause of death. Back braces may be useful in correcting the abnormality in young patients. In selected more advanced cases surgical correction is beneficial. In severe deformity treatment is more often directed toward alleviating symptoms.

Ankylosing spondylitis, with vertebral joint immobilization and ossification of paravertebral ligaments, is characterized by symmetrical reduction in mobility of the bony thorax. Diaphragmatic motion is little affected, and uniformity of lung function is unchanged. Rib fixation and increased stiffness of the chest wall result in mild restrictive impairment, but symptomatic respiratory insufficiency is uncommon in the absence of associated bronchopulmonary disease.

Pectus excavatum, or funnel chest, is a congenital deformity in which the lower end of the sternum is attached to the spine by fibromuscular bands. This deformity is rarely associated with significant pulmonary dysfunction and, if subjective complaints are present at all, they are usually attributable to cardiac displacement. The defect is readily amenable to surgical correction early in life, but the indications for such surgery are usually cosmetic rather than functional.

Thoracoplasty is a surgically induced depression of the thoracic cage. The fixed deformity is a result of skeletal regeneration from the periostea left in situ following surgical resection of ribs. Since the procedure is performed for an underlying lung disease, subsequent pulmonary dysfunction is usually more closely related to the original disease than to the chest wall deformity.

READING LIST

Birath G., Soderholm B.: Bronchospirometric investigations before and after a small thoracoplasty. *Am. Rev. Tuberc.* 75:724–729, 1957.

Documents that loss of pulmonary function after thoracoplasty is primarily due to preexisting lung disease.

Kafer E.R.: Respiratory and cardiovascular functions in scoliosis and the principles of anesthetic management. *Anesthesiology* 52:339–351, 1980.

A review of respiratory and cardiovascular problems in kyphoscoliosis.

Maloney J.V., Jr., Schmutzer K.J., Raschke E.: Paradoxical respiration and "pendelluft." *J. Thorac. Cardiovasc. Surg.* 41:291–298, 1961.

Disproves the existence of pendelluft in flail chest.

Sankaran S., Wilson R.F.: Factors affecting prognosis in patients with flail chest. *J. Thorac. Cardiovasc. Surg.* 60:402–410, 1970.

Demonstrates that prognosis in flail chest is influenced by concomitant nonrespiratory injuries.

Travis D.M., Cook C.D., Julian D.G., et al.: The lungs in rheumatoid spondylitis: gas exchange and lung mechanics in a form of restrictive pulmonary disease. *Am. J. Med.* 29:623–632, 1960.

A study of pulmonary function in patients with ankylosing spondylitis.

Webb A.K.: Flail chest—management and complications. *Br. J. Hosp. Med.* 20:406–411, 1978.

A review of the management of flail chest.

Weg J.G., Krumholz R.A., Harkleroad L.E.: Pulmonary dysfunction in pectus excavatum. *Am. Rev. Respir. Dis* 96:936–945, 1967.

A review of pulmonary function in patients with pectus excavatum.

Wilson R.F., Murray C., Antonenko D.R.: Nonpenetrating thoracic injuries. *Surg. Clin. North Am.* 57:17–36, 1977.

A review of the major causes of nonpenetrating thoracic trauma.

23

Diseases of the Pleural Space

NORMALLY, the visceral and parietal pleural surfaces are in apposition, gliding over each other during respiratory movements and lining what is only a potential space. Under abnormal conditions, the pleural space may be invaded by air, fluid, or organized fibrous tissue. A suppurative process in the pleural space may be localized empyema or generalized pyothorax. As such a process heals, or when blood in the pleural cavity organizes, fibrous tissue is laid down, resulting in fibrothorax. The pleura may also be the site of metastatic tumors or of primary mesotheliomas.

Pneumothorax

Air may enter the pleural space spontaneously from pulmonary structures or be introduced either deliberately or as a result of trauma. The most common cause of traumatic pneumothorax is penetration of the lung by a fractured rib.

Acute spontaneous pneumothorax is a potentially serious complication of many parenchymal lung diseases such as tuberculosis, emphysema, primary or metastatic pulmonary malignancies, and a number of interstitial lung diseases, especially eosinophilic granuloma, lymphangioleiomyomatosis, and pulmonary tuberous sclerosis. It may also occur in patients receiving mechanical ventilation with PEEP. However, it occurs most commonly in otherwise healthy young adult males as a consequence of rupture of small subpleural blebs. Such blebs are usually multiple and situated over the apex of the lung. In young persons who have had a spontaneous pneumothorax, there is a 10% likelihood of pneumothorax occurring later on the opposite side and a greater chance of recurrence on the same side. Spontaneous pneumothorax is also common between the ages of 45 and 65, presumably because of the high prevalence of emphysema in this age group.

Surgically induced pneumothorax is a part of every thoracotomy or penetrating chest wound. An open defect in the chest wall allows free passage of air and has been called a "sucking wound." Some degree of pneumothorax also may occur with thoracentesis. Although this is often ascribed to inward leakage of air through the thoracentesis needle, it is probably as often a result of puncture of the lung during the procedure.

Chest pain of sudden onset is the most common symptom of spontaneous pneumothorax. The pain usually subsides in a few hours, and, unless the pneumothorax is large, the dyspnea that often accompanies the pain disappears after 24 hours even in the absence of significant lung reexpansion.

Physical signs in a large pneumothorax include tracheal deviation and unilateral tympany over the chest. A decrease in vesicular sounds and some faint bronchial breathing may be noted over the affected side. In patients receiving mechanical ventilation and PEEP, the only clue to the development of a pneumothorax may be a sudden decrease in Pa_{O_2} or an increase in the peak inspiratory airway pressure.

A definitive diagnosis is generally made from chest roentgenograms. A small pneumothorax is difficult to diagnose from physical examination and may even be missed on routine upright inspiratory roentgenograms. The abnormality may be more obvious on a roentgenogram taken on expiration. Bullous disease of the lung may be confused with pneumothorax and may require special radiologic techniques, such as tomograms, to clarify the diagnosis.

Since pleural pressure is negative with respect to pressure within parenchymal air spaces, rupture of the lung surface permits air to leak into the pleural space. The lung is then allowed to collapse due to its own elastic recoil. The air leak will continue until the decrease in lung size is adequate to allow closure of the leak. Thus, the degree of lung collapse and mediastinal shift is related to the size of the leak. Continued leak of air into the pleural space may lead to chronic pneumothorax.

Physiologic consequences of pneumothorax depend on its size and on the integrity of the underlying lung. Acute hypoxemia occurs as a result of perfusion of the poorly ventilated collapsed lung. This tends to improve in a matter of hours as perfusion of the collapsed lung diminishes. Serial observations of pulmonary function in otherwise healthy adults with spontaneous pneumothorax show a loss of lung volume, decreased lung compliance, decreased diffusing capacity, poor intra-alveolar distribution of inspired gas, and some degree of physiologic shunting. All of these functional alterations improve as the collapsed lung reexpands. In otherwise healthy young adults, these changes are of relatively little consequence, and a small pneumothorax may be asymptomatic. But in the patient with severe chronic respiratory insufficiency, the additional dysfunction associated with the pneumothorax may be sufficient to precipitate severe hypoxemia and hypercapnia. In such cases, prompt diagnosis and treatment are essential.

Occasionally, a ball-valve mechanism allows air to be pumped into the pleural space, particularly during the effort of coughing, resulting in progressively increasing intrapleural pressure. In such a "tension pneumothorax," the mediastinal shift toward the opposite side may be pronounced, compromising function of the opposite lung and leading to severe respiratory distress. With the increase in intrathoracic pressure, venous return is impeded, leading to circulatory collapse as well. In an open pneumothorax due to trauma or "sucking chest wound," large amounts of air may be entrained through the defect in the chest wall, thereby preventing any inflation of the ipsilateral lung. This may result in severe, life-threatening hypoxemia.

A small, relatively asymptomatic pneumothorax may be allowed to absorb spontaneously. Bilateral or tension pneumothoraxes should be decompressed without delay, initially by needle aspiration and then by chest intubation. Chest intubation and continuous suction will hasten the resolution of a large pneumothorax; such therapy is imperative in patients with severely compromised lung function. Use of a chest tube not only hastens removal of the air but also results in enough pleural irritation to induce some adhesions, lessening the probability of recurrent episodes. Occasionally, persistent leak of air from the lung requires surgical closure of the lung rupture.

Because of the likelihood of continued recurrences of spontaneous pneumothorax, creation of pleural symphysis must be considered in patients with recurrent episodes. This usually involves scarification of the pleural surface or parietal pleurectomy together with resection of subpleural blebs.

In a large, life-threatening, open pneumothorax, the chest wall defect should be occluded immediately. Surgical closure of the chest wall defect and repair of any lung parenchymal injuries should then be undertaken, followed by chest intubation and continuous suction.

Occasionally, especially after prolonged pneumothorax, adequate reexpansion of the lung is prevented by adhesions, pulmonary fibrosis, or obstructive atelectasis from mucus impaction. With absorption or removal of air, very negative pressures may occur in the pleural cavity, usually leading to pleural effusion. When the underlying problem cannot be corrected, it may be necessary to perform a thoracoplasty to eliminate the persisting pleural space. In general, this is indicated primarily when there is a frank bronchopleural fistula resulting in empyema, a condition often seen in tuberculosis prior to effective chemotherapy. Even in the absence of infection, inability of the collapsed lung to expand (common in the past when pneumothorax was used in the treatment of tuberculosis) leads to effusion, fibrin deposition, and fibrothorax after the pneumothorax absorbs.

Considerable information can be obtained from measurements of intrapleural pressure in patients with persistent pneumothorax. High negative pressures indicate inability of the lung to expand despite closing of the air leak. Persistence of pressures near atmospheric indicates a persisting leak. When continuous suction through a chest tube is being applied and pressures remain near atmospheric, the rate of leak from the lung must exceed the rate of aspiration of air. Additional or larger tubes may be needed, or surgical intervention may be indicated.

Fibrothorax

In the creation of pleural symphysis, the visceral and parietal pleurae are fused, but simple obliteration of the pleural space has not itself been shown to impair lung function. Even a degree of fibrous thickening of the pleura in the costophrenic angle, quite common following any pleural inflammation, does not seriously impair lung function. Development of more extensive fibrothorax, however, can lead to significant respiratory insufficiency. Such extensive fibrosis is most often the late result of organization and resolution following tuberculous effusion, healed empyema, or traumatic hemothorax. Progression and contracture reduce mobility, narrow intercostal spaces, reduce the volume of the hemithorax, and displace the mediastinum toward the affected side.

Physical findings of a fixed, contracted hemithorax with markedly diminished breath sounds and dullness to percussion, together with a history of a predisposing event, suggest the diagnosis of fibrothorax. Roentgenographic evidence of pleural thickening is characteristic. However, the functional importance of the lesion should not be judged from the degree of radiopacity it produces. Functional impairment is more closely related to the amount of contraction and restriction of motion of the involved hemithorax.

The confining fibrous layer produces a restrictive ventilatory abnormality with loss of lung volume and diminished VC. Surprisingly, perfusion is usually reduced out of proportion to the reduction in ventilation. Arterial blood gas composition is either normal or reveals mild hypoxemia. In patients with bilateral lung disease, the distribution of ventilation and perfusion found on bronchospirometry or lung scanning may help to decide how much of the overall functional abnormality is a result of the fibrothorax.

If the underlying lung parenchyma is normal, early decortication with removal of the fibrous peel and reexpansion of the lung results in marked improvement in ventilation, gas exchange, and pulmonary artery pressure. If the fibrothorax has been present for many years, immediate improvement following decortication is less dramatic, but function may continue to improve for many months following operation. The degree of anticipated improvement is related to the extent of previously existing parenchymal disease. Thus, the functional improvement following decortication in patients with tuberculosis may be disappointing, whereas decortication for traumatic hemothorax is usually attended by good functional recovery.

Pleural Effusion

Normally, there is only a small amount of fluid present in the pleural space at any time, and this fluid is constantly being exchanged. The forces which govern fluid movement in the pleural space have been described in chapter 5. Pleural effusions develop when these forces are disrupted and are usually a result of one of the following four basic mechanisms: (1) increased hydrostatic pressure in the systemic circulation, (2) decreased colloid oncotic pressure of the blood, (3) lymphatic obstruction, or (4) increased pleural capillary permeability secondary to inflammatory or neoplastic involvement of the pleura.

The characteristic physical signs of pleural effusion are dullness or flatness to percussion and diminished breath sounds over the area of fluid accumulation. A pleuritic type of pain occurs only if there is some inflammatory change in the pleura, but a more constant type of discomfort is present not infrequently in any large pleural effusion. In the absence of underlying respiratory impairment, 2,000 ml or more of fluid may accumulate before the patient begins to experience dyspnea. On chest roentgenogram there are the characteristic findings of diffuse opacification in the dependent portion of the affected hemithorax with blunting of the costophrenic angle.

The minimum unilateral accumulation of pleural fluid that can be detected on the standard chest roentgenogram is probably about 250 ml, although smaller volumes may be detected in the lateral decubitus position or by special radiographic techniques. Considerably larger volumes are usually needed for the effusion to be detected on physical examination. In the presence of loculation of the fluid, however, it may be difficult to differentiate an effusion from other types of radiopacities without special radiographic studies.

Fluid in the intrapleural space acts as a space-occupying mass. The result is a decrease in lung volume on the involved side proportional to the size of the fluid collection. The effusion causes a mediastinal shift toward the contralateral side with decrease in lung volume of that side as well. The result is a restrictive ventilatory abnormality. Both ventilation and perfusion shift away from the affected side. Presumably by reflex vasoconstriction, blood flow through the partially collapsed lung under the effusion is usually reduced in proportion to ventilation, but varying changes in gas exchange have been described, dependent on the degree of $\dot{V}_A/\dot{Q}$ ratio alterations. When fluid is removed either mechanically or by absorption, pulmonary mechanics and gas transfer return to normal.

The diagnostic approach to a pleural effusion starts with a careful analysis of the clinical history and findings on physical examination, which may provide clues to implicate one of the common causes of pleural effusion shown in Table 23-1. If clinically indicated, the next step should be to obtain a sample of pleural fluid via thoracentesis to characterize it as exudate or a transudate. When the disease process is associated with inflammation, tissue destruction, or lymphatic obstruction, the fluid is an exudate. Exudates usually meet one of the following criteria: (1) pleural fluid to serum protein ratio greater than 0.5, (2) pleural fluid to serum lactic dehydrogenase (LDH) ratio greater than 0.6, or (3) absolute pleural fluid LDH greater than 200 IU. Transudates rarely are associated with any of the above criteria and are caused by diseases that increase capillary hydrostatic pressure, such as congestive heart failure, or that decrease blood oncotic pressure, such as the nephrotic syndrome.

In addition to determining the values of pleural fluid LDH and protein, analysis of the fluid usually includes a cell count, glucose measurement, Gram stain, and culture. Bloody effusions are commonly seen after trauma, pulmonary infarction, and with malignancy. Neutrophilic predominance suggests an infectious etiology which may be confirmed on Gram stain or culture. Lymphocytic and eosinophilic effusions, however, have been associated with a

TABLE 23–1.—COMMON CAUSES OF PLEURAL EFFUSIONS

TRANSUDATES
Congestive heart failure
Cirrhosis
Nephrotic syndrome
Hypoproteinemia
EXUDATES
Bacterial pneumonia
Tuberculosis
Fungal infection
Malignancy
Pancreatitis
Systemic lupus erythematosus
Rheumatoid arthritis
Trauma
Pulmonary infarction
Pneumothorax
Subphrenic abscess

number of disease processes and are nonspecific. A low pleural fluid glucose level is observed with empyemas, and it is strikingly low in effusions due to rheumatoid arthritis. Recently, determination of the pleural fluid pH has been shown to yield important diagnostic and therapeutic information. A pH of less than 7.30 is usually associated with one of six conditions: (1) parapneumonic effusion or empyema, (2) malignancy, (3) collagen vascular disease, (4) tuberculosis, (5) esophageal rupture, or (6) hemothorax. Furthermore, evidence suggests that a parapneumonic effusion with a pleural fluid pH <7.20 will not resolve spontaneously and requires chest tube drainage. Other tests on the pleural fluid may also be of value in the appropriate clinical situations. Pleural fluid amylase levels are elevated in pancreatic effusions. Complement levels are low in systemic lupus erythematosus (LE) and rheumatoid arthritis, and detection of LE cells in the pleural fluid is thought to be highly specific. If malignancy is being considered, cytologic examination should be performed.

If the diagnosis is not apparent after pleural fluid analysis, closed pleural biopsy is often useful in evaluating effusions secondary to coccidioidomycosis, tuberculosis, and malignancy. In some cases, thoracoscopy (pleuroscopy) may also be helpful. Thoracotomy may be necessary, however, in a few cases in which the diagnosis is uncertain after performing other less invasive procedures.

Treatment must be directed at the cause of the effusion. Palliation is obtained by aspiration of the fluid, allowing reexpansion of the underlying lung. If the effusion is recurrent or persistent, closed chest-tube drainage may be required; therapy is also directed at the underlying cause. If such measures still prove unsuccessful, it may be necessary to consider pleural symphysis to obliterate the pleural space permanently.

Chylothorax

Damage to the thoracic duct by trauma, inflammation, or malignant involvement produces chylothorax. This type of effusion achieves the characteristics and composition of chyle. The diagnosis is suspected when milky fluid is aspirated from the pleural space, and confirmed when elevated triglyceride levels are found in the fluid. Physiologic changes in pulmonary function are those of serous pleural effusions. Since chyle is bacteriostatic, empyema does not occur, but fibrous deposition from the chronic chylous effusion occurs, and fibrothorax may follow. Treatment depends on the cause. Radiation or chemotherapy may be helpful when malignancy is present. Surgical intervention may be required where the cause is related to mechanical disruption of the thoracic duct and where more conservative measures have failed.

Primary Pleural Neoplasms

Diffuse malignant mesothelioma occurs primarily in middle-aged men and has a high correlation with exposure to asbestos. Frequently, the disease may not develop until 20 or more years after exposure. The presenting symptoms are usually chest pain and dyspnea. Pleural thickening and pleural effusion are seen on chest roentgenogram. The diagnosis is difficult to make cytologically or with a closed pleural biopsy and generally requires a thoracotomy. Although an occasional long survival occurs after radical surgery, most patients exhibit a rapid downhill course despite any therapy.

In contrast to the diffuse variety, solitary fibrous mesotheliomas are almost always benign lesions which arise from the visceral pleural. They usually present as unknown thoracic mass lesions. Surgical excision is both diagnostic and curative.

READING LIST

Good J.T., Tarlye D.A., Maulitz R.M., et al.: The diagnostic value of the pleural fluid pH. *Chest* 78:55–59, 1980.

Demonstrates the usefulness of pH determinations in evaluating pleural fluid.

Greene R., Mcloud T.C., Stark P.: Pneumothorax. *Semin. Roentgenol.* 12:313–325, 1977.

A review of the radiologic and pathophysiologic features of pneumothorax.

Hughes R.L., Mintzer R.A., Hidvegi D.F., et al.: The management of chylothorax. *Chest* 76:212–218, 1979.

Discusses the pathogenesis and management of chylothorax.

Legha S.S., Merggia F.M.: Pleural mesothelioma: clinical features and therapeutic implications. *Ann. Intern. Med.* 87:613–617, 1977.

A review of the clinical features and treatment of mesothelioma.

Light R.W., MacGregor I., Luchsinger P.C., et al.: Pleural effusions: the diagnostic separation of transudates from exudates. *Ann. Intern. Med.* 77:507–513, 1971.

A classic article proposing the criteria for differentiating transudates from exudates.

Turton C.W.G.: Pleural effusions. *Br. J. Hosp. Med.* 23:239–249, 1980.

A review of the diagnostic evaluation of pleural effusions.

24

Localized Parenchymal Disease

THE EFFECT of localized parenchymal processes on lung function depends on the amount of lung involved; the nature, type, and duration of involvement; the state of the remaining lung; and ultimately the extent to which the process itself is amenable to resolution. Some types of lesions produce no significant dysfunction, although they produce spectacular abnormalities on chest roentgenogram; others that are radiologically unimpressive produce profound alterations in lung function. In general, acute changes lead to more severe dysfunction than those that occur insidiously, and effects are least severe when the process affects both regional perfusion and ventilation to similar degrees. In the present discussion, four categories of localized lesions will be distinguished: (1) atelectasis, (2) localized parenchymal infiltrates, (3) solid masses, and (4) air containing lesions.

Atelectasis

Atelectasis is a dimunition of volume or collapse of lung units. Such a decrease of volume may ensue when a portion of the lung is impinged upon by a space-occupying lesion. It may also occur with contraction of fibrous tissue in some lung region. In these situations, the functional abnormalities are not distinctive and usually depend on the nature of the underlying disease.

Atelectasis may also result from a localized airways obstruction ("resorptive" atelectasis) or from changes in alveolar stability associated with surfactant abnormalities. These latter types of atelectasis may produce distinctive types of functional alterations. Resorptive or "obstructive" atelectasis results when lung units are deprived of ventilation. Because the oxygen tension in pulmonary arterial blood is much lower than in the isolated alveoli, oxygen is rapidly absorbed from a nonventilated lung region. Nitrogen, being less soluble, is absorbed more slowly. With complete airways obstruction, absorption of all of the gas in a previously air-filled lung unit may be complete in several hours. Gas absorption, and therefore lung collapse, will occur more rapidly if an oxygen-enriched atmosphere was breathed before occlusion of the lung unit and may take only a few minutes after breathing 100% oxygen. This potential hazard must be borne in mind when administering oxygen therapy. When high concentrations of oxygen are inhaled, atelectasis may develop beyond a mucus plug before the patient can clear his secretions.

Whether atelectasis follows complete obstruction of an airway depends on the site of the obstruction and the availability and patency of channels for collateral ventilation of the obstructed lung unit. Obstruction of a lobar bronchus results in lobar atelectasis, but airway occlusion beyond the level of segmental bronchi may not be followed by complete absorption of gas peripheral to the obstruction because of the availability of collateral channels. Anastomotic communications between respiratory bronchioles, bronchioalveolar channels between lobules, and alveolar pores of Kohn are potential pathways for collateral ventilation. (There is evidence to suggest that the pores of Kohn normally are not open and that they may not even be present before 10 months of age.) When airway occlusion is peripheral to segmental bronchi, the availability of collateral channels usually permits continued aeration of the obstructed unit. Resorptive atelectasis, then, results only when the obstruction is in a major bronchus or when, because of disease, peripheral obstruction is accompanied by nonavailability of collateral channels of ventilation.

As air is absorbed from the obstructed lung unit, some degree of intra-alveolar edema occurs. The accumulation of intra-alveolar fluid diminishes the magnitude of volume loss and contributes to the radiologic density characteristic of this condition. If the atelectasis is permitted to persist, the edema fluid will be absorbed, and the minimal volume of the lung unit will be achieved. A chronic total collapse of a lobe may be difficult to see on chest roentgenogram and is often detected only because of visible compensatory hyperinflation of the remaining lung.

The symptoms and signs of acute atelectasis due to bronchial obstruction depend on the distribution of the abnormality and the total amount of lung involved. Dyspnea is a common symptom and rapid shallow breathing is characteristic. When involvement is extensive, cyanosis may appear. With collapse of an entire lung or a major portion of one lung, mediastinal structures shift toward the affected side, and the hemidiaphragm is elevated. These anatomical displacements may be detected on physical examination. Vesicular breath sounds are also diminished over the collapsed lung. Roentgenographically, the atelectatic lung appears as a zone of increased density originating at the hilus and extending peripherally. Mediastinal shift, elevation of the ipsilateral hemidiaphragm, hilar displacement, and compensatory hyperinflation of the remaining normal lung are common roentgenographic abnormalities associated with massive atelectasis.

Following occlusion of a bronchus, blood flow to the affected area persists for a time though ventilation has ceased. The hypoxemia resulting from this right-to-left shunting may be resistant to correction by supplemental oxygen. Hyperventilation of the unobstructed lung often occurs, leading to a fall in Pa_{CO_2}.

In contrast, chronic atelectasis or atelectasis of a chronically diseased lung produces few blood gas alterations. Blood flow to the chronically atelectatic lung is appropriately diminished, and hypoxemia, if present, will be mild. Hyperventilation is not observed and, if the remaining lung is normal, ventilatory impairment resulting from diminution of lung volumes may be slight. The most common cause of chronic atelectasis in adults is an endobronchial carcinoma obstructing a lobar or segmented bronchus.

The object of therapy is to remove the obstruction, if possible, and to reexpand the collapsed lung. When massive atelectasis occurs from impingement of a foreign body or mucus impaction, vigorous bronchial hygiene measures should be attempted. If these fail, bronchoscopy with direct aspiration of the obstructing material should be carried out.

Patchy atelectasis may be observed on a chest roentgenogram as bilateral radiopaque areas, easily confused with pneumonic lesions. The pathogenesis is not always clear. Patchy atelectasis may occur with mucus impactions or in areas where regional compliance has been altered. Changes in alveolar surfactant, which may play a part in the pathogenesis of the adult respiratory distress syndrome (ARDS), result in alveolar instability and patchy atelectasis. This is discussed more fully in chapter 28.

Atelectatic patches may occur in otherwise healthy lungs. The normal individual, although usually unaware of it, periodically sighs, hyperinflating the lung. In the absence of such periodic hyperinflation, poorly inflated portions of the lung, usually at the lung bases, become less and less compliant. Ultimately, such areas may become atelectatic. This type of patchy atelectasis is likely to occur whenever periodic deep breathing is prevented, as during prolonged mechanical ventilation, during anesthesia, in the postoperative period, in the presence of chest wall injury, or during coma. To prevent this complication, periodic deep inspirations or sighs are provided by modern mechanical ventilators, induced by the anesthesiologist during surgery, or encouraged in patients following surgery or chest wall injury. (Incentive spirometry is sometimes used to encourage deep breathing.) During long-term mechanical ventilation, atelectasis is prevented by using larger than normal tidal volumes.

Parenchymal Infiltrates

Localized infiltrates may result from a wide variety of etiologic agents and are noted as pulmonary manifestations of a variety of systemic diseases. The most common cause is an acute infectious process. Three basic types of inflammatory infiltrates may be identified: (1) inflammatory alveolar edema, which spreads through the air spaces of adjacent lung units, producing an alveolar type of parenchymal consolidation; (2) inflammatory reaction primarily involving interstitial tissues, and (3) inflammation initially involving airways, which may spread to surrounding parenchyma, producing bronchopneumonia.

Chills and fever, together with tachypnea, cough, sputum production, and pleuritic pain, are characteristic of acute bacterial pneumonia. The clinician should look for the physical signs of rales, dullness to percussion, and diminished breath sounds. Often, symptoms or physical signs are minimal, although the chest roentgenogram reveals an extensive pneumonic process. This is especially true in mycoplasma pneumonia and in chronic infections.

The chest roentgenogram will reveal localized parenchymal infiltrates varying in extent and distribution. The alveolar type of parenchymal consolidation is often discrete and localized. It may progress to complete lobar involvement, but this has diminished in frequency since the advent of early antibiotic therapy. Since this type of pneumonia originates in airspaces, the parenchymal consolidation is usually adjacent to a pleural surface, and radiolucent bronchi may be visible in the involved area (air bronchogram). Interstitial pneumonias usually present a more patchy distibution, whereas bronchopneumonias are often diffuse. Since the latter involve airways, consolidation often shows a segmental distribution, and atelectasis may occur secondary to accumulation of inflammatory exudate in airways.

Pathophysiologic manifestations associated with localized inflammatory infiltrates vary with the distribution and magnitude of the disease process and the rate of development of the abnormality. Slowly developing abnormalities such as tuberculosis produce minimal physiologic alterations, unless they are extensive or result in marked distortion of lung architecture. In these chronic disease processes, both ventilation and perfusion are reduced in areas of disease so that neither significant venous admixture nor significant increase in alveolar dead space generally occurs. The reduction in lung volume is roughly proportional to the amount of lung involved by the disease.

Acute pneumonias of rapid onset produce more profound pathophysiologic abnormalities. The effects of severe ventilation-perfusion imbalance, or right-to-left shunting caused continued perfusion of consolidated or underventilated portions of lung results in a degree of hypoxemia roughly porportional to the amount of lung involved. Hypoxemia is often of greater magnitude in bronchopneumonia than in alveolar pneumonia. Rapid, shallow breathing with increase in dead space ventilation, together with a decreased compliance of the pneumonic lung, results in increased work of breathing. In the absence of another underlying lung disease, the characteristic tachypnea associated with alveolar hyperventilation of the uninvolved lung results in hypocapnia. Only in terminal stages does carbon dioxide retention occur. When overall ventilatory capacity is limited by a coexisting chronic obstructive disease, however, alveolar underventilation and hypercapnia may ensue early in the course. In patients with very reactive airways, acute pulmonary infection may lead to increased airways obstruction. This results from a combination of smooth muscle contraction, bronchial wall edema, and accumulation of bronchial secretions.

Diffusing capacity is reduced in pneumonia, but usually returns to normal soon after resolution of the disease process. An exception to this is seen following recovery from a viral interstitial pneumonia. In this case, the diffusing capacity abnormality may persist for many months or even years after complete roentgenographic clearing of parenchymal infiltrates and return of the VC to normal. This probably reflects persistence of an interstitial abnormality following this type of inflammatory disease.

Ventilation and perfusion scans may be abnormal in patients with acute pulmonary infections as a result of the abnormal distribution of blood flow and inspired gas. Both ventilation and perfusion are generally decreased in the areas of pneumonic radiopacity. But ventilation and/or perfusion defects may also be noted in areas that appear radiologically normal. These are readily misdiagnosed as areas of pulmonary embolization on pulmonary scans.

Solid Masses

Solid parenchymal masses may be the late result of a resolving chronic inflammatory process or may represent a neoplastic disease. Primary pulmonary neoplasms, metastatic tumors, and residua of granulomatous infections are often first discovered on a routine chest roentgenogram. If peripheral in location, they may produce few symptoms or physiologic derangements. Functional alterations produced are a function of their size. Reduction in lung volume and restriction of volume excursion are produced by any large space-occupying lesion. Unless the mass impinges on an airway, ventilation-perfusion relationships generally remain normal, and the diffusing capacity is usually reduced only in proportion to the loss of lung volume. If the mass is situated in or near an airway, the symptoms and effect on lung function

will depend on the extent to which airways obstruction results, as described in chapter 26.

Nodular residua of old granulomatous infections are rarely symptomatic. In association with malignancies, there may be chest pain and general systemic symptoms, including weight loss. Bronchial adenomas or carcinomas commonly produce hemoptysis. Systemic neuromuscular, endocrine, and metabolic manifestations of bronchogenic carcinoma may occur.

Air-Containing Lesions

The presence of an air-containing parenchymal lesion is usually established by roentgenographic examination. Cavitation of a tumor mass or of an area of lung involved in an infectious disease process appears as an air-filled space. However, it is a secondary phenomenon, and the signs, symptoms, and functional abnormalities will be related to the primary disease. The air-containing lesions of potential functional significance are blebs, bullae, and cysts.

Blebs are subpleural collections of air. They are usually small and produce no significant derangement of function. However, rupture of subpleural blebs has been implicated as a cause of spontaneous pneumothorax (discussed in chap. 23). Occasionally, blebs become large and then may become functionally important.

A bulla, an air-filled space within the substance of the lung, is presumed to result from destruction of alveolar tissue and coalescence of airspaces. Cysts are considered to be congenital and, unlike the bullae they resemble, have a lining of bronchial epithelium. Since congenital cysts are subject to infection, which can alter the character of their epithelial lining, it may be difficult to distinguish them from the residua of acquired lung abscesses. Bullae may occur in many of the diffuse interstitial lung diseases, and air-containing lesions are not uncommon in bronchiectasis, probably as a result of healed peribronchial abscesses.

The physiologic abnormalities and resulting signs and symptoms produced by air-containing lesions depend on the nature of the bronchial communication with such lesions as well as on their size. Often, bullous lesions have markedly impaired bronchial communications and depend on collateral channels for ventilation. Very poorly ventilated lesions produce physiologic abnormalities similar to solid space-occupying lesions. If adequate bronchial communication exists, however, the lesion will be included in lung volume measurements, and inert gas studies will reveal maldistribution of inspired gas.

When giant blebs or bullous lesions are not part of a generalized emphysematous destructive process, they rarely produce blood gas abnormalities or cause significant airways obstruction. They may lead to pulmonary dysfunction, however, by compressing otherwise normal lung. Surgical resection may be indicated for removal of these large space-occupying lesions. When the remaining lung is normal, the benefits of surgical therapy may be substantial.

Bullous degeneration is commonly associated with generalized obstructive disease. In this case, obstructive ventilatory abnormalities, reduced diffusing capacity, and blood gas abnormalities are related primarily to the underlying disease. Contribution of the discernible bullae to the overall dysfunction is difficult to assess in these patients. Surgical removal of bullae or giant blebs is rarely of benefit in the presence of diffuse obstructive emphysema, but may be indicated when there is progressive enlargement, frequent infection, recurrent pneumothorax, or clear-cut evidence of compression of relatively normal lung. Evidence for the latter is best obtained by angiographic studies, which demonstrate intrinsically normal vasculature that is displaced and impinged upon by the air-containing lesions. Significant improvement of lung function from bullectomy in such patients is rare or short-lived, however. (See chapter 12 in regard to functional indications for thoracic surgery.)

READING LIST

Bendixen H.H., Hedley-Whyte J., Laver M.B.: Impaired oxygenation in surgical patients during general anesthesia with controlled ventilation. *N. Engl. J. Med.* 269:991–996, 1963.

A classic study demonstrating that atelectasis with a decrease in oxygenation occurs when sighs are not incorporated during constant tidal volume ventilation under anesthesia.

Benumof J.L.: Mechanism of decreased blood flow to atelectatic lung. *J. Appl. Physiol.* 46:1047–1048, 1979.

Demonstrates that hypoxic pulmonary vasoconstriction is the major cause of decreased blood flow in an acutely atelectatic lobe.

Briggs D.D.: Pulmonary infections. *Med. Clin. North Am.* 61:1163–1183, 1977.

A review of the clinical features, pathophysiology, and treatment of the more common pneumonias.

Carr D.R., Rosenow E.D.: Bronchogenic carcinoma. *Basics RD* 5:1–6, 1977.

A review of the clinical features, roentgenographic manifestations, and diagnosis of bronchogenic carcinoma.

Laurenzi G.A., Turino G.M., Fishman A.P.: Bullous disease of the lung. *Am. J. Med.* 32:361–378, 1962.

Physiologic and clinical characteristics of a series of patients with bullous lung disease are reviewed.

Diffuse Parenchymal Diseases

A HOST OF LUNG DISEASES is characterized by diffuse parenchymal involvement. Many infectious processes caused by bacterial, mycotic, or viral agents may appear in a diffuse miliary form involving the entire lung. Primary or metastatic pulmonary malignancies may also exhibit disseminated bilateral distribution. Even if we exclude infectious and neoplastic diseases, there remains a large number of diffuse parenchymal diseases. Many are difficult to classify and are of uncertain etiology. Because these diseases have certain common features and exhibit similar abnormalities in function, they are discussed as a group in this chapter. Idiopathic diffuse pulmonary emphysema, on the other hand, is included with the discussion of chronic obstructive diseases, since its pattern of dysfunction is different and is closely related to associated airways abnormalities.

In general, the diffuse parenchymal diseases share a pattern of altered lung function that includes diminished lung volumes, reduced diffusing capacity, chronic hyperventilation, and varying degrees of hypoxemia that may be apparent only on exercise. The chest roentgenogram characteristically reveals bilateral, diffuse, but not always uniformly distributed radiopaque densities. Many attempts have been made to differentiate, describe, and characterize the different types, shapes, sizes, and distributions of these densities, but with few exceptions such information has not been of specific diagnostic value. Furthermore, the pattern observed on the chest roentgenogram may change with time as densities fade, increase, or coalesce. There is often

little relationship between the extent of the roentgenographic abnormality and degree of lung dysfunction. There may be marked dysfunction with little radiologic evidence of disease or vice versa.

These diseases may be acute or insidious in onset. They may be rapidly progressive, slowly progressive or static in their course. They may be very responsive to therapy or totally unresponsive.

The terminology describing this group of diseases is often confusing, and classification has been difficult. Dividing these diseases into categories based on whether the parenchymal involvement is acinic or interstitial may help to describe the chest roentgenogram, but often primary alveolar involvement progresses to interstitial fibrosis, and this description helps little to characterize the etiology or pathophysiology. Although at the present state of knowledge any classification must be arbitrary and imperfect, an attempt at such a classification is presented in Table 25–1.

This classification is incomplete, and only the more common of the specific diseases are listed as examples. Though it is not the purpose of this book to attempt to describe fully all of the disease entities to be encountered in pulmonary medicine, certain ones are used as examples of types of diffuse parenchymal disease.

Diseases of Known Etiology

NEOPLASTIC AND INFECTIOUS DISEASES.—
These are included because they may exhibit the

156

TABLE 25–1.—CLASSIFICATION OF DIFFUSE
PULMONARY PARENCHYMAL DISEASES

Diseases of known etiology
  Neoplastic
  Infectious
  Allergic inhalation diseases (''allergic alveolitis'')
    Farmers' lung
    Bagassosis
    Pigeon breeders' lung
    Mushroom workers' lung
    Maple bark disease
    Suberosis, etc.
  Toxic inhalation diseases
    Inorganic dusts and fibers (pneumoconiosis)
      Silicosis
      Asbestosis
      Berylliosis
      Talcosis, etc.
    Gases (irritative bronchoalveolar edema)
      Nitrogen dioxide (silofillers' disease)
      Phosgene, etc.
  Radiation pneumonitis
  Pharmacologic reactions
    Busulfan or bleomycin lung
    Hexamethonium lung, etc.
Diseases of unknown etiology
  Systemic collagen-vascular diseases
    Goodpasture's syndrome
    Necrotizing angiitis (polyarteritis nodosa)
    Wegener's granulomatosis
    Lupus erythematosus
    Rheumatoid lung
    Polymyositis-dermatomyositis
    Diffuse systemic sclerosis (scleroderma)
  Granulomatous diseases
    Sarcoidosis
    Histiocytosis-X
      Letterer-Siwe disease (acute histiocytic
        reticuloendotheliosis)
      Hand-Schüller-Christian disease (lipogranulomatosis)
      Eosinophilic granuloma
  Idiopathic diffuse interstitial and alveolar diseases
    Usual interstitial pneumonia (idiopathic alveolitis)
    Diffuse interstitial fibrosis (fibrosing alveolitis)
    Desquamative interstitial pneumonia (desquamative
      alveolitis)
    Lymphoid interstitial pneumonia (lymphoid alveolitis)
    Primary pulmonary hemosiderosis
    Pulmonary alveolar proteinosis
    Pulmonary alveolar microlithiasis

---

same pathophysiologic and radiologic abnormalities as other diffuse diseases, but often the clinical picture will reflect the underlying disease primarily, and the dysfunction resulting from the diffuse distribution of the disease may be a less important, secondary phenomenon. On the other hand, mycobacterial and fungal infections susceptible to specific therapy and alveolar cell carcinoma may mimic the idiopathic diffuse interstitial diseases.

ALLERGIC AND TOXIC INHALATION DISEASES.—Inhalation of noxious substances is a common cause of diffuse parenchymal lung disease and respiratory dysfunction. This may result from industrial exposure, but not all industrial lung diseases belong in this classification. Some types of industrial exposures (e.g., cotton dust) primarily result in airways abnormalities rather than diffuse parenchymal infiltrations.

Allergic alveolitis is the result of an immunologic reaction to inhalation of organic dusts. Increasing numbers of organic dusts are being implicated as causes of this syndrome. Lung diseases caused by inorganic dust exposure are a result of chronically developing tissue reaction, which vary according to the physical and chemical properties of the inhaled substances. The toxic reaction that follows inhalation of certain gases, on the other hand, is a nonspecific, direct, irritative bronchoalveolar edema. Diseases resulting from inhalation of inorganic dusts are usually considered direct toxic reactions, but allergic mechanisms may also play a role in some patients. For example, the likelihood of lung disease developing from inhalation of beryllium dust varies greatly among those exposed, suggesting that individual sensitivity to the substance may be a significant factor.

Silicosis remains a common disease among workers involved in hard-rock mining, quarrying, sandblasting, and other occupations in which there is exposure to crystalline silica dust. Although silica is ubiquitous and extremely fibrogenic, development of silicosis usually requires a relatively long, intense exposure. The fibrous tissue response to the inhaled particles initially produces a reticular or fine nodular pattern on chest roentgenogram, but the pattern may progress in time to that of conglomerate silicosis, with larger solid fibrous nodules. Conglomerate silicosis is often associated with secondary emphysema and airways obstructive problems. Tuberculosis frequently complicates conglomerate silicosis.

The lung's reaction to inhaled asbestos fibers is to produce a typical interstitial fibrosis. Due to the distribution of the dust, changes usually begin medially at the lung bases. Characteristic asbestos bodies can be identified on histologic examination. Pleural plaques are a unique feature of asbestosis, often leading to a "ground glass" type of radiopacity in the lower lung fields. Unlike silicosis, a clear relationship between length and intensity of exposure has not been established for asbestosis. Of special significance is the carcinogenicity of asbestos fibers; the incidence of bronchogenic carcinoma and malignant pleural mesothelioma in patients with asbestosis is very high.

Other pneumoconioses develop in response to inhalation of particulate beryllium, talc, graphite, cobalt, and other inorganic dusts associated with various industrial processes. The type of response of the lung to these inhaled irritants depends on the solubility of the substance, the duration and intensity of exposure, and to a considerable degree on the sensitivity of the individual. The inhaled particles must be small enough, less than 1 μ in diameter, and deposited in sufficient quantity to overwhelm the lung's defense mechanisms. In general, interstitial fibrosis, often progressive, is the common feature of these pneumoconioses. With the exception of silicosis and asbestosis, increased incidence of tuberculosis or malignancy has not been confirmed.

Inhalation of iron compounds leads to deposition of radiopaque material in lung tissues. This results in a characteristic radiologic abnormality, but, since there is little tissue reaction, no significant dysfunction usually results.

Black lung disease has been very broadly interpreted to mean any respiratory disorder occurring in anyone who has worked in a coal mine, whether or not there is roentgenographic evidence of pneumoconiosis. It includes anthracosilicosis, a modified form of silicosis that has been described in anthracite or hard-coal miners. It also includes a different type of disease that has been described in bituminous or soft-coal miners, an entity termed "coal workers' pneumoconiosis." The latter is characterized by focal aggregations of coal dust in the lung, relatively slight fibrosis, and dilatation of air spaces around the coal dust foci, producing focal emphysema. As this process continues, the end result may be indistinguishable from any other type of emphysema if characteristic radiologic changes do not develop.

Radiologic and physiologic findings are variable in black lung disease. Simple coal workers' pneumoconiosis may exhibit roentgenographic evidence of disease (stippling of the lung) with little functional abnormality. In other cases, progressive massive fibrosis occurs with widespread consolidation of the lung and severe dysfunction. The pattern of dysfunction is related to the loss of functioning lung tissue but, in late stages, is complicated by airways obstructive changes as a consequence of the accompanying emphysema, with eventual ventilatory failure and cor pulmonale. The factors that result in massive fibrosis are uncertain, since not all patients with the simple form of the disease progress to this stage. Indeed, it is unclear how coal dust leads to this unique form of pneumoconiosis. It has been suggested that the total amount of particulate matter, of whatever composition, may be the important factor and that cigarette smoking probably has an important synergistic role in the development of coal workers' pneumoconiosis. There is no specific effective therapy for the disease.

RADIATION PNEUMONITIS.—Radiation therapy to the thorax often results in some degree of pulmonary parenchymal reaction. In the acute phase, pulmonary interstitial edema and lymphangiectasis, tissue necrosis, and alveolar desquamation may occur. This acute radiation pneumonitis is usually followed by recovery. In some cases, chronic pulmonary and pleural fibrosis may result, leaving stiff tissue reduced in volume. The exact role of steroids in management of this problem remains uncertain, although their use during acute radiation pneumonitis frequently results in an improvement in symptomatology. In addition, withdrawal of steroids administered during the period of radiation therapy often unmasks acute radiation pneumonitis.

PHARMACOLOGIC REACTIONS.—Some types of diffuse lung disease have been attributed to response to pharmacologic agents. Interstitial pneumonitis and fibrosis have been described after a use of a variety of cytotoxic drugs including busulfan, bleomycin, cyclophosphamide, methotrexate, and mitomycin. Hexamethonium, mecamylamine, methysergide, and nitrofurantoin have also been incriminated as causing interstitial pneumonitis and fibrosis. The list of pharmacologic agents implicated in producing lung fibrosis continues to grow.

Diseases of Unknown Etiology

A distressing number of the diffuse parenchymal diseases are of unknown etiology. They can be classified only on the basis of their association with findings in other organ systems or on the basis of their characteristic histopathology. Unfortunately, there is an imperfect relationship between morphologic and clinical findings. Indeed, it remains possible that some of the current diagnostic categories represent only different stages in the evolution of the same underlying disorder.

SYSTEMIC COLLAGEN-VASCULAR DISEASES.—Connective tissue or collagen-vascular diseases may involve many different organ systems. The common feature exhibited by these diseases is fibrinoid degeneration of connective tissue with vasculitis of varying degrees. Clear separation of disease entities listed under this category is often difficult. It may depend on the specific histopathology, distribution of lesions, clinical course of the patient, or specific nature of demonstrable autoimmune phenomena.

All of these disease entities are associated with diffuse interstitial pneumonitis and fibrosis of varying degrees. The severity of vasculitis is variable. The chest roentgenogram generally reveals nondescript diffuse parenchymal involvement. Large nodules may be noted, especially in Wegener's granulomatosis. In lupus erythematosus pleural effusion is common.

GRANULOMATOUS DISEASES.—Of the noninfectious granulomatous diseases, sarcoidosis is the most common. The characteristic lesions are noncaseating granulomas usually microscopic and diffusely distributed throughout the lung parenchyma. These sarcoid lesions may be found in spleen, lymph nodes, liver, bone, and skin, as well as lungs, and when clustered, may form yellow-gray nodules. The histopathology itself is nonspecific, but the presence of disseminated noncaseating granulomas, lack of evidence for any of the infectious granulomas, characteristic roentgenographic distribution of lesions and, when available, a positive Kveim skin reaction allow a diagnosis of sarcoidosis. Fibrosis may develop as the granulomas heal.

Recently, analysis of bronchoscopic washings (bronchoalveolar lavage or BAL) in patients with sarcoidosis has provided additional information regarding its pathogenesis. Patients with active sarcoidosis usually have increased numbers of T-lymphocytes in their lavage fluid, suggesting that the granulomatous infiltration in sarcoidosis is related to excess numbers of activated T-lymphocytes.

Because the roentgenographic evidence of sarcoidosis exhibits considerable variation, four types or stages of the disease have been described, based on the appearance of the chest roentgenogram: (1) bilateral hilar lymph node enlargement without apparent parenchymal involvement, (2) a combination of both hilar node and parenchymal involvement, (3) parenchymal infiltrates without lymph node enlargement, and (4) signs of pulmonary fibrosis. There is evidence that these represent evolving stages in sarcoidosis. The likelihood of complete spontaneous clearing is excellent in stage 1 and even in stage 2. But the presence of chronic pulmonary infiltrates, especially when accompanied by evidence of fibrotic changes, makes the prognosis guarded.

Generally, sarcoidosis patients with extensive pulmonary fibrosis are the most severely impaired, with evidence of restrictive ventilatory impairment, reduced diffusing capacity, decreased lung compliance, and exercise-induced hypoxemia. Cor pulmonale is a common complication. Patients with extensive parenchymal infiltrates exhibit similar abnormalities, though usually to a lesser degree. Patients who show only hilar node enlargement with no roentgenographic evidence of parenchymal disease may also show evidence of restrictive disease, decreased compliance, and reduced diffusing capacity, even in the absence of any symptoms, suggesting that their pulmonary lesions are more extensive than indicated by the chest roentgenogram.

Corticosteroid therapy for sarcoidosis often produces clinical improvement and radiologic clearing of pulmonary infiltrates. Ventilatory function may be improved, but the diffusing capacity has been reported to be less susceptible to improvement. Cessation of therapy is often followed by deterioration of lung function. Although serial tests of lung function are important in following the course of patients with sarcoidosis and in regulating steroid therapy, repeated analysis of BAL fluid in conjunction with gallium scanning of the lungs may provide an alternative means of monitoring disease activity in these patients.

A form of histiocytosis involving the lung is commonly called eosinophilic granuloma. The characteristic lesion consists of granulomatous nodules featuring foamy histiocytes and eosinophilic infiltration. These lesions may be confined to the lung or involve other organs. The chest roentgenogram may reveal coarse nodulation, miliary infiltration, or patchy densities. With development of fibrosis, roentgenographic clearing of the diffuse parenchymal densities may be apparent, or multiple small cysts may develop, giving the lung a honeycomb appearance. Complete resolution without fibrosis may also occur. Usually the disorder is self-limiting, and the patient is left with minimal reduction in TLC, diminished diffusing capacity, and mild exercise-induced hypoxemia. Occasionally, however, severe lung dysfunction results, especially when there is extensive pulmonary fibrosis.

Corticosteroid therapy has been used for eosinophilic granuloma with uncertain success. Because the natural history of the disease is unpredictable, the efficacy of therapy is difficult to evaluate.

IDIOPATHIC INTERSTITIAL-ALVEOLAR DISEASES.—A final group of diffuse parenchymal diseases is characterized by varying degrees of alveolar wall inflammation, interstitial fibrosis, alveolar cellular desquamation, accumulation of protein material in alveoli, and alveolar hemorrhage. These diseases have been classified on the basis of their predominant histopathologic features. The term "Hamman-Rich syndrome" has been variably applied to these entities and is best avoided. "Usual interstitial pneumonitis" or "idiopathic alveolitis" describes those diseases in which interstitial pneumonitis predominates, but some fibrosis, desquamation of alveolar lining cells, and hemosiderosis may occur. When fibrosis is prominent and there is less evidence of active inflammatory reaction, "diffuse interstitial fibrosis" or "fibrosing alveolitis" is often diagnosed. Massive proliferation and desquamation of alveolar cells characterize "desquamative interstitial pneumonitis" or "desquamative alveolitis." Bronchoalveolar lavage in patients with interstitial pneumonitis reveals increased numbers of polymorphonuclear leukocytes. On the basis of this data, it has been recently suggested that the initial abnormality in idiopathic interstitial pneumonitis is a diffuse alveolitis produced by increased numbers of polymorphonuclear leukocytes which, if untreated, will eventually produce irreversible fibrosis.

Response to adrenocortical steroids or immunosuppressive therapy is variable in these patients and difficult to predict from either clinical or histopathologic findings. In relatively few patients, marked improvement may be induced. More often, it is difficult to determine if therapy has affected the variable and unpredictable natural course of the disease. Serial use of BAL has been advocated as a means of monitoring therapy and disease activity in these patients. However, its precise role remains to be clarified.

It is important to distinguish scattered dense fibrotic lesions that are the residue of old localized infections from the diffuse interstitial fibrosis mentioned above. Fibrotic residua of old infectious granulomas or of recurrent bacterial infections are not progressive and do not produce the alveolar-capillary block syndrome. In fact, unless they result in marked distortion of lung architecture or are associated with emphysematous changes, such lesions may produce remarkably little pulmonary dysfunction.

Pathophysiology

The common pattern of dysfunction in diffuse parenchymal pulmonary diseases is one of a restrictive impairment, reduced diffusing capacity, and hypoxemia. Usually VC is reduced, RV normal or reduced, and TLC smaller than predicted. Inert gas washout or equilibration studies may reveal some abnormal distribution of inspired air. Static and dynamic compliance is characteristically decreased. Forced expiratory flow, as measured by the FEV_1, is usually well preserved or reduced only in proportion to VC. However, with advanced fibrosis, some disruption of lung architecture may occur, resulting in coalescence of air spaces and cystic degeneration. This can result in the roentgenographic pattern known as honeycomb lung. Frank emphysematous changes accompanied by an obstructive ventilatory abnormality may be superimposed on the restrictive abnormality. This is especially common in coal workers' pneumoconiosis and conglomerate silicosis. Spontaneous pneumothorax is not an uncommon complication of many of the diffuse parenchymal diseases.

Reduced diffusing capacity is a common feature of these diseases. Arterial hypoxemia is a prominent characteristic of advanced disease but, with less severe involvement, may be present only on exercise. The observation of impaired gas exchange in the presence of diffuse parenchymal disease of the types described led to the concept of alveolar-capillary block, as discussed in chapter 13. It was postulated that thickening of the alveolar membrane resulted in impaired diffusion. It is apparent, however, that the thickening of the alveolar membrane is insufficient in magnitude and uniformity of distribution to account for all of the observed hypoxemia. An increase in physiologic dead space and disturbance of $\dot{V}A/\dot{Q}$ ratios have also been demonstrated in these patients. Lung regions with decreased compliance and reduced ventilation would contribute to the $\dot{V}A/\dot{Q}$ abnormalities. Such $\dot{V}A/\dot{Q}$ abnormalities, in combination with the increased resistance to diffusion offered by the thickened membrane, serve to explain the re-

duced diffusing capacity and hypoxemia. Since overall ventilatory capacity is generally well preserved, hypercapnia is uncommon except at the terminal stages of illness. Indeed, patients usually hyperventilate in an attempt to maintain a normal Pa_{O_2}, leading to chronic, well-compensated hypocapnia.

At times, the level of impairment is insufficient to produce subjective symptoms, and the diffuse parenchymal disease is discovered only on a routine chest roentgenogram. On the other hand, significant impairment may be present with minimal radiologic evidence of disease. Therefore, to evaluate the clinical course and efficacy of therapy in patients with diffuse lung disease, it is necessary to use serial pulmonary function tests as well as serial chest roentgenograms.

Differential Diagnosis

There are few more difficult problems in diagnosis than diffuse parenchymal lung diseases. At times, as in the case of frank miliary lesions, the radiologic appearance may suggest a few diagnostic possibilities. More often, the radiologic interpretation simply indicates a nondescript "diffuse fibrosis." On receiving such a radiologic interpretation, it is well to remember that this is only a description of the roentgenogram and not necessarily an anatomical diagnosis. All of the entities listed in Table 25–1 may produce a similar radiologic appearance.

In the majority of patients, definitive diagnosis will eventually require lung biopsy for direct histologic study and for culture. Unless there are reasons to suspect a miliary granuloma or a generalized neoplasm, and in the absence of node enlargement in the areas, neither scalene nor mediastinal node biopsy is likely to be productive.

The need for lung biopsy may be obviated if a specific diagnosis can be made on the basis of one of the following:

1. A history of exposure to a known pulmonary toxin or to a substance capable of inducing allergic alveolitis. The latter diagnosis may then be confirmed by serologic, skin, or provocative

tests. The presence of eosinophilia should suggest an allergic alveolitis.

2. Manifestations that point to a generalized disease susceptible to diagnosis by biopsy elsewhere in the body, as in collagen-vascular diseases, diffuse carcinomatosis, and sarcoidosis.

3. Immunologic or cultural evidence of one of the infectious granulomas.

4. Recent exposure to pharmacological agents known to lead to diffuse fibrosis, such as bleomycin in large doses as cancer chemotherapy.

If a specific diagnosis cannot be made on the basis of such findings, lung biopsy should be performed as soon as possible after the progressive nature of the disease is evident. Otherwise, functional abnormalities may become so severe that biopsy for definitive diagnosis will be excessively hazardous.

READING LIST

Basset R., Corbin B., Spencer H., et al.: Pulmonary histiocytosis X. *Am. Rev. Respir. Dis.* 118:811–820, 1978.

A review of the clinical and pathologic features of 78 cases.

Becklake M.R.: Asbestos-related diseases of the lung and other organs: their epidemiology and implications for clinical practice. *Am. Rev. Respir. Dis.* 114:187–227, 1976.

A comprehensive monograph reviewing asbestosis and related diseases.

Crystal R.G., Gadek J.E., Ferrans V.J., et al.: Interstitial lung disease: current concepts of pathogenesis, staging, and therapy. *Am. J. Med.* 70:542–548, 1981.

An extensive review article which discusses the concept that interstitial diseases are caused by a diffuse alveolitis and that bronchoalveolar lavage and gallium scanning are useful in staging and assessing the response to therapy.

Crystal R.G., Roberts W.C., Hunninghake G.W., et al.: Pulmonary sarcoidosis: a disease characterized and perpetuated by activated T-lymphocytes. *Ann. Intern. Med.* 64:73–94, 1981.

A review of the current theories regarding the immunologic abnormalities in sarcoidosis.

Gross N.H.: Pulmonary effects of radiation therapy. *Ann. Intern. Med.* 86:81–92, 1977.

A comprehensive review of the pulmonary effects of radiation therapy.

Hunninghake G.W., Fauci A.S.: Pulmonary involvement in the collagen vascular disorders. *Am. Rev. Respir. Dis.* 119:471–503, 1979.

This article reviews the pulmonary manifestations of a variety of collagen-vascular or autoimmune diseases.

Jones R.N., Weill H.: Occupational lung disease. *Basics RD* 6:1–6, 1978.

This review includes brief descriptions of occupational lung diseases that produce diffuse parenchymal lung disease.

Kataria Y.P.: Sarcoidosis: an overview. *Clin. Notes Respir. Dis.* 14:2–14, 1975.

A review of the clinical aspects of sarcoidosis.

Morgan W.K.C., Lapp N.L.: Respiratory disease in coal miners. *Am. Rev. Respir. Dis.* 113:531–559, 1976.

A review of coal workers' pneumoconiosis.

Richerson H.B.: Allergic alveolar diseases. *Postgrad. Med.* 60:121–127, 1976.

A brief review of hypersensitivity pneumonitis.

Turner-Warwick M., Burrows B., Johnson A.: Cryptogenic fibrosing alveolitis: clinical features and their influence on survival. *Thorax* 35:171–180, 1980.

Turner-Warwick M., Burrows B., Johnson A.: Cryptogenic fibrosing alveolitis: response to corticosteroid treatment and its effect on survival. *Thorax* 35:593–599, 1980.

Two recent articles on the natural history and prognosis of idiopathic diffuse interstitial lung disease.

Weiss R.B., Muggia F.M.: Cytotoxic drug induced pulmonary disease: update 1980. *Am. J. Med.* 68:259–266, 1980.

A review of drug-induced lung disease caused by cytotoxic agents.

Ziskind M., Jones R.N., Weill H.: Silicosis. *Am. Rev. Respir. Dis.* 113:643–665, 1976.

A comprehensive review of silicosis.

Localized Airways Abnormalities

LOCALIZED AIRWAYS ABNORMALITIES include partial or complete obstruction and pathologic dilatation or bronchiectasis. Localized airways obstructions present features that differentiate them from the more common generalized airways obstruction. This differentiation is essential, since localized abnormalities are often curable. Such localized obstructions may rise from any of three mechanisms: (1) lesions extrinsic to the airway but impinging upon and narrowing the airway, (2) intrinsic airway lesions causing narrowing of the lumen, and (3) intraluminal obstructions arising from retained secretions or aspirated foreign material. The problem caused by localized obstruction depends upon whether the obstruction is above or below the tracheal bifurcation.

Obstruction Above the Tracheal Bifurcation

The extrathoracic air passages are often subject to obstruction. The most common obstruction, nasal congestion, is inconvenient, but of little consequence to respiratory function. A number of lesions of the trachea and larynx can result in partial obstruction. The obstruction may be fixed or variable and either intrathoracic or extrathoracic. The resulting dysfunction is discussed in chapter 13.

Extrinsic lesions such as an enlarged thyroid may constrict the trachea. Intrinsic lesions, such as polyps or tumors of the trachea, larynx, or vocal cords; bilateral vocal cord paralysis; enlarged tonsils; and stenosing or cicatricial lesions secondary to trauma or surgery, may cause obstruction, as may aspirated foreign bodies. Traumatic laryngeal edema, laryngospasm, or the inflammatory laryngeal edema of croup are particularly serious forms of upper airway obstruction. An unusual variety of upper airway obstruction may occur during sleep in obese patients and mimic a hypoventilation syndrome. This has been discussed in more detail in chapter 20.

Tracheal and laryngeal obstructions are generally characterized by inspiratory and expiratory stridor, with the inspiratory component the more prominent. There is moderate to marked increase in resistance to airflow in both phases of respiration. It is often most notable during inspiration and is unresponsive to bronchodilators. The distribution of ventilation, which may be altered in the presence of intrathoracic or diffuse airways obstruction, is normal in the presence of upper airway obstruction. Findings on lung function tests are also discussed in chapter 13.

When obstruction is severe, adequate alveolar ventilation may not be maintained even with an increase in respiratory work. Hypercapnia, arterial hypoxemia, and even pulmonary hypertension may develop.

Stridor, a characteristic spirogram, intercostal retraction during inspiratory efforts, a neck mass, or an abnormal upper airway shadow on radiologic study should suggest the presence of an upper airway obstruction. Definitive diagnosis is most often made on endoscopy, and normal function can be restored on removal of the obstruction.

Obstruction Below the Tracheal Bifurcation

Localized obstruction of intrathoracic airways is a common occurrence. If the obstruction is complete, varying degrees of resorptive ("obstructive") atelectasis may occur, with effects described in chapter 24. If the obstruction is partial, hyperinflation peripheral to the obstruction is not uncommon. Because the bronchial lumen enlarges during inspiration and narrows during expiration, the resistance to flow is greater during expiration than inspiration. As a result, air passes in more easily than out past the obstruction, and the lung peripheral to the partial obstruction becomes overdistended.

The right middle lobe bronchus, arising from the mainstem bronchus at an acute angle, is particularly vulnerable to extrinsic compression from enlarged surrounding lymph nodes, giving rise to the atelectasis known as "middle lobe syndrome." Intrinsic bronchial tumors, benign or malignant, may cause local obstruction that progresses from partial to complete occlusion of the bronchial lumen. Aspiration of a foreign body is a common cause of localized airway obstruction in children. Because the axis of the right main stem bronchus is in a more direct line than the left with the axis of the trachea, aspirated material lodges with greater frequency in the right lung. Aspirated vegetable or protein material swells and stimulates a local inflammatory reaction, with the result that occlusion may become complete and the offending material difficult to dislodge or remove. Mucus impaction may also lead to atelectasis, as described previously. Occasionally, a calcified lymph node erodes into a bronchus and exudes as a broncholith. This may lead to severe hemoptysis and partial occlusion of the airway.

The symptoms of localized intrathoracic airways obstruction vary with the cause and acuteness of onset. Extrinsic constricting or intrinsic obstructive lesions may produce few symptoms, whereas aspiration of foreign material may be followed by choking, coughing, wheezing, and acute respiratory distress. Cough and hemoptysis may be symptoms of a bronchial neoplasm.

Localized wheezing on auscultation is suggestive of a partially obstructed airway. The chest roentgenogram may reveal atelectasis resulting from complete airway occlusion or radiolucency pointing to localized hyperinflation peripheral to a partial obstruction. Enlarged lymph nodes or tumor impinging on a major bronchus may be discerned on the chest roentgenogram. Often, small endobronchial lesions can only be found by bronchoscopy. Bronchoscopy, ventilation and perfusion lung scans, or bronchospirometry may be needed to define the site and effect of a localized obstruction.

When occlusion is complete, the functional abnormalities may be attributed to the resulting atelectasis (see chap. 24). The dysfunction caused by partial obstruction depends on the site of obstruction and the amount of lung peripheral to the obstruction. Some expiratory slowing may be found if the obstructing lesion is centrally located. Abnormal distribution of ventilation can be demonstrated. Hypoxemia may result from continued perfusion of the underventilated portion of lung. It is often difficult or impossible to differentiate the functional abnormality caused by the localized obstruction itself from that caused by an underlying lung disease or by the neoplastic or infectious process that is the primary cause of the obstruction.

The object of treatment is to remove the obstruction. Purely intraluminal obstructions often may be approached bronchoscopically with removal of the foreign body or removal of retained secretions. Occasionally, following complete occlusion of an airway by aspirated vegetable or protein material, inflammation and infection may follow, making endoscopic removal of the obstruction impossible. A limited open surgical resection may be required.

When a neoplasm is the cause of a localized obstruction, simple removal of the obstruction itself is seldom feasible. Usually the treatment for such lesions consists of open thoracotomy with removal of both the obstructing lesion and peripheral lung tissue. Endoscopic removal of benign endobronchial neoplasms is occasionally possible. If the obstruction can be removed or surgical resection limited, good results may be anticipated. If the cause of the obstruction is a malignant neoplasm, the prognosis is related to the type and extent of the malignant process rather than to the obstruction itself. Partial bronchial occlusion from neoplasm may be an indication for radiation therapy.

Bronchiectasis

The term "bronchiectasis," indicating simply a dilatation of the bronchi, is used in a variety of clinical settings. It may merely describe one of the types of residual damage left by an old granulomatous disease. In this instance, the abnormal bronchi are limited in location to sites of old fibrotic lesions. The term is also used to describe localized bronchial abnormalities that occur with partial reinflation of a chronically atelectatic area, as in the middle lobe syndrome. Dilatation of bronchi may also be noted in the course of acute lobar pneumonia; such changes (sometimes called "pseudobronchiectasis") disappear over the ensuing three to six months. The term "bronchiectasis" is sometimes used to describe the cylindrical dilatation of airways seen on full inspiration in patients with severe generalized chronic bronchitis. In most such cases, bronchial caliber diminishes markedly on expiration, and the changes appear to reflect only an increase in compliance of airways. Bronchiectatic changes are also noted in pulmonary aspergillosis, a consequence of a local Arthus type of reaction to the allergenic focus of infection.

In all of the conditions thus far mentioned, the term "bronchiectasis" is appropriately used to describe a feature of the underlying disorder. When used as a primary diagnostic term, however, it should refer to a more distinctive clinical syndrome in which bronchi are pathologically dilated as a result of suppurative disease in their walls. Most often, this appears to be a consequence of a severe respiratory infection in early childhood. This problem, once among the most common chronic respiratory disorders, has decreased markedly in frequency since the advent of effective antimicrobial therapy.

In this syndrome, bronchiectatic changes tend to be most severe at the lung bases. Symptoms result from accumulation of secretions, chronic endobronchial infection, and recurrent acute pneumonias. Repeated hemoptysis can be a major problem. Recurrent infections lead to chronic inflammatory and fibrotic changes in the involved areas of the lung. With persistence of infection, a diffuse bronchitis often complicates the picture, leading to a generalized airways obstructive problem.

Bronchiectasis should be suspected in patients with recurrent lung infections, recurrent hemoptysis, or persistent production of large quantities of purulent sputum. Expectorated blood is of bronchial arterial origin and characteristically bright red. The three-layered green sputum once considered typical of the disease is rarely found now that infection can be controlled. The chest roentgenogram may be normal or reveal evidence of chronic inflammatory change, usually most marked at the lung bases. Large dilated bronchi traversing chronically inflamed portions of lung may present a honeycomb appearance.

Definitive diagnosis depends on bronchography, which allows assessment of the severity and extent of the bronchial disease. Such studies have been of great importance in the past when lung resection was recommended in order to remove infected areas of lung. With newer therapy, lung resection is almost never required except for severe hemorrhage. In fact, since the present major risk for these patients is development of respiratory insufficiency and cor pulmonale, every effort should be made to avoid lung resection, since this reduces pulmonary reserve. Unless it is needed to resolve a diagnostic dilemma, bronchography should not be performed. It occasionally leads to symptomatic exacerbations of disease and often causes a temporary increase in airways obstruction.

The physiologic changes in bronchiectasis are related to both the extent and severity of parenchymal inflammatory changes and the severity of associated diffuse airways obstruction. Stiffening of the lung and reduction of lung volumes are noted. Striking increases in bronchial arterial flow occur in areas of chronic inflammation. As a result of anastomoses between the bronchial and pulmonary arteries, there may be considerable left-to-right shunting of blood, with a consequent strain on the left ventricle. Variable physiologic shunting with hypoxemia is also noted.

When airways obstruction is superimposed, the physiologic alterations closely resemble those of chronic obstructive bronchitis described in chapter 27. Death may result from progressive respiratory insufficiency and cor pulmonale. Effective treatment depends on improving bronchial hygiene and controlling infection. Postural drainage procedures should be appropriate for the areas of lung involved. There is little point, for example, in a prone, head-down position for patients with anterior segment disease. The general measures used in these patients are otherwise similar to those used for severe chronic bronchitis, as described in chapter 27.

An association between chronic sinusitis and bronchiectasis has been claimed. It is doubtful that infected nasal sinuses can actually lead to bronchiectatic changes in the lung, however, and treatment of the sinuses should be undertaken only as indicated by the local disease process. The frequent association of sinusitis and bronchiectasis is probably a result of impaired resistance to infection throughout the respiratory system in some individuals. An association of sinusitis, bronchiectasis, and situs inversus is known as Kartagener's syndrome. It is associated with ciliary dysfunction, which is described further in chapter 27.

READING LIST

Jaffe H.J., Katz S.: Current ideas about bronchiectasis. *Am. Fam. Physician* 7:69–76, 1973.

A relatively recent general review of bronchiectasis and its treatment.

Ochsner A.: Bronchiectasis, disappearing pulmonary lesion. *N.Y. State J. Med.* Sept.: 1683–1689, 1975.

A historical perspective on the disease which appears to have become much less common than it was 20 years ago.

27

Generalized Airway
Obstructive Diseases

THIS CHAPTER DEALS with chronic or recurrent disorders which affect airway structure or function and which are not localized to a single area of the lung. It covers asthma, the chronic bronchitis syndromes, and emphysema. The most important consequence of these diseases is an *obstructive ventilatory abnormality*. We will continue to use this terminology instead of the proposed alternative "airflow limitation" (see chap. 13). As noted in chapters 6 and 13, this abnormality may result from an increase in airways resistance (secondary to intrinsic disease of the airways) or from loss of lung recoil (a characteristic of emphysema). Cystic fibrosis and the immotile cilia syndrome are also discussed briefly as special types of chronic obstructive bronchitis.

Definitions and
Interrelationships of Syndromes

As depicted in Figure 27–1, the bronchopulmonary system may react in several ways when exposed to noxious stimuli. The type of reaction depends on inherent host susceptibility as well as on the nature and severity of the stimulus.

When a subject with hyperreactive ("twitchy") airways is exposed to any of a variety of provocations, bronchospasm may occur. There is constriction of bronchial smooth muscle, often accompanied by mucus hypersecretion and mucosal edema. Recurrent episodes of bron-

chospasm of sufficient severity to cause symptoms are diagnosed as *asthma*.

A different response occurs when there is chronic low-grade exposure to bronchial irritants in a subject without airways hyperreactivity. After sufficient exposure, almost all subjects will develop mucous hypersecretion leading to chronic productive cough. This syndrome, called *simple chronic bronchitis,* is accompanied by impaired mucociliary clearance and increased susceptibility to bronchopulmonary infection.

Many subjects react to prolonged exposure to irritants, especially cigarette smoke, by developing inflammatory and obliterative changes in their small airways, those less than 2 mm in diameter. Clinically significant airflow limitation occurs only when these changes become very extensive. The factors which cause some subjects but not others to develop severe small airways changes remain unclear. Despite the fact that bronchioles as well as small bronchi may be involved, the conventional name for this entity, *chronic obstructive bronchitis,* will be used in this chapter.

The final disorder, *emphysema,* is characterized by a dilation of airspaces distal to the terminal bronchiole with destruction of alveolar walls. This results in a loss of alveolar surface area and in a decrease in lung recoil. As with chronic obstructive bronchitis, there appears to be considerable variability in susceptibility to emphysema. Subjects with a severe protease-in-

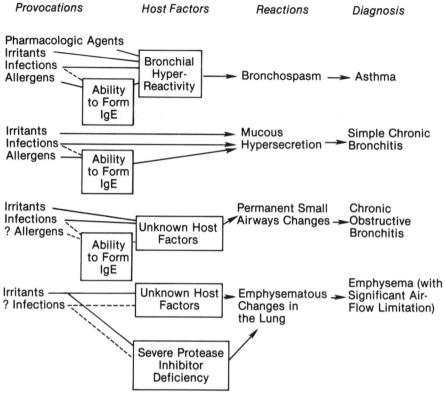

Fig 27–1.—The relationships of provocative agents and host susceptibility to bronchopulmonary reactions and diseases. *Dashed lines* indicate uncertain pathways.

hibitor deficiency are especially at risk, as described later in this chapter.

Unfortunately, these syndromes are by no means mutually exclusive. Indeed, in view of their common causative factors, they frequently coexist. Furthermore, they may predispose to one another. Some combinations are so frequent that they have been given special names, such as "wheezy bronchitis" in children and "asthmatic bronchitis" in adults. Chronic obstructive bronchitis and emphysema also often coexist, and their relative importance in producing severe persistent airflow obstruction may be difficult to determine. It was suggested some time ago that such cases be included under the term "chronic obstructive pulmonary (or lung) disease," and the acronyms COPD and COLD became popular. However, since these terms are now being used to cover an even wider variety of disorders and their meanings vary from one institution to the next, their use is no longer recommended.

In clinical practice, one generally uses the single diagnosis that best describes the patient's overall problem. This should not be interpreted to mean that related problems do not coexist and should not limit one's therapeutic efforts. A diagnosis of emphysema does not exclude the possibility that bronchoconstriction or bronchial secretions might be aggravating the patient's symptoms. All aspects of the patient's disease should be considered in deciding on a therapeutic program, not only those which determine the primary diagnosis.

Asthma

Approximately 3% of the general population has asthma. It often begins within the first three years of life, and it is 1.5 to 2 times more common in boys than in girls. The disease often remits in adolescence, and only about 25% of patients continue to have serious symptoms in early adult life. However, many others continue to have mild wheezing problems, and the rate of recurrent overt disease later in life is uncertain. An onset of disease in early adulthood is also relatively common. As will be discussed, new diagnoses of asthma after the age of 35 are not usual, but disease that develops late in life differs somewhat from that seen in childhood.

PATHOPHYSIOLOGY

The vast majority of cases diagnosed before the age of 35 occur in allergic individuals. However, even when there is clear evidence that many of the attacks have an allergic origin, other factors may provoke attacks. These include infections, exercise, nonspecific bronchial irritants, bronchoconstrictor medications, and perhaps even emotional factors, an indication of the nonspecific "twitchiness" of the airways.

The mechanisms which cause some airways to be hyperreactive remain unclear. Theories include the characteristics of the bronchial anatomical nervous system (e.g., β-receptor insensitivity), the number or characteristics of bronchial mast cells, and the contractile characteristics of the bronchial muscles themselves. While often assumed to be an inherited trait, bronchial hyperreactivity can also be acquired. It has been demonstrated to persist for weeks following a viral respiratory tract infection. It is possible that the bronchial hyperreactivity seen in some atopic subjects is a result of previous subclinical allergic bronchoconstriction and that the bronchi have been "trained" to overreact. This would explain the apparent connection between atopy and bronchial reactivity, as well as the diminished bronchial reactivity of asthmatic patients after the disease goes into remission.

To develop allergic bronchospasm, the patient must inhale an allergen capable of inducing a bronchial reaction, and that allergen must traverse the bronchial mucosa. It must then bridge two IgE molecules which are specific for the allergen and which are bound to the wall of a bronchial mast cell. When this occurs, the mast cell is induced to form active mediators from precursors and to release them, as well as preformed mediators, by degranulation. Mast cell reactions are depicted in Figure 27–2.

Mediators released include histamine, slow-reacting substance of anaphylaxis (SRS-A), eosinophil chemotactic factor of anaphylaxis (ECF-A), and an increasing variety of other substances, including prostaglandins and kallikreins. The relative importance of the various mediators and their interactions remain unclear. Histamine is relatively less important than in some other allergic reactions, and antihistamines are generally ineffective for treating asthma. The released mediators cause constriction of smooth muscle and mucous secretion.

Mediator activation and release as well as smooth muscle contraction are under control of the adenyl cyclase cAMP (3′,5′-cyclic adenosine monophosphate) system. High levels of cAMP inhibit both mast cell reactions and the constriction of smooth muscles. Thus, one mechanism for the effect of theophylline may be to inhibit phosphodiesterase, which prevents the breakdown of cAMP. The resulting increase in cAMP would relieve bronchoconstriction. Stimulation of β$_2$-adrenergic receptors (adenyl cyclase) leads to increased cAMP production and has similar effects.

Vagal effects appear important in modulating attacks in the experimental animal but are of questionable importance in humans. On the other hand, though little used yet in clinical practice in the United States, anticholinergic agents such as atropine are effective bronchodilators in some patients.

Attacks can be generated by direct stimulation of irritant receptors in the airway. Presumably, such receptors are involved in attacks resulting from inhalation of irritants, cold air, or exercise. It is currently believed that bronchoconstriction with exercise or cold air is related to excess heat exchange across the bronchial wall. It is not known whether the mast cells are involved in these types of attacks.

When an allergic asthmatic is challenged with an offending allergen, an "immediate" reaction

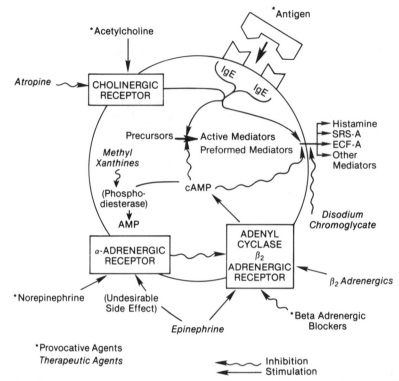

Fig 27–2.—Reactions in the mast cell regulation release of mediators. Provocative factors are indicated by an *asterisk* and therapeutic agents by *italics*. A *straight* or smoothly *curved line* indicates stimulation, while *wavy lines* are used to indicate inhibition.

occurs within minutes of the challenge. These "immediate" bronchospastic reactions can be promptly reversed by inhaling β_2-adrenergic agonists and prevented by prior inhalation of such agents or by cromolyn, which apparently stabilizes mast cells (see Fig 27–2). Curiously, however, these reactions are not prevented by use of adrenocortical steroids, which are the most effective antiasthmatic agents in clinical practice. This apparent paradox can be understood if one appreciates that there is more to asthma than the dramatic, readily reversed immediate reaction just described.

Even if untreated, the immediate reaction tends to improve over a few hours, and lung function may return to normal or near-normal levels. A second, late-phase reaction may then be seen six to ten hours after the initial provocation. This can be more severe than the immediate reaction and can last up to 24 hours. It responds only partially to bronchodilator medications.

At one time, this late-phase reaction was considered to be an Arthus reaction involving IgG antibodies. It now appears to represent an inflammatory reaction in the airway induced by the earlier "immediate" attack. If the immediate reaction is prevented by cromolyn, the late-phase reaction is eliminated. In contrast, corticosteroids prevent the late-phase reaction even after a severe immediate reaction to an antigen challenge.

CLINICAL FEATURES

In children and young adults, recurrent attacks of the immediate type may be the predominant complaint. These are usually easily controlled. Subjects with more persistent disease appear to have a prolonged, delayed-phase type of disease. Immediate reactions induced by acute allergen exposures or exertion may be superimposed on more chronic fluctuating symptomatology. In such patients, bronchodilator drugs may produce only partial relief, and corticosteroids may be needed to obtain a full remission. It is easy to understand why the immediate response to àn inhaled bronchodilator during spirometric testing would be of limited use in assessing the reversibility of the disease in such patients.

What has been said thus far can also be applied to subjects with an onset of asthma after the age of 35, but with some modifications. One can rarely demonstrate immediate hypersensitivity (IgE-mediated type 1 allergy) as a cause of asthma in such subjects. Indeed, in some studies, they show no more allergy skin test reactivity than the general population. Recurrent respiratory infections may be a major cause of exacerbations. There is often a chronic productive cough, justifying a diagnosis of chronic bronchitis. Indeed, there is no clear-cut distinction between chronic obstructive bronchitis with periodic exacerbations and persistent asthma. The term "asthmatic bronchitis" is sometimes used to describe such conditions, which vary greatly in the degree of reversibility of airways obstruction. The presence of sputum or blood eosinophilia strongly suggests significant reversibility. At times, differentiation of asthma from chronic obstructive bronchitis is made only by demonstrating improvement of airflow with corticosteroid therapy. The long-term prognosis of these "overlap" cases is uncertain, but complete remission appears to be unusual.

DIAGNOSIS

Except in its more persistent forms, there is rarely a problem in the diagnosis of asthma. The recurrent attacks of wheezing dyspnea are characteristic, especially when they occur at rest. The chest roentgenogram is normal except during attacks, when some hyperinflation may be seen. Spirometric studies show severe expiratory slowing during attacks and improvement with administration of a bronchodilator. Between ep-

isodes, standard spirometric tests may show mild persisting expiratory slowing or be entirely within normal limits. More sensitive indices of nonuniform distribution of lung function often reveal a mild persisting abnormality even when spirometric studies are normal. During a severe episode of bronchospasm, the VC is reduced and RV markedly increased. A temporary increase in TLC may be noted during an attack.

The major problem in the diagnosis of asthma is exclusion of other conditions that may lead to episodes of wheezing dyspnea, such as recurrent pulmonary emboli, anatomical airway lesions (e.g., foreign bodies, tumors, specific infections), fluctuations of symptoms in a chronic airways obstructive disorder, and episodes of acute left ventricular failure, especially when they occur as paroxysmal nocturnal attacks. Perhaps the most difficult entity to distinguish is the hyperventilation syndrome. The absence of wheezing, lack of response to therapy, and perfectly normal spirometric test results of such patients should make one suspicious.

If there is a question about the diagnosis and the patient cannot be observed during an attack, one may do bronchial challenge tests to demonstrate airways hyperreactivity (see chap. 13). Overall bronchial reactivity can be measured by determining the dose of an inhaled bronchoconstrictor agent (e.g., methacholine or histamine) required to induce a given decline in lung function. In children, exercise provocation is commonly used, and recently cold air challenge has been recommended to demonstrate hyperreactivity of airways.

While the atopic status of the subject can be readily assessed by a battery of allergy skin tests or measurements of serum IgE, the relationship of specific allergens to attacks may be difficult to ascertain. Antibodies to a wide variety of environmental substances, including foods, molds, and pollens, develop in these individuals. There are also a variety of occupational exposures which can provoke attacks. Common causes of occupational asthma are listed in Table 27–1.

In attempting to identify specific allergens, allergy skin testing is often used. Intradermal or scratch tests may yield some nonspecific reac-

TABLE 27–1.—SOME COMMON CAUSES
OF OCCUPATIONAL ASTHMA

Inorganic materials
   Platinum
   Nickel
   Vanadium
   Tungsten
Other chemicals
   Isocyanates
   Formaldehyde
Solder flux
Natural organic materials
   Grain
   Animal danders
   Castor bean
   Cotton or hemp dust
   Enzymes in detergents

Note: Not all of these have been shown to induce their bronchoconstrictive effects by classic allergic mechanisms.

tions, and the less traumatic prick test is more reliable. Prick testing shows a closer relationship to specific IgE as determined by radioallergosorbent test (RAST). But even when prick tests reveal the presence of antibodies to a specific antigen or when specific IgEs are identified by the RAST technique, this antigen may be of no importance in provoking bronchospasm. To produce a symptomatic attack, the antigen must reach the bronchial mucosa in a state in which it can react with local antibodies, and its specific IgE must be bound to mast cells in the bronchial wall. For these reasons, there is an imperfect relationship between skin test results and identifiable causes of attacks. This is most obvious with regard to foods.

Significant aeroallergens are more reliably identified by inhalation challenge, a relatively difficult and somewhat dangerous procedure. Even inhalation allergen challenges are not totally reliable, since the state of bronchial reactivity to a given antigen may be influenced by other factors, such as the state of irritation of the bronchial tree, infections, medications, and possibly even emotional factors. Also, challenges are usually performed with higher doses of allergen than are normally encountered in the environment. Inhalation challenges are most useful in identifying occupational provocations. In most other cases, identification of specific anti-

gens responsible for attacks of bronchospasm depends on a careful history considered together with simple immunologic test procedures.

MANAGEMENT

Patients with asthma experience great variety in the frequency, severity, and duration of their episodes. In some, all attacks occur in relationship to exposure to one or two specific antigens, and symptoms may be controlled simply by avoidance of these allergens. In such patients, bronchodilator medications are needed only occasionally, when accidental exposure to an allergen occurs. When allergens cannot be avoided but exposure is predictable and periodic, as with seasonal ragweed pollen allergy, bronchodilators and adrenal corticosteroids may be used during the period of exposure to prevent attacks. There may be a role for hyposensitization in patients whose symptoms are not readily controlled by simpler therapeutic measures.

Management of the disease is more difficult when there are frequent or prolonged attacks, when patients have nearly continuous low-grade symptoms, and when episodes are related to factors other than exposure to allergens. In such patients it is essential to recognize that the asthmatic tendency is a continuing problem, even though the symptoms may be intermittent. Most of these patients show some degree of functional abnormality even between symptomatic episodes. Principles of therapy include the following:

1. A serious effort must be made to identify the multiple factors that provoke exacerbations of disease and to avoid these factors as far as possible. Exacerbations should be treated early and vigorously. Antibiotic therapy should be started promptly at the onset of a lower respiratory tract infection.

2. Prescribing medication only to relieve acute attacks represents inadequate therapy. In severe asthma, a regular program of bronchodilators is needed to normalize lung function between attacks and to prevent periodic exacerbations. Therapy is generally begun with a long-acting oral theophylline preparation and the dose

adjusted to give a blood level close to 15 mg/L. Long-acting inhaled β₂-adrenergics are given concurrently. For subjects unable to use a metered-dose inhaler, jet nebulization can be used. The place of oral β-adrenergic agents is uncertain, but some patients appear to improve further with oral therapy even after receiving maximum doses of inhaled medication. The mechanisms of action of these agents and cromolyn sodium at the mast cell level are depicted in Figure 27–2. Similar reactions involving cAMP also occur in the smooth muscle, but there the outcome is muscle relaxation instead of mediator inhibition.

3. Regular inhalation of cromolyn sodium often is effective in preventing asthmatic attacks. It is especially useful in young patients with very intermittent symptoms. In them, cromolyn may obviate the need for steroids. A minimum trial of four to six weeks of regular therapy is required to evaluate the treatment. Since cromolyn is not a bronchodilator and seems to act only by preventing mediator release, it should not be given during an exacerbation.

4. Adrenal corticosteroids are used when airways obstruction cannot be controlled with maximum tolerable doses of bronchodilators. When prescribed, they should be given in moderately high doses (e.g., 30–60 mg of prednisone per day) for a short period to obtain rapid control of symptoms. The dose is then tapered over a one-to-two–week period, and an attempt made to discontinue this medication. When continuous steroid therapy is needed, the maintenance dose should be kept as low as possible, and an effort should be made to use an alternate-day program with a short-acting agent such as prednisone. Use of inhaled beclomethasone may help wean patients from oral steroids. This poorly absorbed inhaled steroid must be used regularly, two puffs four times daily, to be effective, and it should not be started during an exacerbation. It is best used in patients who have achieved good control with low doses of oral steroids in an attempt to discontinue the systemic medication.

5. Aspirin and aspirin-containing compounds should be avoided in asthmatic subjects, since they sometimes precipitate bronchospasm. Antihistamines are not advised because they tend to cause inspissation of secretions. Direct bronchoconstricting drugs should be avoided and β-blockers (e.g., propranolol) should be used with caution, if at all.

6. Patients must be taught to live as normally as possible within the limits imposed by their disease. They should be encouraged to take regular physical exercise, should be provided with medications to deal with milder symptomatic exacerbations, and should be assured that professional care will be readily available if a serious attack occurs. Every effort should be made to avoid dependence on complicated mechanical apparatus or on other types of treatment that require frequent visits to a medical facility.

STATUS ASTHMATICUS

A severe, persistent attack of bronchospasm, called status asthmaticus, is life-threatening. Early in the episode, patients are apt to hyperventilate, but nevertheless show some degree of hypoxemia. This hypoxemia may be aggravated by bronchodilator therapy and should be carefully monitored. Worsening of hypoxemia from bronchodilators appears to result from further deterioration of already disturbed ventilation-perfusion relationships. If the attack is not terminated promptly, and particularly if sedatives or narcotics have been administered, ventilation becomes increasingly difficult to maintain, and acute ventilatory failure may ensue. True respiratory muscle fatigue also occurs with prolonged status asthmaticus (see chap. 21).

Treatment of status asthmaticus includes a bolus of aminophylline given IV and a continuous IV drip to maintain an adequate blood level within the therapeutic range (10–20 mg/L). Beta₂-adrenergic agents should be given parenterally and by nebulization. Aerosolized bronchodilators should be followed by bronchial hygiene measures if there is a secretion problem (see subsequent sections).

The importance of prompt and vigorous treatment of status asthmaticus cannot be overemphasized. Persistence of severe airways obstruction increases the likelihood of respiratory muscle fatigue and acute ventilatory failure. A significant rise in Pa_{CO_2} in an asthmatic patient indicates the need for ventilator management.

The goal of therapy is complete elimination of the airways obstructive problem, not just symptomatic relief. If patients are discharged from the hospital with persisting mild bronchospasm, they are likely to require rehospitalization within a few days. At the time of hospital discharge, doses of steroids should be increased temporarily rather than decreased, and full doses of bronchodilators should be maintained.

SPECIAL FORMS OF THE DISEASE

A triad of asthma, nasal polyps, and aspirin sensitivity has been described. In fact, reactions to aspirin and related compounds are common in asthmatic patients. This appears to result from interactions with the prostaglandin system and is not immunologically mediated. Both allergic rhinitis and nasal polyps are also common in asthmatic patients, and both can occur with or without aspirin intolerance. Thus, the "asthma triad" is probably only the concurrence of common features of the disease.

Pulmonary allergic reactions may be associated with bronchospastic disease. These have been thought to represent type 3 (Arthus) or even type 4 (delayed) reactions, but uncertainty remains. An interesting example of this type of disease is "allergic aspergillosis." Here, organisms growing in bronchial mucous plugs may elicit apparent Arthus-type as well as type 1 allergic reactions. The Arthus type of allergy is characterized by circulating precipitating antibodies, a somewhat delayed skin test reaction to antigen (4 to 12 hours), and a tissue-damaging response rather than a simple wheal and erythema. When such a reaction occurs in the airway, local damage may lead to a characteristic proximal bronchiectasis. Pulmonary fibrosis may result from recurrent episodes of allergic pneumonitis. The associated bronchospasm is likely to be quite persistent and require continuous steroid therapy for its control. Diagnosis is confirmed by demonstrating an Arthus-like as well as an immediate type 1 skin reaction to an aspergillus antigen or by the finding of very high levels of total and aspergillus-specific IgE in a subject with a positive allergy prick test to an aspergillus antigen. The disease should be suspected whenever asthma is associated with recurrent allergic pneumonitis or with proximal bronchiectasis.

Many other causes of allergic alveolitis have been reported. As indicated in the section on allergic alveolitis (see chap. 25), these are associated with varying degrees of bronchospasm.

Finally, asthma may occur as part of a generalized immunologic disease and is occasionally seen in collagen-vascular diseases in association with vasculitis.

Simple Chronic Bronchitis

PATHOPHYSIOLOGY

Chronic irritation of the airways, especially by cigarette smoke, leads to an increase in mucus-secreting cells and an increase in the size of mucous glands. This is sometimes assessed by the ratio of gland to total wall thickness, the Reid index. There is mucous hypersecretion, and the resulting mucus may have an abnormal character. In addition, ciliary action is impaired, and cough becomes the major mechanism by which the excess secretions can be cleared. Any retained secretions provide an excellent breeding ground for bacteria. This, plus a direct adverse effect of cigarette smoke on macrophage function, allows the normally sterile bronchial system to harbor a mixed flora of organisms. These usually resemble bacteria found normally in the mouth, but *Hemophilus influenzae* is often present as well.

When there is any further insult to airways function (such as superimposed viral infection), organisms multiply more rapidly, and the sputum may become frankly purulent. Such episodes often last for several weeks and can be serious if there is concomitant airflow limitation from asthma, chronic obstructive bronchitis, or emphysema.

The simple presence of secretions in the airway can lead to mild ventilatory abnormalities, but, unless secretions are extremely viscid or occur in a patient with an ineffective cough, they rarely lead to severe airways obstruction. Except for patients with severe airways obstructive diseases, life-threatening problems from secretions are seen primarily in postoperative cases and in patients with concurrent neuromuscular diseases. In these settings, segmental or even lobar atelectasis secondary to mucous plugs are common.

CLINCIAL FEATURES

The majority of cases of simple chronic bronchitis occur in long-term cigarette smokers and consist of little more than coughing up a small amount of mucoid secretion each morning. The same problem may occur with occupational or environmental exposure to irritant gases, fumes, or dust. Mucous hypersecretion may also occur from bronchial allergic reactions, and there may be little accompanying bronchoconstriction if the airways are not excessively "twitchy." An allergic basis for chronic cough should be suspected when there is eosinophilia of blood or sputum. Such cases may also show an increase in the FEV_1 in response to bronchodilator agents, unmasking their mild bronchoconstriction.

Physical findings may be normal, or there may be varying degrees of coarse crackles, rhonchi, and wheezes. The last are sometimes elicited by a forced expiration, which may also induce a paroxysm of coughing.

DIAGNOSIS

The diagnosis is essentially one of exclusion. Other causes for chronic productive cough must be excluded. Parenchymal lung lesions are ruled out radiologically. If there is any reason to suspect a localized endobronchial disease (e.g., relatively short history of severe symptoms or hemoptysis), bronchoscopy may be needed as well. As noted, the presence of eosinophilia of blood or sputum or a mild airflow limitation responding to bronchodilators suggests an immunologic basis for the disease.

When chronic productive cough is noted in a child or young adult or when symptoms are un-usually severe, one should suspect either an immotile cilia syndrome or cystic fibrosis, which are discussed briefly later in this chapter.

COURSE AND PROGNOSIS

The prognosis of simple chronic bronchitis is quite variable. Available data suggest that mucous hypersecretion occurs independently of both the emphysematous and small airways lesions, which may also be induced by smoking. The presence of simple chronic productive cough does not necessarily imply that a smoker will have an unusually rapid decline in ventilatory capacity. Symptoms tend to fluctuate greatly in severity and often disappear when the inhaled irritant is removed.

In some cases, there are frequent purulent exacerbations requiring antibiotic therapy. Following such therapy, the bacterial flora of the sputum may change, with resistant organisms such as staphylococci or Pseudomonas predominating.

MANAGEMENT

If there is no serious airways obstruction and the patient can cough adequately, the main therapy is avoidance of irritants. For most patients, this means giving up cigarettes. The patient should also be advised to keep well hydrated.

Purulent exacerbations are generally treated with a seven- to ten-day course of a broad-spectrum antibiotic, such as tetracyline or ampicillin.

When an allergic basis for the disorder is suspected or when mild bronchoconstriction appears to be present, antiasthmatic therapy, described in the previous section, may be effective. Even without evidence that there is an asthmatic component, a trial of bronchodilator medications may be worthwhile, especially if there are severe episodes of paroxysmal coughing.

Much more vigorous therapy is necessary when there is airways obstruction or when the patient's ability to cough is otherwise impaired. Regular bronchial hygiene measures may be needed in such cases. After inhaling a bronchodilator and bland mist, the patient lies down, takes a few deep breaths, and makes a deliberate effort to cough out retained secretions. This may be more effective if various head-down positions are tried. Percussion or vibration of the chest while doing postural drainage may be efficacious and especially important when there is an ineffective cough.

When there is atelectasis secondary to retained secretions, the above bronchial hygiene measures should be applied vigorously and often. If they are not effective in relieving the atelectasis, bronchoscopy with suctioning and irrigation of the affected area may be needed.

When the sputum is especially viscous and there is an acute problem with retained secretions, acetylcysteine inhalation or instillation into the bronchus may be of use. It is not recommended, however, as routine treatment.

Chronic Obstructive Bronchitis and Emphysema

These diseases, characterized by chronic airways obstruction, are the most common causes of respiratory insufficiency. They are second only to heart disease as reasons for disability benefits under the Social Security Administration and are increasingly important causes of mortality.

A large fraction of cigarette smokers have mild functional abnormalities, reflecting changes in their small airways, and some degree of anatomical emphysema is found in at least half of consecutive autopsies on older men. These conditions tend to coexist, but with a regularity that is uncertain. Mild degrees of anatomical emphysema are not necessarily associated with significant respiratory symptoms. Whereas mild to moderate degrees of peripheral airways dysfunction may be detected by tests described in chapter 13, most subjects with such abnormalities do not have clinically significant impairment of lung function. In a minority of subjects, the small airways abnormalities or emphysema or both become sufficiently severe to lead to disabling airways obstruction that is resistant to therapy.

PATHOPHYSIOLOGY

The slowing of forced expiration observed in these patients results from some combination of: (a) loss of lung recoil, allowing excessive narrowing of airways during expiration; and (b) intrinsic bronchial changes (consisting of inflammatory lesions in small airways and sometimes mucous gland hypertrophy, inflammation and accumulation of secretions in larger bronchi) which lead to mechanical obstruction to airflow. Regardless of the mechanism for the airways obstruction, there is slowing of forced expiration, with markedly reduced FEV_1 and FEV_1/VC ratio. With severe emphysema, inspiratory airways resistance may be normal despite the marked narrowing of airways that occurs on forced expiration. With severe intrinsic bronchial disease, inspiratory as well as expiratory resistance tends to be elevated.

When emphysematous changes are severe, premature airways closure causes marked trapping of gas, leading to a large increase in RV. As a result of decreased lung recoil, TLC is also increased, but TLC does not change in proportion, and the RV/TLC ratio is elevated.

In patients with severe bronchial disease, recurrent pulmonary infections frequently develop, leading to some degree of localized atelectasis and fibrosis. In this case, instead of the loss of lung recoil and increase of compliance characteristic of emphysema, lung compliance may be normal or even decreased. As a result of occlusion of airways at small lung volumes, trapping of gas and some increase in RV occur, but TLC may be normal or even reduced. The combination of a moderately increased RV and a normal or low TLC leads to a high RV/TLC ratio even in the absence of extensive emphysema.

In all patients variations in mechanical properties in different lung regions lead to a marked nonuniformity in the distribution of ventilation, as reflected in abnormal inert gas washout curves. In the presence of intrinsic bronchial disease, ventilation is apt to be impaired to areas of lung that are still relatively well perfused (low ventilation/perfusion ratios), leading to severe venous admixture and hypoxemia. Resting hypoxemia may be less severe in the emphysematous type of disease in which the most underventilated areas tend to be those with the most severe emphysema in which blood flow is also reduced. A marked exertional fall in Pa_{O_2} may occur in severely emphysematous patients, however, possibly related to their very limited diffusing capacity.

Some portions of lung have little blood flow but well-maintained ventilation (high ventilation/perfusion ratios). The ventilation to such areas is partially wasted in terms of gas exchange, resulting in increased physiologic dead space. If adequate alveolar ventilation is to be maintained, overall minute volume must increase to compensate for this wasted ventilation. In late stages of the disease, when overall hyperventilation is limited and there is a large physiologic dead space, alveolar hypoventilation and hypercapnia develop. Chronic hypercapnia usually occurs later in patients with a purely emphysematous disorder than in those with intrinsic bronchial disease since, in severe emphysema where lung compliance is high, patients can assume an efficient, slow, deep pattern of breathing, minimizing their anatomical dead space ventilation. The faster, shallow breathing pattern of patients with a bronchial type of disease is more conducive to early development of alveolar underventilation. An early development of hypercapnia is also noted in subjects with reduced ventilatory drive, a trait inherited by a reasonable fraction of the population. Recent studies also suggest that severe blood gas abnormalities which occur during sleep in some subjects may be of importance in precipitating secondary effects of hypoxemia, such as erythrocytosis and pulmonary hypertension. These sleep apnea problems may be the major causes of the "blue bloater" syndrome described below. These issues are described in more detail in chapter 20.

In patients with extensive emphysema but without severe resting hypoxemia, the cardiac output tends to decrease with increasing severity of the disease. As a result, pulmonary artery pressures are only moderately increased despite a markedly increased pulmonary vascular resistance. With severe hypoxemia this reduction in cardiac output does not occur, pulmonary hypertension is more severe, and right ventricular hypertrophy may be marked.

In an early attempt to point out that patients with persistent airways obstruction varied in both their anatomical and clinical findings, two types of disease were described, type A (emphysematous) and type B (bronchial). Since type A patients are apt to show relatively deep breathing and maintain blood gases close to normal, they have been characterized as "pink puffers." Type B patients, who are apt to be severely cyanotic and have congestive heart failure, have been called "blue bloaters." These artificial distinctions no longer appear meaningful. If emphysematous changes are obvious radiologically, or if the lung is huge and there is a marked reduction in diffusing capacity, a diagnosis of emphysema is justified. Otherwise, chronic obstructive bronchitis is the appropriate diagnosis. The detailed studies of lung mechanics needed to evaluate how much of the slowing of forced expiration results from loss of recoil and how much from intrinsic airways disease are rarely justified clinically.

INHERITED FORMS OF CHRONIC AIRWAYS OBSTRUCTIVE DISEASE

Three genetic defects predispose to chronic airways obstruction.

CYSTIC FIBROSIS.—Patients who are homozygotes for cystic fibrosis (mucoviscidosis) often have a severe nonemphysematous type of obstructive respiratory insufficiency in childhood. An increasing number of these children now survive beyond their teens, and this disorder should be suspected in any young adult with severe bronchitic symptoms and chronic airways obstruction. Characteristically, these patients have recurrent acute respiratory infections and show widespread pulmonary infiltrates on chest roentgenogram.

Bronchopulmonary infection with a characteristic mucoid Pseudomonas is very common. Patients may give a history of gastrointestinal symptoms related to an accompanying pancreatic insufficiency. The diagnosis is confirmed by finding an excessively high sweat chloride level.

ALPHA$_1$-ANTITRYPSIN DEFICIENCY.—In homozygotes for α_1-antitrypsin deficiency, emphysema with chronic airways obstruction develops, with an onset of symptoms in middle age. Such patients account for 1%–2% of patients with severe airways obstruction. This diagnosis should be suspected in patients under 50 years of age with extensive anatomical emphysema (especially if it is most severe at the bases), in patients with a family history of obstructive airways diseases, and in females or nonsmoking males with severe chronic airways obstruction. Serum trypsin inhibitory capacity, or serum α_1-globulin levels are readily measured, and specific protease inhibitor (Pi) phenotyping by crossed immunoelectrophoresis may be done if there is any doubt about the diagnosis. Most severely deficient patients will have only Z genes (Pi Z) instead of inheriting the normal gene M from each parent (Pi M phenotype). The genetic alleles for the α_1-antitrypsin system include A, S, F, I, P, W, and X, as well as M, but only the Z variant has been clearly associated with emphysema.

It has been suggested that milder degrees of α_1-antitrypsin deficiency, reflecting a heterozygotic state (e.g., a Pi MZ phenotype), are also associated with a high prevalence of chronic airways obstruction. While this may be true in some families, epidemiologic studies have failed to show that Pi MZ subjects in general are at higher risk of developing emphysema.

IMMOTILE CILIA SYNDROMES.—There is a spectrum of recently described syndromes which are characterized by abnormal ciliary function. This leads to impairment of defense mechanisms in both the upper and lower airways, with consequent sinusitis, chronic bronchitis, and even bronchiectasis. Severe chronic obstructive bronchitis may result.

These syndromes are often accompanied by sterility and by dextrocardia or situs inversus. They should be considered when severe upper and lower airways disease occurs in young or sterile individuals. The fully manifested disorder with the triad of situs inversus, chronic sinusitis, and bronchiectasis has been long recognized and designated as Kartagener's syndrome.

PATHOGENESIS

The connection of α_1-antitrypsin status with pulmonary emphysema fits current theories of the genesis of this disorder. Several components of cigarette smoke and of polluted air reduce the ability of the macrophage system to the lung to clear inhaled microorganisms. It is possible that in patients exposed to cigarette smoke or air pollutants, recurrent low-grade pulmonary infections with leukocytic infiltration develop. The leukocytes involved in such infections release proteolytic enzymes, which may lead to local tissue destruction. The severity of emphysema produced would depend on the ability of the individual to inhibit proteolysis, a function of α_1-antitrypsin status. Although fitting many experimental and epidemiologic observations, this mechanism has not been proved to be the genesis of human emphysema. All that is certain is that emphysema occurs in subjects with severely impaired antiproteolysis mechanisms and that chronic bronchitis, emphysema, and chronic airways obstruction are related to cigarette smoking and probably related to exposure to air pollutants.

CLINICAL FEATURES

In most series of patients with clinically significant chronic airways obstruction, males are affected nine to ten times as often as females, and most cases are first diagnosed when patients are age 45 to 65. Dyspnea is the most common chief complaint, but some patients first consult a physician because of cough, wheezing, recurrent or unusually severe acute respiratory infections, or even weakness or weight loss. The dyspnea is usually insidious in onset and steadily progressive, though some patients are aware of shortness of breath only during periodic exacerbations of disease. In such patients, if persistence of ventilatory insufficiency is not appreciated, an inappropriate diagnosis of asthma may be made. Most patients admit to some expectoration when they are questioned directly, but this may consist only of a clearing of the chest shortly after awakening. In other patients the cough is more severe, and there is copious and sometimes purulent sputum. Occasionally, the first symptoms are a consequence of congestive heart failure secondary to cor pulmonale.

Physical findings in patients with chronic airways obstruction are extremely variable. In early stages thoracic examination may be entirely normal except for slowing of *forced* expiration. This maneuver should be a routine part of all physical examinations. Other physical findings occur with increasing frequency as the disease progresses. There may be gross pulmonary hyperinflation with low diaphragm, labored breathing, stooped posture, and use of accessory muscles of respiration. In patients with severe emphysema, vesicular breath sounds are decreased, the area of cardiac dullness is diminished, and there may be a faint high-pitched wheeze at the end of expiration. In patients who have more problems with bronchitis, the chest is often noisy, with wheezes and crackles of varying intensity.

Radiologic findings also are variable. The chest roentgenogram may be entirely normal or show only evidence of hyperinflation. It may reveal evidence of previous inflammatory disease, interpreted as fibrosis, chronic pneumonitis, or localized honeycombing. Bullae are seen in some patients. In advanced emphysema, frank attenuation of vascular markings with localized radiolucency may be noted. Cinebronchography shows excessive bronchial collapse during exhalation and may reveal areas of bronchiectasis or bronchiolectasis. Radioactive lung scans reveal uneven perfusion and ventilation, and pulmonary angiograms allow visualization of irregular vascularization of the lungs and attenuation of small arteries.

It must be emphasized, however, that radiologic findings are not reliable criteria for diagnosis of obstructive lung diseases. A diagnosis of emphysema should not be based solely on an appearance of hyperinflation of the lungs. Many normal lungs have this appearance.

DIAGNOSIS

Diagnosis depends on demonstration of slowing of forced expiration that persists despite prolonged and intensive medical management. It also depends on exclusion of specific diseases that might lead to the same pattern or physiologic abnormality. The chest roentgenogram excludes diffuse parenchymal lung diseases that can produce clinical and physiologic findings resembling those of emphysema and chronic obstructive bronchitis. It is more difficult to exclude a specific disease within the large airways. Clinical features of upper airway obstructions are discussed in chapter 26, and lung function tests, which help distinguish upper airway lesions from the present diseases, are reviewed in chapter 13.

It is essential to distinguish patients with a persistent form of asthma, since such patients have a potentially reversible disease and a much better prognosis. Features which should make one suspicious are listed as indications for a steroid trial in the section on Management below. Blood eosinophilia is an especially important finding in this regard.

COURSE AND PROGNOSIS

When patients with persistent airways obstruction first seek medical attention, they are often in a mild exacerbation of their disease. With adequate therapy, considerable initial improvement may be noted, but the long-term outlook is less favorable. After initial treatment, ventilatory function generally declines at a slow rate, the FEV_1 falling an average of 50 to 75 ml per year. Most other subjective measurements and most clinical features also show progressive worsening, but cough may improve with medical management, especially if cigarette smoking is terminated. Severe respiratory failure and cor pulmonale are characteristic of the last few years of illness.

Prognosis is closely related to the severity of expiratory slowing. Table 27–2 presents a rough guide for predicting survival. Over a 5-year period, mortality rates are not much greater than normal in patients who have relatively mild expiratory slowing ($FEV_1 > 1.35$ L) and no other adverse features, but survival is generally short in patients with severe obstruction, especially when it is accompanied by hypercapnia or cor pulmonale. The prospects for survival for more than 10 years are poor even for patients with FEV_1 in the 1.3–1.7 L range at the time of diagnosis.

It is important, however, to emphasize the variability in the disease. Some patients have long survivals despite very low initial FEV_1. Also, overall survival may have improved since the data in Table 27–2 were collected. This certainly appears to be true for severely hypoxemic patients receiving continuous oxygen therapy.

Symptomatic exacerbations occur frequently in these patients. These are generally associated with an increase in sputum purulence and are considered to be infectious, although they may result as often from a breakdown of host defense mechanisms with overgrowth of existing bacterial flora as from exposure to new pathogenic microorganisms. Some exacerbations can be ascribed to pulmonary emboli, mucus impaction with atelectasis, pneumothorax, or bronchospasm secondary to exposure to irritants or aller-

gens. In late stages of disease when cor pulmonale has developed, worsening of symptoms may reflect only poorer control of chronic congestive failure.

MANAGEMENT

It is essential to exclude directly remediable causes of airways obstruction before embarking on a therapeutic program. Upper airway neoplasms or foreign bodies may be susceptible to surgical removal. Endobronchial infections such as tuberculosis may respond dramatically to specific therapy. Therapy has the following goals in patients with chronic airways obstruction, asthmatic patients whose symptoms persist despite attempts to avoid provocative factors, and patients with irremediable specific lung diseases associated with airways obstruction:

1. Relief of any reversible component of the airways obstruction. Although airway collapse secondary to emphysema is irreversible, many patients have some degree of retention of secretions, mucosal edema, and smooth muscle spasm that may be relieved by appropriate therapy.

2. Relief of cough. The goal is not to suppress cough, but to assist in raising of secretions.

3. Eradication and prevention of bronchopulmonary infection that may contribute to the airways obstructive problem.

4. Avoidance of irritants or allergens that may precipitate acute attacks or aggravate symptoms in patients with chronic disease. Elimination of cigarette smoking is of paramount importance.

5. Improved exercise tolerance to the limits allowed by the patient's permanent physiologic impairment. Injudicious limitation of activity causes excessive disability in many patients by leading to a deterioration of their general physical condition.

6. Treatment of complications of the disease, including control of excessive hypoxemia, elimination of congestive heart failure, and prevention of episodes of acute ventilatory failure.

7. Avoidance of factors that may aggravate

TABLE 27–2.—PROGNOSIS IN PATIENTS WITH CHRONIC AIRWAYS OBSTRUCTION

FEV_1	OTHER ADVERSE FINDINGS*	APPROXIMATE % MORTALITY			
		1 YR	3 YR	5 YR	10 YR
<0.75	Present	30	60	90	95
	Absent	20	40	60	80
0.75–0.95	Present	20	40	60	80
	Absent	10	30	40	70
0.95–1.35	Present	10	30	40	70
	Absent	5	20	30	60
>1.35	Present	5	20	30	60
	Absent	<5	10	15	50

*Includes $Pa_{CO_2} > 45$ torr, diffusing capacity <50% predicted, resting pulse > 100/min, or clinical evidence of cor pulmonale.

the disease, such as elective surgery, excessive sedatives, and narcotics.

8. Relief of the depression and anxiety that so often accompany a disabling chronic disease.

Even when the airways obstruction cannot be completely reversed, symptoms are often markedly ameliorated, patients allowed to lead more active and satisfying lives, premature disability and death avoided, and the number of hospital admissions reduced by appropriate therapy. Although most patients with severe chronic airways obstruction continue to show a slow progression of ventilatory impairment despite treatment and have a poor prognosis in late stages of the disease, this should not lead the physician to a nihilistic attitude toward therapy.

Increased numbers of patients with mild, even subclinical airways obstruction are now being discovered as a result of detection by routine lung function studies (see chap. 13). It is to be hoped that vigorous treatment and cessation of smoking at this stage of the disorder will prevent progression to disability and death. It must be admitted, however, that there is little documentation of this at the present time.

The degree of reversibility cannot always be determined with precision when the patient is first seen. Whereas a favorable response to a single dose of bronchodilator in the pulmonary function laboratory indicates that a good therapeutic response is possible, irreversibility of the obstruction in the laboratory does not necessarily indicate that there will be no response to an intense and prolonged therapeutic program. Initial therapy should include: (1) use of bronchodilators in maximum doses and evaluation of their effects with serial spirometric tests, (2) cessation of smoking and avoidance of other bronchial irritants, (3) expectorant therapy, (4) a trial of chest physiotherapy and postural drainage when there are retained secretions, (5) a regular program of physical exercise, (6) treatment of any existing bronchial infection and prescription of antibiotics for recurrent infection, (7) blood gas measurements at rest and exercise with consideration of oxygen therapy, (8) evaluation of cardiac status with consideration of the need for therapy of heart failure, (9) evaluation

of possible allergic factors in the disease, including advice on avoiding possible antigens, and (10) frank discussion with the patient and family concerning expectations of treatment and side effects of therapy.

After response to initial treatment has been observed, the physician must decide which portions of the program should be continued and whether there is sufficient likelihood of further reversibility of the disease to justify the addition of adrenocortical hormones.

BRONCHODILATOR AGENTS.—Theophylline and β_2-adrenergic agonists are given as described in the management of asthma. When initial therapy leads to significant improvement in ventilatory function, an attempt is made to maintain a maximum bronchodilator program without causing undue side effects. When no significant improvement is obtained by initial therapy, and if there are no indications for corticosteroids, a maintenance program of β_2-adrenergic agents and/or theophylline is usually prescribed to prevent periodic worsening of the airways obstruction.

CORTICOSTEROIDS.—The following features suggest that a trial of adrenocortical hormones may be worthwhile:

1. Greater than 20% improvement in spirographic abnormalities following a single dose of bronchodilator medication.

2. Greater than 20% improvement of functional abnormalities over several weeks of intensive bronchodilator therapy.

3. Noisy or wheezy chest on physical examination.

4. History of acute bronchospastic episodes or at least of considerable fluctuation in severity of symptoms.

5. Chest roentgenogram that does not suggest extensive anatomical emphysema.

6. Evidences of atopic predisposition, including peripheral eosinophilia.

Corticosteroids should be used only after a maximum bronchodilator program has been tried, and bronchodilators should be maintained at full doses while steroids are given. Medication should be discontinued if the patient fails to show objective improvement in lung function tests during a three- to four-week trial of at least 20 mg prednisone per day. If the medication is continued despite the hazards of long-term steroid therapy, dosage is tapered gradually to the lowest level that will maintain the induced improvement in ventilatory function. Isoniazid should be prescribed if there is any evidence of an underlying quiescent tuberculous infection.

ANTIBACTERIAL THERAPY.—In most instances, the presence of bacterial infection in the lower respiratory tract is manifest only by purulence of sputum. An attempt should be made to achieve and maintain mucoid secretions. For patients with recurrent infections, continuous tetracycline or ampicillin therapy is recommended by some authorities. Others use these medications for two- to three-week courses each month. An effective therapeutic regimen involves the use of antibiotics in a prolonged course for initial clearing of purulent sputum and additional courses of medications at the onset of acute respiratory infection or with recurrence of purulent sputum.

TREATMENT OF COUGH AND SECRETIONS.— This is discussed in the management of simple chronic bronchitis.

AVOIDANCE OF BRONCHIAL IRRITANTS.—Cessation of cigarette smoking is of the greatest importance and generally leads to improvement of cough. Obvious other sources of dusts and noxious fumes should also be avoided. Effects of exposure to dusts and cold air may be minimized by breathing through a face mask or woolen scarf. Dust suppression measures, air filtration, or wearing of a special mask may be useful in persons who are especially sensitive to dust inhalation.

CLIMATE.—A change in climate or locale is often recommended for severely disabled patients. A change in residence may be recommended for hypoxemic patients who live at altitudes above 4,000 ft or for those who live in areas of excessive air pollution. Marked temporary improvement may be obtained in persons who are allergic to one or more environmental pollens that do not exist in another area. Unfortunately, many of these individuals subsequently show reactions to inhalants in their new environment.

Many patients consider moving to escape the cold winters of northern areas. Some find relief in warm, humid climates; others are less symptomatic in dry desert areas. It is uncertain that the overall course of the disease is altered by a move to either type of climate.

EXERCISE PROGRAMS.—Unless contraindicated by a concomitant cardiac disorder, a graded regular exercise program should be prescribed. This usually results in improved exercise tolerance even if lung function remains unaltered. In most instances an appropriate program can be prescribed by the physician, although there are advantages in beginning exercise training under the direction of a trained physiotherapist in severely disabled patients or in those requiring supplemental oxygen during exercise training. Exercise programs should have a specific goal that is meaningful to the patient, such as a walk to a neighborhood store.

It is uncertain that breathing training or breathing exercises result in more than psychological benefit. Attempts to train the patient to breathe more slowly are usually successful only in anxious patients who have excessive tachypnea.

OXYGEN THERAPY.—Low-flow oxygen by nasal cannula may be used during exercise in patients with severe exertional hypoxemia, especially as a part of a graded exercise program. Marked erythrocytosis or recurrent heart failure despite only moderate resting hypoxemia suggests a severe nocturnal oxygen deficit. If this is confirmed, use of low-flow oxygen during sleep may greatly improve the patient's status. When severe chronic hypoxemia is present, continuous oxygen therapy may be needed to maintain cardiac compensation. Finally, some patients with very severe chronic hypoventilation cannot maintain a Pa_{O_2} compatible with life without continuous supplemental oxygen. Recent evidence suggests that survival is better with continuous oxygen therapy than with only 15 hours of oxygen per day for patients with resting Pa_{O_2} persistently below 55 torr.

Use of oxygen to treat episodes of dyspnea is almost never indicated. Patients become habituated to oxygen used in this manner, enhancing their invalidism. Routine use of intermittent oxygen, often prescribed in conjunction with IPPB treatments, is unjustified and potentially dangerous.

TREATMENT OF ALLERGIES.—When clear-cut environmental allergens can be identified, every attempt should be made to avoid them. Corticosteroid management may also help control symptoms in atopic individuals. When one or two offending antigens can be identified with certainty (based on a combination of history and allergy test results), there may be a rationale for a hyposensitization program, but this is most unusual in patients with chronic airways obstruction. Hyposensitization programs prescribed solely on the basis of multiple skin test reactions are almost invariably unsuccessful in these individuals.

TREATMENT OF EDEMA AND HEART FAILURE.—Pedal edema is common even in the absence of other evidences of congestive heart failure. It is usually readily controlled by small doses of diuretics. Recurrent or persistent chronic congestive heart failure secondary to cor pulmonale is a much more difficult problem. In addition to the usual treatment for congestive heart failure, phlebotomies may be needed to maintain the hematocrit near 55, and all therapy may be unsuccessful unless hypoxemia is controlled with oxygen administration. Digitalis preparations must be used with great caution in these patients. Digitalis toxicity with arrhythmias commonly results, presumably as a consequence of the fluctuating blood gas and electrolyte values.

CHRONIC HYPERCAPNIA.—Chronic, well-compensated carbon dioxide retention occurs frequently in late stages of obstructive lung diseases. Although it requires no specific treatment, it indicates the need for avoidance of sedatives, caution in the use of oxygen, and careful monitoring of symptomatic exacerbations. Respiratory stimulants and mechanical assistance to ventilation should not be used in patients with chronic, stable hypercapnia.

SURGICAL THERAPY.—Large bullae may require resection either because they compress relatively normal portions of lung, are rapidly expanding, lead to recurrent pneumothorax, or are persistently infected. But attempts to improve lung function by removal of the most emphysematous portions of lung are usually unsuccessful and should not be undertaken without careful, detailed preoperative assessment (see chap. 12).

TREATMENT OF EXACERBATIONS OF OBSTRUCTIVE LUNG DISEASES.—Mild exacerbations of disease are common. They are often associated with respiratory infections and are usually treated effectively by vigorous application of the measures mentioned above. Measurements of arterial blood gas tensions should be made and cardiovascular status reevaluated during serious exacerbations or when there is symptomatic worsening in a patient with severe chronic impairment. Indications of increasing hypercapnia, hypoxemia, or incipient heart failure point to the need for immediate hospitalization and intensive treatment. Sedatives and high concentration oxygen must be avoided, since they may turn a mild exacerbation into life-threatening acute respiratory failure. Severe exacerbations are treated identically to status asthmaticus, as described in the section on asthma. Since most acute exacerbations appear to be associated with intercurrent infection, it should be assumed that antibiotic management is needed unless there is evidence to the contrary. Mild exacerbations are handled satisfactorily with tetracycline, ampicillin, or trimethoprim-sulfamethoxazole. Severe purulent exacerbations should be treated with ampicillin, cephalothin, or even chloramphenicol. Penicillin is a poor choice of antibiotic in this clinical setting unless there is a pneumococcal pneumonia. Sputum smear and culture are of relatively little help in deciding initial therapy. However, if a prompt therapeutic effect is not obtained, results of culture and sensitivity tests will be needed to decide on a more appropriate antibiotic regimen.

The patient's blood gas status must be evaluated at the onset of a severe exacerbation and periodically throughout hospitalization to determine the level of hypoxemia, degree of hypercapnia, and acid-base status. Treatment of respiratory failure and its complications has been discussed in chapter 17. In patients with known severe progressive chronic obstructive bronchitis or emphysema or both, mechanical ventilation should be avoided unless there is a clear and quickly remediable cause for their exacerbation.

Exacerbations are often precipitated or complicated by heart failure secondary to cor pulmonale. Management of this problem is discussed in chapter 16. Other complications that may be associated with or even precipitate an acute exacerbation include pulmonary embolism, pneumothorax, and obstructive atelectasis. The diagnosis of pulmonary embolism in this clinical situation is exceedingly difficult, especially in the absence of evidence of peripheral venous thrombosis. Frequently, anticoagulant management must be initiated on the basis of a strong suspicion of the problem. In patients with severe airways obstruction, pneumothorax should be treated promptly with continuous intrapleural suction.

Specific Diseases Associated with Generalized Airways Obstruction

A variety of pneumonoconioses are accompanied by chronic airways obstruction. In its later stages, conglomerate silicosis is associated with emphysematous changes in the lungs and severe expiratory slowing. Coal workers' pneumoconiosis may present a clinical picture indistinguishable from ordinary chronic obstructive bronchitis and emphysema, except for the history of dust exposure. These problems are discussed in greater detail in chapter 25.

Far advanced pulmonary tuberculosis and other far advanced infectious granulomas are often associated with emphysematous changes and chronic airways obstruction. Indeed, respiratory insufficiency and cor pulmonale are common causes of death in patients with these diseases even if the infectious aspects of the problem can be controlled. Also, noninfectious granulomas, such as sarcoidosis and berylliosis, generally associated with a restrictive type of functional disorder, are occasionally accompanied by persistent airways obstruction.

Exposure to certain industrial air pollutants can, in sensitive individuals, cause symptoms of generalized airways obstruction. Because symptoms are most prominent on fresh exposure to the irritants, the phenomenon of "Monday morning dyspnea" is characteristic. Byssinosis, affecting workers involved in the initial processing of cotton, flax, and hemp, begins with a reversible asthma-like syndrome but may, after long exposure to these organic dusts, progress to a state indistinguishable from chronic obstructive bronchitis. Workers in the polyurethane foam and varnish industries exposed to toluene diisocyanate vapor show similar symptoms, and evidence is accumulating that permanent progressive deterioration in lung function may also occur in these workers.

READING LIST

Afzelium B.A.: Immotile-cilia syndrome and ciliary abnormalities induced by infection and injury (editorial). Am. Rev. Respir. Dis. 124:107–109, 1981.

A recent review of this interesting syndrome.

Chai H., Farr R.S., Froehlich L.A., et al.: Standardization of bronchial inhalation challenge procedures. J. Allergy Clin. Immunol. 56:323–327, 1975.

This is a committee recommendation in regard to methods for assessing bronchial reactivity.

Hilman B.C.: Cystic fibrosis: not just a pediatric disease. J. Resp. Dis. 2:83–97, 1981.

A brief review of cystic fibrosis, emphasizing its diagnosis and treatment in adults.

Lichtenstein L.M.: An evaluation of the role of immunotherapy in asthma (editorial). Am. Rev. Respir. Dis. 117:191–197, 1978.

A critical appraisal of immunotherapy by an expert in the field.

Macklem P.T.: Obstruction in small airways—a challenge to medicine. Am. J. Med. 52:721–724, 1972.

A classic article calling attention to the importance of small airways abnormalities.

Nocturnal Oxygen Therapy Trial Group. Continuous or nocturnal oxygen therapy in hypoxemic chronic obstructive lung disease. Ann. Intern. Med. 93:391–398, 1980.

A report of a multicenter trial comparing survival

of subjects with a 15-hour/day vs. continuous O₂ supplementation. Survival was better with continuous therapy.

Pepys J., Hutchcroft J.: Bronchial provocation tests in etiologic diagnosis and analysis of asthma (State of the Art). *Am. Rev. Respir. Dis.* 112:829–859, 1975.

An excellent review of the uses of challenge tests to identify provocative factors, especially in occupational asthma. Early- and late-phase reactions are described in detail.

Symposium on obstructive lung disease. *Med. Clin. North Am.* 65:453–706, 1981.

This symposium consists of 12 articles covering many aspects of airways obstructive diseases. It is highly recommended reading and has an extensive list of references to original papers.

Thurlbeck W.M.: *Chronic Airflow Obstruction in Lung Disease.* Philadelphia, W.B. Saunders Co., 1976.

Although somewhat dated, this remains the most exhaustive review of clinicopathologic relationships in chronic airways obstruction.

28

Respiratory Distress Syndromes

INFANT RESPIRATORY distress syndrome (IRDS) is a major cause of neonatal mortality which is primarily related to immaturity of the lungs at birth. A similar form of respiratory failure observed in adults is due to multiple etiologies and has been designated the adult respiratory distress syndrome (ARDS). Though the circumstances under which the two diseases occur are different, many of the pathophysiologic mechanisms are similar.

Infant Respiratory Distress Syndrome

IRDS, or hyaline membrane disease, is an affliction of newborn infants, usually premature and of low birth weight, which is characterized by neonatal respiratory distress and hypoxemia. The incidence of IRDS appears to be directly related to the degree of prematurity at birth. However, other factors including perinatal asphyxia, cesarean section without labor, maternal diabetes, and maternal hemorrhage have also been implicated as predisposing to a greater risk.

PATHOGENESIS AND PATHOPHYSIOLOGY.—A deficiency of surfactant in the lungs of these premature infants is the major pathophysiologic factor contributing to the clinical findings in IRDS. Without the stabilizing effect of surfactant, airspaces are more liable to collapse. In the absence of alveolar pores of Kohn as pathways for collateral ventilation, microatelectasis results. There is a subsequent appearance of a hyaline membrane lining the alveoli. One factor in the development of the hyaline membrane may be the use of high airway pressures from mechanical ventilation. It may be that without the protective alveolar lining layer, cellular injury occurs, contributing to the formation of this membrane. Pulmonary hypoperfusion, aspiration of amniotic fluid, asphyxia, or a fibrinolytic enzyme defect may also play an etiologic role. As a result of atelectasis, FRC and crying VC are reduced. Lung compliance is markedly decreased.

These infants exhibit a normal or increased minute ventilation and decreased V_T, resulting in an increase in dead space ventilation. Further increase in dead space ventilation can also occur as a result of poor perfusion of ventilated portions of the lung. At the same time, perfusion of nonventilated atelectatic portions of the lung contribute to the profound hypoxemia characteristic of this syndrome. As a result of immaturity of the pulmonary vasculature, pulmonary vascular resistance and pulmonary artery pressures remain high after birth. This may produce shunting of venous blood through a patent foramen ovale or ductus arteriosus. Therefore, right-to-left intracardiac shunting may also contribute to the observed hypoxemia.

CLINICAL FEATURES.—Symptoms first occur within the first six to eight hours of life and often appear in the delivery room. If therapy is unsuccessful, death usually occurs within 72 hours. Clinical manifestations include increased respiratory rate with retraction of the soft tissue of the chest wall, grunting respirations, harsh breath sounds and fine crackles, systemic hypotension, and hypothermia. Oxygen desaturation is a prominent feature. The chest roentgenogram characteristically reveals air bronchograms contrasted against a diffuse reticulogranular infiltrate filling the lung fields.

PATHOLOGIC FINDINGS.—The lungs at necropsy are airless and liver-like. Postmortem histologic examination of the lung usually reveals widespread atelectasis and eosinophilic hyaline membranes lining aerated portions of the lung. Although the term "hyaline membrane disease" is synonymous with IRDS, the membrane is often absent from the lungs of infants who die within a few hours of birth and is not pathognomonic for this syndrome. The membrane is composed of fibrin and cellular debris derived from blood and injured epithelium and appears to be a secondary development common to a variety of respiratory insufficiency states.

TREATMENT.—Treatment is largely supportive and includes primarily oxygen supplementation, assisted ventilation, continuous distending airway pressure (CDAP), and general supportive measures. Research using artificial surfactant is promising and provides hope that a specific therapy may some day be available.

Supplemental oxygen is usually administered to raise the Pa_{O_2} to between 50 and 70 torr. An excessively high Pa_{O_2} will lead to the development of retrolental fibroplasia. Therefore, frequent monitoring of arterial blood samples or use of a transcutaneous oxygen analyzer is necessary.

Use of CDAP will increase FRC, decrease atelectasis, and improve oxygenation. CDAP can be applied as either a continuous negative pressure around the thorax (CNEP) or as continuous positive airway pressure (CPAP). Since infants are obligate nasal breathers, CPAP may be applied nasally and does not necessarily require an endotracheal tube. When CO_2 exchange is impaired, mechanical ventilation is required in addition to CDAP. High airway pressures and inspired oxygen concentrations associated with mechanical ventilation may contribute to the development of bronchopulmonary dysplasia (see chap. 30) in IRDS survivors. The major adverse effect of CDAP and mechanical ventilation is barotrauma, which may occur in 30% of cases.

General supportive measures in IRDS are often as important as respiratory support. Adequate nutrition is a major concern, as is providing an optimum thermal environment. Jaundice related to hepatic immaturity frequently occurs and must be appropriately treated. With careful management, the overwhelming majority of infants survive the acute episode, but unfortunately many progress to a more chronic form of lung disease, bronchopulmonary dysplasia (see chap. 30).

Recent advances have been made in the prevention of IRDS. Determination of lecithin-sphingomyelin (L/S) ratios in the amniotic fluid have proved useful in predicting fetal lung maturity. Premature labor can sometimes be arrested using sympathomimetic agents. One of the most promising developments has been the demonstration that maternal administration of corticosteroids prior to a premature delivery will accelerate lung maturation and decrease the incidence of IRDS.

Adult Respiratory Distress Syndrome

The adult respiratory distress syndrome (ARDS) is characterized by the rapid onset of clinical signs of respiratory distress and hypoxemia, usually following an acute event which results in lung injury. Acute respiratory distress following shock and trauma has been known to physicians since World War II. However, it was not defined as a syndrome until 1967, when a group of adults with clinical and pathologic findings resembling IRDS were described. Subsequently, there has been increased awareness of this entity, with an estimated incidence of 250,000 cases per year in the United States and a mortality of approximately 50%.

PATHOGENESIS AND PATHOPHYSIOLOGY.—The clinical features observed with ARDS are a result of diffuse damage to the lungs. The mechanisms which produce the diffuse lung injury can be divided into two categories. First, inhalation or aspiration of certain gases or chemicals is directly toxic to the alveolar epithelium, producing destruction and increased permeability of the alveolar capillary membrane. Second, damage to the lung can be initiated in the pulmonary microvasculature. The presence of platelet and fibrin microemboli in pathologic specimens has suggested that accelerated intravascular clotting is often present. Thrombin activation and concurrent fibrinolysis leads to increased levels of fibrin degradation products which may cause microvascular injury. The glycoprotein fibronectin is depleted in many patients with ARDS. Fibronectin is a nonspecific opsonin which is necessary for optimum phagocytic function. It has been suggested that lack of fibronectin resulting from as yet undetermined factors allows fibrin degradation products to circulate longer, thereby increasing lung injury. There is also increasing evidence implicating complement activation and uncontrolled neutrophil protease activity in producing lung microvascular damage. Clinical observations have confirmed that complement activation can occur in potential ARDS producing situations, such as sepsis and multisystem trauma. Activation of complement in the lung microvasculature could attract neutrophils with subsequent release of proteolytic enzymes and liberate free radicals leading to lung injury. In addition, disturbances in the production of prostaglandins, and activation of the bradykinin system may also contribute to the production of ARDS.

Irrespective of the initial mechanism, the primary pathologic consequence of diffuse lung injury is an increase in the permeability of the alveolar capillary membrane for both plasma and red blood cells. Fluid flux ($\dot{Q}_f$) across the alveolar capillary membrane is governed by the Starling equation. It describes the relationships among the oncotic and hydrostatic pressures of the pulmonary capillary and interstitial space, and the permeability of the alveolar capillary membrane for both fluid and solutes (Fig 28–1). Normally, the alveolar capillary membrane is relatively impermeable to both fluid and solutes. The summation of all the Starling forces does, however, result in a small net movement of fluid out of the pulmonary capillaries into the lung interstitium. Accumulation of excess extravascular lung water is prevented by the action of the pulmonary lymphatics. An increase in permeability results in pulmonary edema from leakage of plasma and red blood cells into the

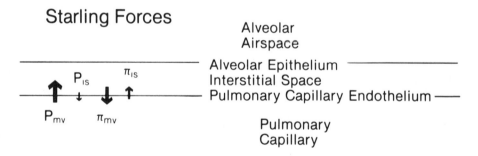

$$Q_f = K_w[(P_{mv} - P_{is}) - \sigma_s(\pi_{mv} - \pi_{is})]$$

Fig 28–1.—Schematic representation of a normal alveolar capillary membrane. Factors governing fluid flux are shown in the Starling equation and graphically illustrated by appropriate arrows. Q_f = fluid flux; K_w = filtration coefficient of water; Pmv = pulmonary capillary hydrostatic pressure; Pis = interstitial space hydrostatic pressure; π mv = pulmonary capillary oncotic pressure; π is = interstitial space oncotic pressure; σ_s = reflection coefficient of solute (describes permeability of membrane to solute—range of σ is 0 to 1.0). Under normal conditions, there is a small degree of net fluid movement into the interstitial space, which is removed by pulmonary lymphatics. When K_w is increased or there are changes in the other factors so that fluid movement into the interstitial space is increased, the lymphatics may be overwhelmed, resulting in pulmonary vascular congestion or edema. Note that when the membrane becomes increasingly permeable to solutes (σ approaches 0), Q_f is determined primarily by the differences in hydrostatic pressures.

interstitium and alveoli, even though the plasma oncotic pressures and the pulmonary capillary hydrostatic pressures are normal. Therefore, ARDS is often referred to as noncardiogenic or increased permeability pulmonary edema. It follows from the Starling equation that an abnormally high pulmonary capillary hydrostatic pressure will further increase fluid flux out of the vascular space into the lung and worsen the pulmonary edema. In contrast, the effects of plasma proteins on changing fluid flux are further governed by the value of the reflection coefficient for solutes (σ). ARDS increases the permeability of the alveolar capillary membrane for solutes, thereby decreasing σ. From the Starling equation (see Fig 28–1), it can be seen that as σ decreases, $\dot{Q}_f$ becomes primarily determined by the differences in microvascular and interstitial hydrostatic pressures. Therefore, increasing the plasma oncotic pressure in ARDS may not appreciably alter fluid movement into the lungs.

Similar to IRDS, although it is not the primary factor, surfactant depletion participates in the pathogenesis of ARDS by contributing to the development of atelectasis. Damage to the type 2 pneumocyte results in deficient surfactant production. Use of high inspired oxygen concentrations and mechanical ventilation with large tidal volumes to treat ARDS further impairs surfactant production.

The primary physiologic abnormalities of the diffuse lung injury observed with ARDS are hypoxemia and a reduction in FRC and lung compliance. Pulmonary edema and surfactant depletion result in an increase in lung elastic recoil. Therefore, FRC and lung compliance are reduced, and many alveoli become atelectatic. Hypoxemia is produced by a number of interrelated factors. First, in dependent lung areas, some alveoli may close during expiration and not fully participate in gas exchange. This occurs because closing capacity may be now greater than the reduced FRC. Second, right-to-left intrapulmonary shunting occurs through atelectatic lung areas. Third, even in the absence of frank atelectasis, many alveoli receive inadequate ventilation, and there are many areas

TABLE 28–1.—COMMON DISORDERS ASSOCIATED WITH ARDS

Infection
  Septicemia
  Viral pneumonia
  Pneumocystis pneumonia
  Bacterial pneumonia
  Fungal pneumonia
Trauma
  Lung contusion
  Fat emboli
  Head injury
Aspiration
Inhalation
  Toxic gases (NO_2, chlorine, phosgene)
  Smoke
Drugs
  Salicylates
  Narcotics
Shock
Pancreatitis
Disseminated intravascular coagulation
Massive blood transfusions

where $\dot{V}_A/\dot{Q}$ ratios are markedly reduced. Last, there may be an increase in the barrier to the diffusion of oxygen as a result of pulmonary edema.

Although early in the development of ARDS hypercarbia is not observed, there are many areas in the lung which receive proportionally more ventilation than perfusion, leading to an increase in physiologic dead space. However, an increase in minute ventilation usually provides adequate compensation to prevent hypercarbia. Later in the course of the illness, disordered reparative processes may further increase the V_D/V_T. At this stage, minute ventilation may not rise in proportion, and Pa_{CO_2} will increase.

CLINICAL FEATURES.—The clinical manifestations of ARDS invariably occur within 24 hours of an acute event which results in lung injury. A variety of medical and surgical conditions has been reported to produce ARDS (Table 28–1). Some of these conditions, such as aspiration of gastric acid, viral pneumonia, or lung contusion, injure the lung directly. Others, such as septic shock, disseminated intravascular coagulation, or fat emboli, probably produce indirect lung injury mediated by circulating lung toxins. In some instances, as with head trauma or drug ingestions, the mechanism of injury has not been clearly defined. It should be emphasized, however, that almost any condition that results in shock or trauma to the lung can result in ARDS, and that in many cases of ARDS a number of causal factors can be identified.

The initial clinical manifestations consist of dyspnea, tachypnea, and hyperpnea. In some cases there may be labored respiration with intercostal retraction and use of the accessory muscles of respiration. There is usually absence of adventitious lung sounds on auscultation of the chest. Chest roentgenograms show diffuse bilateral alveolar and interstitial infiltrates which may be indistinguishable from cardiogenic pulmonary edema. Arterial blood gases reveal progressive hypoxemia which is not easily corrected by use of supplemental oxygen, and therefore suggests the presence of right-to-left intrapulmonary shunting. The Pa_{CO_2} is usually reduced as a result of an increase in minute ventilation. However, late in the course of severe ARDS, hypercapnia may be observed, reflecting a marked increase in physiologic dead space. This is usually an ominous prognostic sign. More sophisticated pulmonary function studies reveal a reduction in FRC and lung compliance.

PATHOLOGIC FINDINGS.—The pathologic features observed in the lung depend on the duration of illness, but usually do not show any findings specific for the initial factors producing the lung injury. Grossly, the lungs are heavy and have areas of hemorrhage on the surface which become confluent as the disease progresses. Cut surfaces appear hemorrhagic and congested. Within 24 hours, microscopic examination shows interstitial and intra-alveolar edema and hemorrhage resulting in alveolar collapse. Intravascularly, there are often platelet and fibrin microemboli. Ultrastructural studies reveal that the initial injury produces extensive damage to the alveolar capillary membrane. Hyaline membranes are present by 48 hours. By 72–96 hours, if the patient survives, evidence of early fibrosis is present.

TREATMENT.—Therapy for ARDS consists of five general aspects: (1) treatment of factors responsible for initiating the syndrome, (2) ventilatory support, (3) appropriate fluid management, (4) appropriate respiratory and hemodynamic monitoring, and (5) meticulous general medical care.

Specific therapy or removal of causal factors should be initiated if possible. If septicemia and bacterial pneumonia are suspected, they should be treated with antibiotics. Fat embolism syndrome is often responsive to corticosteroids, and severe hemorrhagic pancreatitis may benefit from peritoneal lavage. Use of heparin and corticosteroids in all cases of ARDS has been advocated, but there is little evidence that they are efficacious.

Mechanical ventilation with a volume constant ventilator using supplemental oxygen is necessary in most cases of ARDS to avoid hypoxemia. Use of PEEP is indicated to minimize the possibility of oxygen toxicity if adequate arterial oxygenation is not obtained with an inspired oxygen concentration of less than 40%–50%. The detrimental effects and the criteria which are used to obtain the optimum level of PEEP are discussed in chapter 18.

In the presence of an increase in alveolar-capillary membrane permeability, overaggressive administration of fluids will worsen pulmonary edema. Volume replacement must therefore be given judiciously. For this reason, and because of the necessity of measuring cardiac outputs during PEEP therapy, placement of a thermodilution pulmonary artery catheter is usually indicated. This device can be easily inserted at the bedside, and will allow determination of a number of important cardiorespiratory parameters including cardiac output, pulmonary artery, and pulmonary artery occlusion (wedge) pressures (PAOP). The PAOP should be kept as low as possible consistent with an adequate cardiac output. If the cardiac output is inadequate in spite of a normal PAOP, use of vasopressors such as dopamine or dobutamine should be considered. Whether to use crystalloid or colloid for fluid administration in ARDS is a source of ongoing controversy. Since there are little data to suggest any clinical advantage of colloid solutions, use of crystalloids is probably preferable.

Most patients with severe ARDS are clinically unstable and require continuous hemodynamic and respiratory monitoring to detect changes in their condition before a sudden deterioration occurs. As previously discussed, insertion of a pulmonary artery catheter is usually indicated. In addition, an arterial catheter should be placed to facilitate sampling for arterial blood gases, and to monitor arterial pressure continuously. Recently, transcutaneous (Tc) measurements of P_{O_2} and P_{CO_2} have been suggested as a noninvasive monitoring technique. Changes in the TcP_{O_2} and TcP_{CO_2} reflect either alterations in respiratory gas exchange or blood flow, and thus they may be useful in detecting subtle changes in the hemodynamic or respiratory status of the patient. With the use of computer technology and mass spectrometry, it is now possible to monitor continuously inhaled and exhaled respiratory gases, and also to make in vivo measurements of extravascular lung water. The clinical usefulness of these new techniques remains to be determined.

Patients with ARDS require meticulous attention to the proper function of all organ systems. Mortality from ARDS often results from complications of intensive care or are related to failure of organ systems other than the lungs. Intravenous or alimentary nutrition should be started early in the course. Vigilance is required to prevent and treat gastrointestinal bleeding, nosocomial infection, and renal insufficiency.

Although the immediate mortality from all forms of ARDS ranges from 40% to 60%, long-term sequelae in survivors are relatively few. Approximately 40% of survivors have abnormal pulmonary function consisting of various combinations of mild restrictive lung disease, impairment of the DL_{CO}, exercise oxygen desaturation, and airflow obstruction. Since recovery of lung function is surprisingly good, aggressive therapy of patients with ARDS is usually justified.

READING LIST

Farrell P.M., Avery M.E.: Hyaline membrane disease. *Am. Rev. Respir. Dis.* 111:657–688, 1975.

This is a comprehensive review of all facets of IRDS.

Hallman M., Teramo K., Kankaanpaa K., et al.: Prevention of respiratory distress syndrome: current view of fetal lung maturity studies. *Ann. Clin. Res.* 12:36–44, 1980.

The current status of the usefulness of L/S ratios is discussed.

Hopewell P.C., Murray J.F.: The adult respiratory distress syndrome. *Annu. Rev. Med.* 27:343–356, 1976.

This article is a concise summary of the pathogenesis and treatment of ARDS.

Hyers T.M.: Pathogenesis of adult respiratory distress syndrome: current concepts. *Semin. Respir. Med.* 2:104–108, 1981.

In this article the current theories regarding the pathogenesis of ARDS are reviewed.

Petty T.L.: Adult respiratory distress syndrome: historical perspective and definition. *Semin. Respir. Med.* 2:99–103, 1981.

The historical background and current definition of what constitutes ARDS is discussed.

Pontoppidan H., Geffin B., Lowenstein E.: Acute respiratory failure in the adult. *N. Engl. J. Med.* 287:690–698; 743–752; 799–806, 1972.

This is the classic review article discussing the pathophysiology and treatment of ARDS.

Rinaldo J.E., Rogers R.M.: Adult respiratory distress syndrome: changing concepts of lung injury and repair. *N. Engl. J. Med.* 306:900–909, 1982.

A summary of some current theories regarding the development of ARDS.

Saldeen T.: The microembolism syndrome. *Microvasc. Res.* 11:227–259, 1976.

The relevance of microembolic disease to ARDS is discussed in extensive detail.

Shapiro D.L.: Respiratory distress syndrome. *N.Y. State Med. J.* 80:257–259, 1980.

A concise summary of the current status of the treatment and prevention of IRDS.

Pulmonary Vascular Diseases

CONGESTIVE HEART FAILURE, congenital heart diseases, and acquired valvular diseases may have secondary effects on the pulmonary circulation and on lung function. In addition to such secondary involvement, the pulmonary vasculature may be the site of a primary or intrinsic disorder. Pulmonary vascular diseases will be discussed under four headings: (1) pulmonary thromboembolic diseases, (2) anatomical intrapulmonary shunts, (3) primary pulmonary hypertension, and (4) pulmonary vascular changes secondary to hemodynamic abnormalities.

Pulmonary Thromboembolic Disease

Pulmonary thromboembolic disease is defined as the pathophysiologic derangement that results when a pulmonary arterial channel is occluded by clotted blood. It is estimated that pulmonary embolism is the third most common cause of death in the United States and is said to account for about 5% of sudden deaths. It is also one of the most important causes of morbidity and mortality in a general hospital population. In autopsy series, the incidence of pulmonary emboli has been reported to be as high as 64%, suggesting that many cases are clinically unrecognized. However, the reported incidence is greatly influenced by the characteristics of the population studied. The incidence in children for example, is lower than in debilitated elderly adults. Furthermore, the clinical significance of small emboli found at autopsy is difficult to assess.

Pulmonary emboli most commonly result from detached fragments of thrombi originating in the deep veins of the lower extremity above the knee. Venous thrombi below the knee do not appear to be sources of emboli. However, they can extend superiorly, and thereby become an embolic threat. Emboli also occasionally may arise from veins of the upper extremity, pelvis, or the right heart. Rarely, obstruction of a pulmonary artery results from a nonthrombotic embolus or occurs as a result of spontaneous in situ thrombosis.

Three factors place patients at risk for the development of pulmonary thromboembolism: venous stasis, hypercoagulability of the blood, and damage to blood vessel walls. Venous stasis occurs in clinical situations where there is prolonged bedrest or immobilization of the lower extremities. Therefore, pulmonary embolism is a frequent complication in patients with congestive heart failure or following major surgical procedures. Fractures of the lower extremities, pregnancy, carcinoma, and polycythemia rubra vera predispose to intravascular clotting, and emboli emanating from the right side of the heart are often associated with atrial fibrillation or endocarditis. Trauma to the lower extremities may result in vascular injury, and also may predispose to thrombosis. Although the physician must be alert to the possibility of pulmonary thromboembolism in clinical situations that may predispose to its development, the diagnosis should be made with caution and indiscriminate use of anticoagulants avoided. On the other hand, pulmonary thromboembolism may be life-threatening, necessitating accurate diagnosis with rapid institution of therapy.

The signs and symptoms of pulmonary thromboembolism are extremely variable. The frequent finding of emboli at autopsy in patients in whom the condition was not suspected indicates that pulmonary thromboembolism may be clinically silent. In a patient with signs of peripheral deep-vein thrombophlebitis, the classic syndrome associated with a moderate-sized embolus consists of chest pain of sudden onset, dyspnea, hyperpnea, hemoptysis, and fever. The pain may be substernal but is usually pleuritic, and a pleural rub may be heard on auscultation. The patient frequently expresses profound apprehension. Massive pulmonary thrombosis may result in a sudden shocklike state, and with occlusion of major vessels, death rapidly follows. Frequently, however, the symptoms of thromboembolism are subtle, such as unexplained fever or worsening of a preexisting cardiac or cardiopulmonary disorder. Recurrent small pulmonary emboli may be unnoticed until development of right ventricular hypertrophy (RVH) or congestive heart failure directs attention to the pulmonary vasculature.

Alterations in gas exchange and respiratory function have been described in pulmonary thromboembolism, but the reasons for many of them are far from clear. Experimental transient occlusion of a major pulmonary vessel or ligature of a main pulmonary artery in the course of surgical resection is well tolerated and is not attended by the profound consequences of thrombotic occlusion. Therefore, all of the effects of acute pulmonary thromboembolism cannot be explained by simple mechanical occlusion of the vessels.

Recent evidence suggests that the blood gas abnormalities observed with pulmonary embolism are a result of an increase in ventilation-perfusion mismatching. Perfusion of poorly ventilated alveolar units leads to hypoxemia. Ventilation of portions of lung deprived of their blood supply results in increased dead space ventilation. However, there is a marked compensatory increase in minute ventilation, so that the Pa_{CO_2} actually decreases. Any involvement

of a major portion of the lung may be detected by an increased difference between arterial and end-tidal carbon dioxide tensions, but this abnormality seldom persists after the first 72 hours following thromboembolism. The VC is commonly reduced, probably the result of the decreased compliance that follows small airway constriction and altered surfactant production.

Frequently observed is bronchoconstriction manifested by wheezing and a reduction in FEV_1. This occurs early in the thromboembolic episode and is usually transient. It can be reversed by inhalation of isoproterenol aerosol and also by IV administration of heparin. The bronchoconstriction is probably mediated in part by release from the lung or platelets in the thrombus of humoral agents such as histamine, serotonin, or prostaglandins.

Although a pulmonary embolus may obstruct a large portion of the pulmonary vascular bed, infarction is a relatively rare event. Oxygen supplied via the bronchial circulation and the airways protects the pulmonary parenchyma from ischemia. Therefore, it is not surprising that infarction occurs primarily in patients who also have preexisting cardiopulmonary impairment such as congestive heart failure. The diagnosis of pulmonary infarction is commonly made on the basis of the observation on chest roentgenogram of a wedge-shaped density, its apex pointing toward the hilus. However, intrapulmonary hemorrhage peripheral to the vascular occlusion is commonly the cause of the radiologic lesion, and resolution of the lesion within ten days is suggestive of postembolic hemorrhage rather than tissue death.

DIAGNOSTIC TESTS IN PULMONARY EMBOLISM

The diagnosis of pulmonary embolism is often difficult to confirm even when clinical suspicion is quite high. Although emboli produce both an increase in dead space ventilation and perfusion of areas with low ventilation/perfusion ratios, normocapnia or hypocapnia is usually present. Furthermore, despite previous data to the contrary, it is now generally recognized that lack of hypoxemia does not exclude pulmonary embolism. Pulmonary function tests are nonspecific, especially if there is preexisting cardiopulmonary disease, and often are impractical to perform in an acutely ill patient. Blood counts and serum chemistry studies are likewise of little value. The presence of an acute right heart strain pattern on ECG supports the diagnosis of embolism, but usually the ECG is normal or shows merely a sinus tachycardia. A pulmonary infiltrate may be observed on chest roentgenogram if there is concomitant infarction or hemorrhage, but is not specific for embolism. Similarly, roentgenographic evidence of oligemia in an area of lung is neither specific nor sensitive.

When the clinical situation is highly suspect for pulmonary embolism, documentation of deep-vein thrombosis may provide enough evidence to initiate therapy. Although radiocontrast venography is the reference standard for the diagnosis of deep-vein thrombosis, it is invasive, and there is the risk of a contrast medium reaction and exacerbating or producing phlebitis. Recently, venous Doppler examination, venous plethysmography, radioactive fibrinogen leg scanning, and radionuclide venography have been shown to be useful in demonstrating the presence of deep-vein thrombosis. None of these indirect tests, however, is completely sensitive and specific, and pulmonary embolism does not necessarily arise solely from veins in the lower extremity.

The most useful noninvasive screening test for the diagnosis of pulmonary embolism is the perfusion lung scan, which is highly sensitive for the detection of pulmonary emboli. A normal perfusion lung scan excludes the diagnosis of pulmonary embolism. However, an abnormal perfusion scan is nonspecific, since a perfusion deficit can be produced by many other conditions besides occlusion of a pulmonary artery by an embolus. Ventilation lung scanning is often combined with perfusion scanning to increase the latter's specificity. It is based on the principle that abnormalities in perfusion caused by emboli should be normally ventilated, whereas other causes of perfusion deficits will have ventilation abnormalities as well. Although the probability of a correct diagnosis is enhanced with the combination ventilation-perfusion lung scanning, false positives and negatives do occur, especially when severe preexisting lung disease is present.

Pulmonary angiography is generally regarded as the definitive test to diagnose pulmonary embolism. Although it is invasive, mortality with angiography is less than 1%, and morbidity less than 5%. The recent development of IV pulmonary angiography using computer contrast enhancement techniques has shown some promise and is less invasive than conventional pulmonary angiography. Angiography usually should be performed in the following situations: (1) when the clinical suspicion of pulmonary embolism is high, but the lung scan is not consistent with the diagnosis, (2) when vena caval interruption or use of thrombolytic agents is being considered, and (3) when there is severe preexisting cardiopulmonary disease where lung scanning is difficult to interpret. Both angiography and lung scanning should be performed within 48 hours of suspected onset, since resolution of emboli may occur after longer delays.

DIFFERENTIAL DIAGNOSIS IN SUSPECTED PULMONARY EMBOLISM

Any of the following signs or symptoms may lead to suspicion of the presence of pulmonary embolism: (1) roentgenographic evidence of a pulmonary infiltrate of unknown etiology; (2) symptoms of chest pain, hemoptysis, or dyspnea in a patient with a normal chest roentgenogram; (3) worsening of symptoms in a patient with a chronic cardiorespiratory disorder; (4) sudden development of a shocklike state; or (5) right ventricular hypertrophy (RVH) of uncertain etiology. The diagnostic approach will depend on which of these manifestations is present.

ROENTGENOGRAPHIC EVIDENCE OF PULMONARY INFILTRATE.—The radiologic observation that most often raises the question of pulmonary embolism is a nondescript infiltrate or multiple infiltrates. Differential diagnosis is usually between an infectious process and pulmonary thromboembolism with infarction. The latter is particularly suspected when there is little fever, no purulent sputum, and a normal white blood cell count. Pulmonary embolism is also suspected when symptoms begin suddenly without a prodrome of malaise and fever or when hemoptysis or chest pain is an early symptom. The presence of peripheral venous disease or a clinical setting in which embolism is common (e.g., congestive heart failure, post trauma, or post surgery) strengthens the likelihood of embolism.

There are few diagnostic tests that specifically distinguish an infarction from a pneumonic infiltrate. Radioactive perfusion scans will be abnormal in the area of the infiltrate in either case. Lung scans are more meaningful if they reveal areas of impaired perfusion in parts of the lung that are not involved by the radiologic abnormality. The latter findings suggest additional emboli that have not resulted in infarction. But the physician must be cautious in interpreting these tests. Localized emphysematous changes or reactive changes in the vasculature of the lung contralateral to pneumonitis may produce an abnormal contralateral lung scan. Definitive diagnosis depends on angiographic demonstration of emboli.

ACUTE SYMPTOMS IN A PATIENT WITH A NORMAL CHEST RADIOGRAM.—Pulmonary embolism is included in the differential diagnosis when acute chest pain, hemoptysis, or dyspnea develops in a patient without chronic cardiopulmonary disease and without a discernible radiologic pulmonary abnormality. The presence of peripheral venous thrombosis, characteristic ECG changes, or a clinical setting in which thromboembolism is especially common lends support to the diagnosis. A positive lung perfusion scan may be sufficiently diagnostic in this situation.

Some patients exhibit a short-lived episode of bronchospasm early in the pulmonary embolic episode. The physician should suspect that an episode of bronchospasm has been induced by embolism in patients otherwise prone to thromboembolism when there has been no preceding asthmatic tendency or when there is accompanying hemoptysis. Ultimate differentiation usually depends on angiograms, since lung scans may be abnormal even in ordinary asthma.

EXACERBATION OF SYMPTOMS OF CHRONIC CARDIOPULMONARY DISEASE.—The cause of sudden worsening of symptoms in patients with chronic cardiopulmonary disorders is often difficult to discern, and acute pulmonary embolism must always be considered when no other obvious explanation can be found. Unfortunately, definite diagnosis is very difficult. Hemoptysis in the absence of purulent sputum is suggestive, and the presence of peripheral venous thrombosis greatly increases the probabilty of embolism. ECGs are of limited use, since evidence of increased strain of the right side of the heart may occur with exacerbations of any cause in patients with advanced pulmonary insufficiency.

Lung scans and pulmonary function tests are also of limited use, since perfusion abnormalities and lung function abnormalities from emboli cannot be distinguished from changes caused by the patient's chronic disease. Angiograms provide the most specific information, but the physician may be reluctant to perform this test in patients with severe chronic lung disease. Since emboli occur frequently in these patients, it is sometimes necessary to use anticoagulant therapy when there is only a strong suspicion of thromboembolic disease.

SUDDEN SHOCK-LIKE STATE.—Massive pulmonary embolism may lead to sudden death or to the abrupt development of low cardiac output, severe hypotension, and vasomotor collapse. The clinical picture may resemble severe myocardial infarction, and differentiation of these conditions may be extremely difficult. When there are reasons to suspect massive embolism, such as preexisting peripheral thrombophlebitis, development of symptoms in the early postoperative period, or occurrence of the syndrome in a young woman, prompt angiographic studies may be justified to confirm the diagnosis, especially if thrombolytic therapy is to be used should massive embolism be confirmed. If more conservative therapy would be elected in any case, the patient may be treated with anticoagulants and supportive measures even without a secure diagnosis. Differentiation of myocardial infarction from massive embolism may become apparent from the evolution of the ECG and chest roentgenogram. Finding a markedly elevated physiologic dead space may also point to the diagnosis of embolism. If necessary, lung scans or angiograms or both may be done when the patient's clinical condition improves.

RIGHT VENTRICULAR HYPERTROPHY.—Recurrent, often "silent" emboli may lead to slowly developing RVH. The resulting syndrome is almost indistinguishable from primary pulmonary hypertension, described below. The differential diagnosis of RVH is discussed in chapter 16.

TREATMENT OF
PULMONARY EMBOLISM

Treatment of acute embolism is primarily supportive, including control of anxiety and pain, correction of hypoxemia with oxygen, and support of blood pressure in patients with shock. Anticoagulants should be started immediately with a bolus dose of 5,000–10,000 units of IV heparin followed by a continuous infusion of approximately 1,000 units/hour. The dose should be adjusted subsequently to keep the activated partial thromboplastin time or activated clotting time 1½ to 2½ times the control value. The continuous infusion method has been associated with fewer bleeding complications than intermittent IV administration. When the patient is stable, oral anticoagulation with a coumarin derivative is started with the dose adjusted to keep the prothrombin time 1½ to 2½ times the control value. Heparin is continued since these agents take five to seven days to become completely effective. Oral anticoagulant therapy is continued for approximately six weeks, but may be continued indefinitely when there is a history of recurrent embolization or continued presence of factors predisposing toward thromboembolism.

The thrombolytic agents streptokinase and urokinase have been shown to produce faster angiographic resolution and hemodynamic improvement than heparin therapy. Although no improvement in survival has been documented, use of these agents may be indicated where massive embolism is present and there is severe hemodynamic compromise. Emergency surgical embolectomy has been used in the past for similar indications, but now has little role with the introduction of thrombolytic agents.

Surgical interruption of the inferior vena cava or placement of an inferior vena caval umbrella or "filter" is occasionally recommended, particularly when anticoagulants cannot be used or when recurrent emboli originating in lower extremities occur despite anticoagulant treatment. In patients at high risk for development of thromboembolic disease, prophylactic use of low-dose subcutaneous heparin therapy, 5,000 units every 12 hours has been shown to decrease the incidence of thromboembolic disease. In some clinical situations, antiplatelet agents such as dextran and aspirin, and physical measures such as elastic stockings may also prevent the development of thromboembolism.

Anatomical Intrapulmonary Shunts

Left-to-right shunting causes oxygenated blood to be supplied to the lung. It does not result in arterial blood gas abnormalities. Such shunts are usually detected as a consequence of the hemodynamic abnormalities or murmurs they produce. They are diagnosed either angiographically or, in the case of intracardiac lesions, on the basis of cardiac catheterization studies, which reveal a sudden increase in blood oxygen concentration as the catheter is advanced from the vena cava through the right side of the heart. In contrast, an anatomical right-to-left shunt causes poorly oxygenated blood to reach the peripheral arterial circulation. Its presence is established by an abnormally large alveolar-arterial oxygen difference that cannot be abolished by breathing 100% oxygen.

Normally, a small amount of poorly oxygenated blood reaches the left ventricle through normal anatomical structures, including thebesian, anterior cardiac, and bronchial veins. Intracardiac defects from congenital heart diseases are the most common causes of clinically important anatomical shunting. True intrapulmonary shunts also occur occasionally, either through a congential malformation or an acquired abnormal vascular channel.

CONGENITAL PULMONARY SHUNTS.—Left-to-right shunts may occur as a result of abnormal pulmonary venous drainage causing oxygenated pulmonary venous blood to enter the right atrium. Congenital pulmonary arteriovenous (AV) fistulas can be the source of right-to-left shunts. These lesions are often multiple, and larger ones may be visible on the chest roentgenogram. Angiograms provide a definitive diagnosis. Many patients with pulmonary AV fistulas have similar vascular communications elsewhere in the body as a part of the entity known as hereditary hemorrhagic telangiectasia. Right-to-left shunts may also occur with congenital pulmonary hemangioma.

ACQUIRED PULMONARY SHUNT.—The development or opening of anatomic communications between the systemic and pulmonary circulations constitutes an acquired form of shunt. The hypoxemia of hepatic cirrhosis is believed to be largely on the basis of acquired right-to-left shunt. Here, portopulmonary communications allow venous blood from the portal system to enter the pulmonary veins. Dilatation of peripheral pulmonary arteries with pleural spider nevi and intrapulmonary shunts have also been described in these patients. Pulmonary malignancies or chronic inflammatory processes derive their blood supply from the bronchial circulation. Large left-to-right shunts may develop through bronchial artery-pulmonary vein communications as a residual of chronic granulomatous disease, especially with bronchiectasis.

Primary Pulmonary Hypertension

In this rare disorder, primarily affecting children and young adults, there is progressive pulmonary hypertension and RVH of undetermined etiology. The pathologic changes noted in the pulmonary vascular bed include arterial muscular hypertrophy, fibrous occlusion of small vessels and even necrotizing angiitis. In some instances there are changes compatible with an organized thrombus, causing this entity to be virtually indistinguishable from chronic recurrent thromboembolism.

Diagnosis is made by exclusion of all other causes for severe pulmonary hypertension. Although previously there has been no effective treatment for this disorder, recent experience with vasodilating agents such as diazoxide, isoproterenol, and calcium channel blockers such as nifedipine have been promising.

Secondary Pulmonary Vascular Changes

When the pulmonary vasculature is subjected to high pressures during birth, as in certain congenital heart diseases, the prominent media of smooth muscles of fetal vessels fail to regress normally. In acquired pulmonary hypertension, intimal proliferation precedes medial hypertrophy. Later, the vessels narrow, and increasing intimal fibrosis may lead to vascular occlusion. Necrotizing angiitis finally occurs.

These nonspecific changes, which may be a consequence of any underlying disease leading to pulmonary hypertension, eventually result in an increase in pulmonary vascular resistance independent of the underlying disorder. For example, in long-standing mitral stenosis, secondary changes in the pulmonary vascular bed may cause pulmonary hypertension to persist for weeks or months following successful valve surgery. The fact that pulmonary vascular resistance slowly falls toward normal after relief of mitral stenosis indicates that some of the changes noted above are potentially reversible.

READING LIST

Clagett G.P., Salzman E.W.: Prevention of venous thromboembolism. *Prog. Cardiovasc. Dis.* 17: 345–366, 1975.

A discussion of the various methods used to prevent thromboembolic disease.

Dalen J.E., Alpert J.S.: Natural history of pulmonary embolism. *Prog. Cardiovasc. Dis.* 17:259–270, 1975.

A review of the epidemiology of pulmonary embolism.

Dines D.E., Arms R.A., Bernatz P.E., et al.: Pulmonary arteriovenous fistulas. *Mayo Clin. Proc.* 49:460–465, 1974.

A review of 63 cases of pulmonary arteriovenous fistulas.

Heath D., Smith P.: Pulmonary vascular disease. *Med. Clin. North Am.* 61:1279–1307, 1977.

The pathogenesis of pulmonary arterial disease is discussed.

McNeil B.J.: A diagnostic strategy using ventilation perfusion studies in patients suspect for pulmonary embolism. *J Nucl. Med.* 17:613–616, 1973.

A proposal for the use of ventilation lung scanning in the diagnosis of pulmonary embolism.

Moser K.: Pulmonary embolism. *Am. Rev. Respir. Dis.* 115:829–852, 1977.

A comprehensive review of pulmonary embolism.

National Cooperative Study: The urokinase pulmonary embolism trial. *Circulation* 47(suppl. 2):1–108, 1973.

The results of the cooperative study concerning the use of urokinase in pulmonary emboli.

Pittman D.C.: Primary pulmonary hypertension. *Angiology* 30:756–766, 1979.

A brief discussion of primary pulmonary hypertension.

Robin E.D.: Overdiagnosis and overtreatment of pulmonary embolism: the emperor may have no clothes. *Ann. Intern. Med.* 87:775–781, 1977.

A devil's advocate approach to the use of lung scanning in pulmonary emboli.

Rosenow E.C., Osmundson P.J., Brown M.L.: Pulmonary embolism. *Mayo Clin. Proc.* 56:161–178, 1981.

A review of pulmonary embolism.

Sherry S.: Preventing pulmonary embolism with heparin in low doses. *Postgrad. Med.* 56:80–84, 1976.

The efficacy of low-dose heparin in the prophylaxis of pulmonary emboli is discussed.

30

Miscellaneous Causes of Respiratory Insufficiency

Near Drowning

Death from drowning is due either to aspiration of water or to asphyxiation secondary to reflex laryngospasm. Near drowning constitutes a medical emergency. The diagnosis is usually all too obvious, and certain historical factors, such as length of submersion, temperature of the water, age of the patient, and the degree of metabolic acidosis, will influence the ultimate prognosis.

Submersion without aspiration of water occurs in 10%–15% of drowning victims. Reflex laryngospasm prevents entry of water into the lungs in these individuals. If the length of submersion is not prolonged, so that permanent neurologic damage does not occur, complete and rapid recovery can usually be expected with appropriate resuscitation.

Unfortunately, 85%–90% of drowning victims aspirate water, resulting in pulmonary edema and hypoxemia in many cases. Hypoxemia occurs irrespective of the type of water aspirated. With massive aspiration of hypertonic sea water, pulmonary edema results because of movement of vascular fluid down an osmotic gradient into the alveoli. When massive amounts of fresh water are aspirated, there is rapid uptake of fluid into the circulation. Pulmonary edema then occurs from circulatory overload. Fresh water aspiration also leads to loss of the surface tension lowering properties of surfac-

tant, resulting in alveolar instability and atelectasis, and further contributing to hypoxemia. Regardless of the type of fluid aspirated, foreign material such as mud, sand, and algae often find entry into the lungs, provoking an intense inflammatory response. This may increase the permeability of the alveolar capillary membrane and exacerbate the pulmonary edema.

Metabolic acidosis is common, and a pH of less than 7.0 is a poor prognostic sign. Hematologic and electrolyte changes have been overemphasized in the past, and rarely present a problem in management. Arrhythmias are not infrequent and are related to the degree of hypoxemia and acidosis. Neurologic findings are variable, caused by hypoxemia and cerebral edema. Although hypoxic brain damage is thought to occur within a few minutes of submersion, survival without neurologic sequelae has been reported after a cold water submersion of up to 40 minutes.

Treatment is largely supportive and includes use of ventilatory support and supplemental oxygen (see chap. 18). There is no evidence that empiric use of corticosteroids or antibiotics is efficacious.

Pulmonary Problems Related to Congestive Heart Failure

ACUTE PULMONARY EDEMA.—Normally, the balance of hydrostatic and plasma oncotic pressures plus lymphatic drainage keep the airspaces free of fluid. These relationships are described by the Starling equation (see chap. 28). Pulmonary edema occurs when fluid leaves the capillaries faster than it can be removed by the lymphatics.

The most common cause of pulmonary edema is an increase in pulmonary capillary pressure secondary to left ventricular failure. With acute failure of the left side of the heart and increase in pulmonary venous pressure, arteriolar constriction of dependent vessels of the lung (where pulmonary hypertension is most severe) results in a shift of blood flow to more superior lung regions. This arteriolar constriction reduces mean capillary pressure at the lung bases, delaying pulmonary edema. Peripheral vasoconstriction is also present, resulting in an increase in central blood volume. As pulmonary venous and mean pulmonary capillary pressures increase with worsening of heart failure, transudation of fluid occurs.

Pulmonary edema may be of sudden or gradual onset. Paroxysmal nocturnal dyspnea and wheezing may indicate mild, relatively slowly developing pulmonary edema. When fully developed, dyspnea, wheezing, and cough with expectoration of profuse amounts of frothy pink-stained sputum appear. Breathing is noisy and gurgling, and moist bubbling rales can be heard on auscultation. The chest roentgenogram reveals confluent patchy opacifications usually sparing the periphery of the lung fields.

Lung volumes and expiratory air flows are reduced, the work of breathing is increased, and Pa_{O_2} is diminished. In severe cases, hypoxemia may be profound with obvious cyanosis, and carbon dioxide retention may occur.

Treatment consists of correcting hypoxemia by supplemental oxygen, reducing central blood volume and improving left ventricular function. Intravenous furosemide produces rapid venodilation with a decrease in left ventricular preload even before its diuretic effect occurs. In very acute conditions, a small phlebotomy may have dramatic results. Morphine is helpful not only in allaying anxiety but also in producing some relief of systemic vasoconstriction and block of pulmonary reflexes. Rapid administration of digitalis may be needed, especially if the episode was precipitated by atrial fibrillation with a fast ventricular response. In severe cases, left ventricular afterload reduction with nitroprusside may be indicated. If hypoxemia cannot be corrected promptly, continuous positive airway pressure or mechanical ventilation with PEEP should be used.

DIFFERENTIATING CONGESTIVE HEART FAILURE FROM INTRINSIC LUNG DISEASE AS A CAUSE OF RESPIRATORY INSUFFICIENCY.—Tachycardia, mild dependent edema, and basal rales occur frequently in patients with chronic lung disorders even in the absence of congestive heart failure. When a dyspneic patient shows these features, it is easy to ascribe the findings to a cardiac disorder. This may seem to be confirmed by distention of the jugular veins if it is not recognized that venous distention is present only during expiration, reflecting elevated expiratory intrathoracic pressure. Cardiomegaly is almost always present with cardiac failure; its absence should cause serious doubt about this diagnosis. Insidiously progressive exertional dyspnea over a period of many years is uncommon in congestive heart failure; it suggests a primary bronchopulmonary disease. A history of orthopnea is of little diagnostic help, since this symptom occurs in intrinsic pulmonary diseases as well as in cardiac disorders.

The pulmonary physiologic abnormalities associated with heart failure vary. A reduction of VC is characteristic, but a variable amount of slowing of expiration may accompany the loss of volume excursion, producing a mixed type of ventilatory abnormality. With severe pulmonary edema, a small lung pattern, hypoxemia, and even hypercapnia are expected, but patients are rarely studied at this severe stage of illness. With lesser degrees of chronic heart failure, RV is variable; the diffusing capacity is usually reduced in proportion to VC but may be quite well preserved; arterial oxygenation is near normal; and there is a tendency to low Pa_{CO_2} from hyperventilation. Pulmonary compliance is markedly reduced in congestive heart failure, perhaps explaining the tachypnea and dyspnea of these patients.

Determination that this nonspecific pattern of dysfunction is due to heart disease must be made on the basis of other clinical and laboratory findings or by observing the effect of treatment on lung function measurements. If necessary, measurement of the pulmonary artery occlusion or wedge pressure will decide whether left ventricular dysfunction is present. When there is serious doubt about the diagnosis, and pulmonary artery catheterization cannot be performed, a course of diuretics may be prescribed. Reduction in heart size, clearing of lung fields on roentgenograms and marked improvement in spirometry following diuresis confirm the diagnosis of primary cardiac disease. Repeated spirometry after complete control of heart failure allows assessment of the severity of any associated pulmonary disorder. Digitalis should not be used for a therapeutic trial in these patients.

It is common to encounter respiratory insufficiency resulting from a combination of intrinsic heart disease and chronic airways obstruction. If reduction in VC is greater than expected for the severity of FEV_1 impairment ("mixed" ventilatory abnormality), an element of heart failure is suggested. Change in heart size following diuresis is the most reliable clinical guide to the presence of myocardial decompensation in patients with severe pulmonary diseases.

EVALUATING RADIOLOGIC ABNORMALITIES IN PATIENTS WITH CONGESTIVE HEART FAILURE.— Occasionally, suspicious pulmonary infiltrates, hilar masses, or mass-like shadows are seen near one of the pulmonary fissures in the chest roentgenograms of patients who are in obvious congestive heart failure. Cardiac compensation should be restored and the chest film reevaluated before undertaking further diagnostic studies. With diuresis, patchy areas of pulmonary edema, markedly dilated hilar vessels that appear to be solid tumors, and localized pleural effusions (pseudotumors) may promptly disappear. In addition, the appearance of real pulmonary lesions may change considerably.

Carbon Monoxide Poisoning

The affinity of hemoglobin for carbon monoxide is approximately 200 times that for oxygen. Therefore, inspiration of relatively low concentrations of carbon monoxide can cause a serious reduction in the oxygen-carrying capacity of the blood by allowing the oxygen-carrying sites on hemoglobin to be occupied by CO instead of O_2 molecules. Furthermore, the presence of carboxyhemoglobin shifts the in vivo oxyhemoglobin dissociation curve to the left (decrease in the P_{50}), thereby impairing the release of O_2 from hemoglobin in the tissues. Heavy cigarette smokers may have carboxyhemoglobin levels of greater than 10%, but are usually asymptomatic unless there is underlying coronary artery disease. In the latter individuals, a decrease in angina threshold may be observed. However, inhalation of 0.05% CO for one hour will produce 20% carboxyhemoglobin in blood and result in a mild throbbing headache. Symptoms of hypoxemia progressively develop at higher levels of carboxyhemoglobin, with coma, convulsions, and death at levels between 50% and 80%. The diagnosis is usually based on a history of exposure, but can be confirmed by carboxyhemoglobin measurements. In spite of the severe hypoxemia, cyanosis is absent. Rather, because of the bright red color of carboxyhemoglobin, the skin may appear redder than normal.

Since high oxygen tensions speed the release of carbon monoxide from hemoglobin, treatment consists of adequate ventilation with 100% oxygen until improvement occurs. When CNS depression is marked and spontaneous ventilation depressed, mechanical ventilatory assistance is necessary. Unless anoxic brain damage has occurred, no residual effects remain following recovery.

Altitude

Although the fractional concentration of atmospheric gases remains constant, atmospheric pressure falls with increase in altitude. Therefore, the partial pressure of oxygen falls accordingly. Through various adaptive mechanisms, man is able to acclimatize and live at altitudes as high as 14,000 ft.

The shape of the oxyhemoglobin dissociation curve allows maintenance of adequate arterial oxygen content in the face of considerable variation in Pa_{O_2}. In addition, increase in erythrocyte 2,3-DPG levels occurs in response to chronic hypoxia. Increased red blood cell production with increase in red cell volume and hematocrit also occurs. In response to low inspired oxygen tensions, minute ventilation increases with resulting hypocapnia. Compensatory renal mechanisms maintain pH at normal levels. Some individuals are unable to tolerate ascent to high altitude, especially if done rapidly, and pulmonary edema or acute mountain sickness develops.

High-altitude pulmonary edema may occur with acute mountain sickness or as a separate process. Susceptibility to high-altitude pulmonary edema appears to vary among individuals. It is more common in individuals who return to high altitude after a short stay at a lower altitude. The signs and symptoms are those seen in pulmonary edema from any cause. However, left ventricular failure is not a feature of the process, although pulmonary arterial hypertension is present. The responsible mechanism is not known. Increased permeability of pulmonary arterioles and capillaries has been suggested. Alternatively, there may be inhomogeneous constriction of the pulmonary arterioles resulting in nonconstricted pulmonary capillaries being subjected to high blood flow and pressure with consequent extravasation of fluid into the interstitium. Treatment includes oxygen administration, rest, and use of diuretics pending removal of the patient to a lower altitude.

Acute mountain sickness begins 6–90 hours after ascent to high altitude, with symptoms of insomnia, headache, nausea, vomiting, dyspnea, and lethargy. Severe forms may include cyanosis, pulmonary rales, papilledema, and other signs of cerebral edema. Hypoxemia, respiratory alkalosis, and fluid retention all play a role in the pathophysiology. Pretreatment with acet-

azolamide, a carbonic anhydrase inhibitor, prevents the syndrome.

Chronic mountain sickness may occur in long-time high altitude residents. Onset is slow with gradual development of symptoms consisting of fatigue, dyspnea, somnolence, and decreased mental activity. Characteristically, patients exhibit the plethora of marked erythrocytosis, cyanosis, clubbing of fingers, and pulmonary hypertension with right ventricular failure. Pa_{CO_2} is higher than that observed in healthy residents at the same altitude. The pathogenesis is not understood, but it seems to be related to a loss of respiratory drive and consequent hypoventilation in relation to the altitude at which these persons live. Moving to sea level eventually brings about complete recovery.

Oxygen Toxicity

Whereas oxygen supplementation may be required to correct hypoxemia, excessive inspired oxygen concentrations may be detrimental. Breathing pure oxygen at ambient pressure can damage pulmonary capillary endothelium. This is followed by thickening of the air-blood barrier due to edema and increase in alveolar cells, especially granular pneumocytes, decrease in surface area of exposed alveolar capillaries secondary to widening of the intra-alveolar septi, and, finally, focal areas of atelectasis and hyaline membrane formation. Animals die from severe respiratory failure after about 70 hours of exposure to 100% oxygen. In man, 100% oxygen breathing results in a fall in diffusing capacity after 3 hours or more, and VC begins to fall after 24–60 hours. When oxygen is breathed at increased pressure, more rapid deterioration of function occurs.

The safe limits of inhaled oxygen concentrations are not clear. However, there is currently no evidence that pulmonary oxygen toxicity develops in man at inspired tensions below 0.4–0.5 atm, even when exposure is prolonged. There are no data to support the contention that significant permanent oxygen toxicity develops in man breathing pure oxygen for less than 24 hours. Finally, there are no conclusive clinical or experimental studies to indicate that patients with preexisting pulmonary diseases are more sensitive to oxygen toxicity than are normal volunteers. However, it is important that the lowest concentration of inhaled oxygen be given to achieve the desired level of Pa_{O_2}.

Treatment of oxygen toxicity is not specific. There is little evidence that corticosteroids either reverse the process or protect patients from it. Once the syndrome of reduced lung compliance, small lung volumes, and focal atelectasis with marked intrapulmonary shunting has developed, the clinical picture resembles that of ARDS (see chap. 28).

Postresection States

Immediately following lung resection, there is a shift of blood away from the side of operation, VC is markedly impaired as a result of chest discomfort, and diffusing capacity is reduced roughly in proportion to the amount of lung removed. All of these changes return toward normal over the following weeks.

By 6 weeks postoperatively, the considerable pulmonary reserve of normal subjects is well demonstrated by their tolerance to resection of up to 50% of the lung. In fact, when lung resection is carried out in infancy, eventual pulmonary function may be nearly normal. In adult life, resection of as much as 20% of lung volume usually results in some permanent change in lung function but, in the case of simple lobectomy, this may involve only a slight decrease in VC.

Functional status following extensive resections, such as pneumonectomy, is variable, depending largely on the functional integrity of the remaining lung. In most subjects there is hyperinflation of the remaining lung. VC is about 60% and RV 80%–90% of predicted. Diffusing capacity is reduced roughly in proportion to volume loss. Forced expiratory flow rates and arterial blood gases remain normal. PAP is normal at rest but increases moderately during exercise, reflecting a decreased distensibility of the vascular bed.

If there are even mild abnormalities in the remaining lung, the consequences of pneumonectomy may be more severe. Resting pulmonary hypertension and cor pulmonale commonly develop and may lead to death in the early postoperative period.

Bronchopulmonary Dysplasia

Bronchopulmonary dysplasia (BPD) is a relatively new disease of infancy that primarily affects survivors of IRDS. Up to 40% of infants who require mechanical ventilation for IRDS will develop BPD. Although the etiology of BPD is not completely clear, certain factors such as degree of prematurity, high airway pressures, high inspired oxygen concentrations, and infection have been implicated.

The clinical manifestations are variable and depend on the severity of the disease. BPD usually begins as an extension of the recovery period of IRDS. There is a continuation of the need for supplemental oxygen, and CO_2 retention may be present. Chronic cough with sputum production, wheezing, tachypnea, and fluid retention are frequently observed. Infants with BPD are more susceptible to the development of lower respiratory tract infections. Cor pulmonale is also a common complication. Hyperaeration is seen on the chest roentgenogram, with areas of radiolucency interspersed among focal areas of atelectasis and fibrosis.

Pathologically, there is interstitial fibrosis, persistent collapse and atrophy of scattered areas of the lung, diminished alveolization, and evidence of obliterative airway disease and pulmonary hypertension.

Treatment is primarily supportive, including supplemental oxygen, bronchodilators, adequate nutrition, fluid and salt restriction, and diuretics when indicated. The prognosis for children with mild BPD is encouraging, many showing resolution of their pulmonary disease after five to ten years. Increased survival of smaller birth weight infants in recent years has led to more severe BPD. The prognosis for these infants is still uncertain.

READING LIST

Clarke E.B., Niggeman E.H.: Near drowning. *Heart Lung* 4:946–955, 1975.

A review of the pathophysiologic mechanisms and clinical findings in near drowning.

Cohn H.N., Franciosa J.A.: Vasodilator therapy of cardiac therapy. *N. Engl. J. Med.* 297:27–31; 254–258, 1977.

A summary of the rationale and the indications for vasodilator therapy in congestive heart failure.

Deneke S.M., Fanburg B.L.: Normobaric oxygen toxicity of the lung. *N. Engl. J. Med.* 303:76–86, 1980.

A review of the pathophysiology and biochemistry occurring in oxygen toxicity.

Hultgren H.N.: High altitude medical problems. *West. J. Med.* 131:8–23, 1979.

This is a review of the medical problems occurring with ascent to altitude.

Jackson D.L.: Carbon monoxide poisoning—a growing hazard. *Medical Times* 106:28–37, 1978.

A review of the pathogenesis and clinical findings in carbon monoxide poisoning.

Kafer E.R.: Pulmonary oxygen toxicity. *Br. J. Anaesth.* 43:687–695, 1971.

A review of the evidence for the occurrence of O_2 toxicity in man.

Modell J.H.: Biology of drowning. *Annu. Rev. Med.* 29:1–8, 1978.

A review of the consequences of drowning.

Nickerson B.G., Taussig L.M.: Bronchopulmonary dysplasia. *Ariz. Med.* 36:743–747, 1979.

In this article the pathophysiologic mechanisms and clinical findings of bronchopulmonary dysplasia are reviewed.

Taghizada A., Reynolds E.O.R.: Pathogenesis of bronchopulmonary dysplasia following hyaline membrane disease. *Am. J. Pathol.* 82:241–264, 1976.

A pathologic discussion of the findings in bronchopulmonary dysplasia.

Index